Ultrasound in Biology and Medicine

Ultrasound in Biology and Medicine

A Symposium sponsored by the Bioacoustics Laboratory of the University of Illinois and the Physiology Branch of the Office of Naval Research. Held at Robert Allerton Park, Monticello, Illinois, June 20–22, 1955.

EDITED BY

ELIZABETH KELLY

PUBLICATION

No. 3

•

1957

AMERICAN INSTITUTE OF BIOLOGICAL SCIENCES

WASHINGTON, D. C.

Library of Congress Catalog Card
Number: 57-11005

PRINTED IN THE UNITED STATES OF AMERICA
BY WAVERLY PRESS, INC., BALTIMORE

Preface

THE PRIMARY PURPOSE of this Symposium was to bring together scientists concerned with various aspects of the field of ultrasound in biology and medicine, in order to discuss both the recent advances and the outstanding problems in this field. Since a detailed knowledge of the field of ultrasound in biology is limited to a relatively small fraction of the scientific population, it is hoped that the publication of these proceedings will be helpful in encouraging a wider interest in this research area. The primary aim of this publication is, however, to provide an indication of the present state of development of this field within the United States.

The Symposium Proceedings were recorded by a court reporter and, in addition, recorded directly on magnetic tape. Except for corrections of English usage and phraseology, and occasionally the elimination of nonconsequential conversations, the discussion is recorded here essentially as it took place at the Symposium. It is my personal opinion, that the discussion is of an importance equal to that of the papers themselves. It may sometimes appear to the reader that some of the questions are of minor significance and could, therefore, have been eliminated. One must realize, however, that a simple question and answer concerning procedure may save some investigator, new in the field, days of trial and error operation. In addition, the discussion emphasizes the present development in the field and some of the remaining problems to be solved.

The Symposium was attended by a small group of scientists, mainly physicists and biologists. No attempt was made to represent the large field of clinical medicine which is concerned with ultrasonic diathermy.

We would like to express our sincere appreciation to the Office of Naval Research for their encouragement of this Symposium and for their financial support of the meeting.

ELIZABETH KELLY
Editor

Table of Contents

Acoustic Properties of Blood and Its Components

E. L. Carstensen [1] and H. P. Schwan

The Moore School of Electrical Engineering, University of Pennsylvania, Philadelphia, Pennsylvania

Very little is known, as yet, about the mechanism of absorption of sound in tissue. We have attempted to simplify this problem by choosing a simple but related medium. Blood is a homogeneous liquid from the acoustic point of view and can be measured with greater accuracy than the tissues. Yet, blood is similar to the tissues in the sense that it contains cells.

In earlier work (Carstensen, Li and Schwan, 1953) we demonstrated that a major part of the absorption of sound in blood can be attributed to the presence of the proteins which it contains, i.e. the absorption to a great extent occurs on a purely molecular level. More recent investigations have shown that there is another small component in the absorption which arises from relative motion between the cells and surrounding liquid.

We shall discuss the two mechanisms which cause the absorption of ultrasonic energy in blood: first, the purely protein or molecular absorption and second, the non-protein, relative motion absorption.

Acoustic Properties of Hemoglobin Solutions

The protein chosen for intensive study was the most abundant of the blood proteins, hemoglobin. Hemoglobin solutions were prepared by treating the concentrated red cells of blood with toluene. This action hemolyzed the cell and made it possible by centrifugation to remove almost all of the stromata from the solution. Measurements of the absorption and velocity of sound have been made on the hemoglobin of several mammalian species at various temperatures, concentrations and over a range of values of pH and concentration of neutral salts.

Fig. 1 shows the absorption of sound as a function of frequency in human hemoglobin at a concentration of 16.5 gm. hemoglobin/100 cc. for temperatures 7°, 15°, 25°, and 35° C. Note that the ordinate is absorp-

[1] Now, Camp Detrick, Maryland.

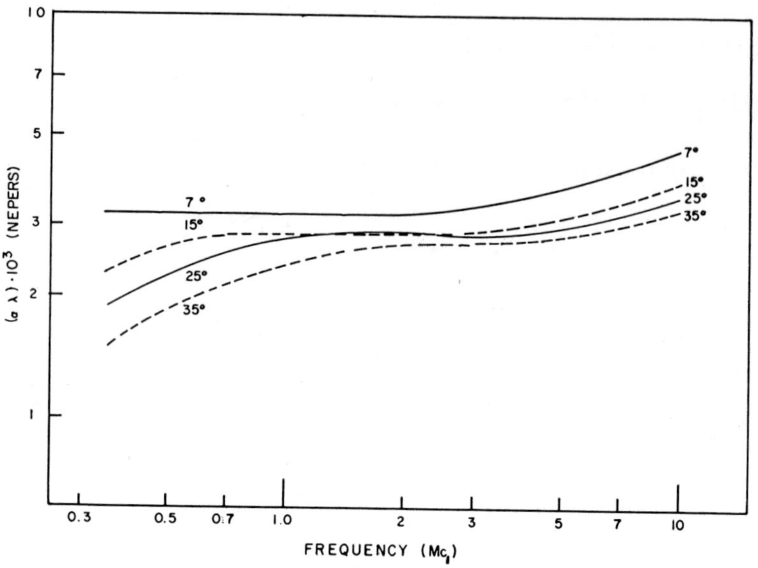

FIG. 1. Influence of Temperature on Solutions of Human Hemoglobin. Absorption per wavelength vs. frequency is given for a concentration of 16.5 gm. Hb/100 cc. Temperature 7°, 15°, 25°, 35° C.

tion per wavelength in nepers. The curves are characterized by a constant middle frequency region, a low frequency region where the absorption falls off with increasing temperature and a high frequency region in which the absorption per wavelength rises over the constant value established in the middle frequency range. The general trend is toward a constant value of $\alpha\lambda$, as is usually reported for tissue, but there are significant departures from that condition. It is tempting to ascribe the absorption to a relaxation process with a broad distribution of relaxing elements. Note that as the temperature increases the curves appear to be shifted toward the higher frequencies as would happen for most relaxation processes.

If a relaxation process is responsible for the absorption, there should be a change in velocity of sound with frequency. Fig. 2 gives the velocity of sound as function of frequency for various concentrations of the human hemoglobin solution above. Measurements were made with a velocity difference technique (Carstensen, 1954a) which has proven sensitive enough to measure the dispersion in the velocity of sound in protein solutions. The existence of dispersion is a strong indication of relaxation processes. However, if a relaxation process is present, a quantitative relationship between absorption and velocity dispersion should be found. This has been demonstrated experimentally (Carstensen, 1954b) for liquids characterized by a single relaxation time. With hemoglobin, however, the problem is compli-

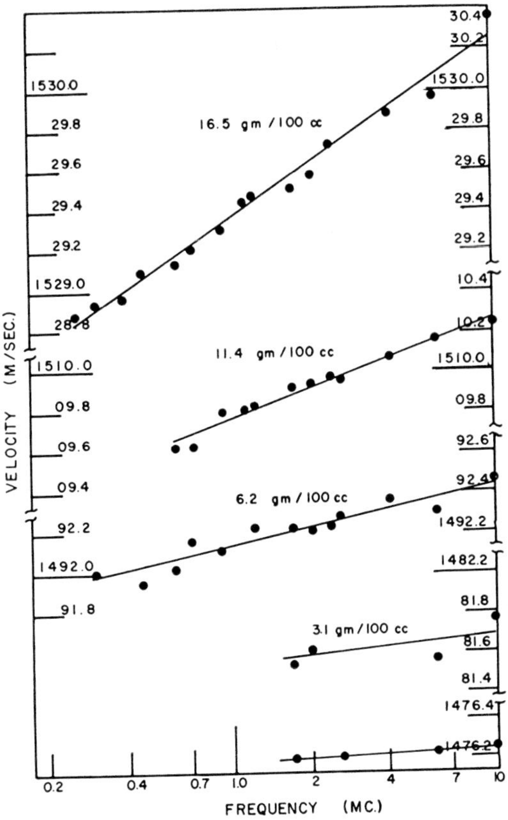

Fig. 2. Dispersion of the Velocity of Sound in Solutions of Human Hemoglobin. Velocity as a function of frequency is given for various concentrations of a hemoglobin solution diluted with distilled water. Temperature 15° C.

cated by a distribution in the characteristic frequency of the relaxing elements. To relate absorption and dispersion without independent knowledge of the distribution of relaxation times is difficult.

There are interesting differences between the absorption of sound in hemoglobin from different species of mammals. As illustrated in Fig. 3, the absorption curve for human hemoglobin has a pronounced plateau in the 1–5 Mc. region. The curve for beef hemoglobin has a continuous slope in the range from 1–10 Mc. but flattens out slightly below 1 Mc. The sheep hemoglobin data are similar to beef, but appear to have a small inflection around 2–4 Mc. These differences are experimentally significant. That is to say that the differences from sample to sample of horse blood, for example, are smaller than the difference between horse and human hemoglobin. In spite of the differences between the various mammalian hemoglobins the

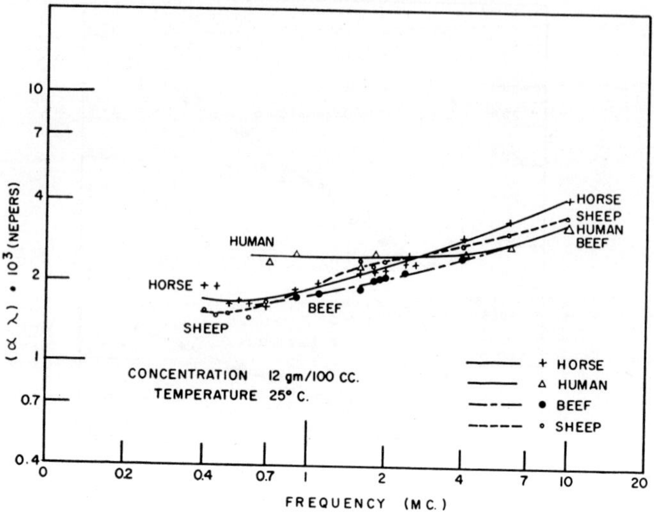

FIG. 3. Absorption of Sound in Solutions of Four Mammalian Hemoglobins. Each solution contains approximately 40 percent of red cells in distilled water. The shapes of the curves are significantly different. Concentration determinations were not accurate enough to detect a significant difference in the absolute level of the various curves. Temperature 25° C.

absorption for any one species was to a great degree independent of its chemical environment. Rather large pH changes and the presence of neutral salts, such as NaCl and $(NH)_2SO_4$, in concentrations great enough to effect changes in solubility had no observable effect on the absorption. However, the absorption of sound in hemoglobin solutions becomes a strong function of concentration above about 15 gm. hemoglobin/100 cc. In Fig. 4 absorption per wavelength per gm. of Hb. is plotted as a function of concentration for two frequencies. Note that the absorption per gram stays nearly constant up to about 15 gm./100 cc.; from there the absorption level increases rapidly with concentration. This implies that at the higher concentrations there is interaction of some form between the molecules.

Absorption of Sound in Blood

The acoustic properties of blood, as related to its protein content and its structure, are discussed next. In Fig. 4, a comparison is presented of the absorption of hemoglobin with the absorption of red cells from beef which have been diluted with distilled water. The data are presented for two frequencies and as a function of concentration. The beef cells have been diluted increasingly with distilled water in order to obtain a variety of concentrations of hemoglobin in the blood. Thus, the concentration level of 30 gm./100 cc. corresponds to packed beef cells, the 20 gm./100 cc. figure

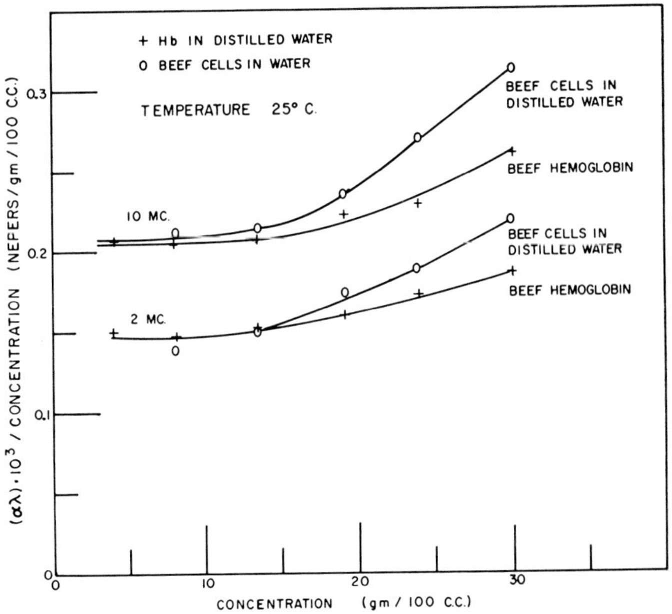

Fig. 4. Absorption of Sound in Solutions of Beef Hemoglobin. Absorption per wavelength per gram of hemoglobin is plotted as a function of concentration (1) for hemoglobin solution (from which approximately 70 percent of the stromata had been removed) and (2) for beef cells progressively diluted with distilled water (all stromata present). Hemoglobin concentration for the two solutions was comparable. The absorption of water in the solution has been subtracted from the observed absorption to show behavior of the protein. Temperature 25° C.

to a dilution of two volume parts packed cells with one part water, etc. The absorption data illustrate that the absorption of sound in the red cells of blood is just that which would be predicted on the basis of the protein which they contain, provided that the cells have been hemolyzed with at least equal volume parts of distilled water. This is shown by comparison of the two curves up to concentrations of 15 gm./100 cc. When the red cells are diluted with distilled water the cell membrane becomes permeable and the hemoglobin is freed so that the concentration inside and outside the cell is roughly uniform. However, if the dilution is less than 1:2, hemolysis is not complete and the local concentration of Hb. in the cells is greater than in the hemoglobin solution at the corresponding dilution. Hence, the data show that blood cells do not add noticeably to the absorption above the level to be expected from their hemoglobin content as long as the concentration of hemoglobin inside and outside the cells is made equal.

For concentration levels in excess of 15 gm./100 cc., the cellular suspensions show higher absorption per gram figures than the hemoglobin solu-

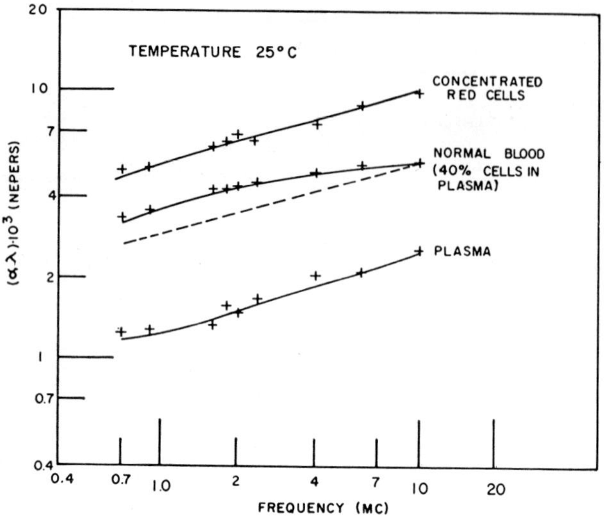

FIG. 5. Absorption of Sound in Beef Blood. Absorption per wavelength ($\alpha\lambda$) is given for the following components of beef blood: (1) the concentrated red cells, (2) plasma, (3) a mixture of cells in plasma in the approximate concentration found in normal blood. Temperature 25° C.

tions of equal concentration. Only a smaller part of the difference can be explained by the fact that the packed cells establish about 90 percent of the total volume and that non-hemolyzed cells contain hemoglobin with a density of 34 gm./100 cc. They must, therefore, absorb more strongly than a hemoglobin solution of the same average concentration due to the rapid increase in the absorption per gram hemoglobin with concentrations demonstrated by the hemoglobin curve.

The absorption of sound in blood is shown in Fig. 5. Here we have shown the cellular and liquid (plasma) components separately, and in between, the absorption as measured for a mixture of two parts concentrated red cells and three parts plasma, which is about the concentration of red cells found in normal blood. The evidence presented so far indicates that the absorption in the packed cells and plasma is a purely molecular phenomena directly related to the concentration of protein present in these substances (Carstensen, Li and Schwan, 1953; Piersol, Schwan, Pennell and Carstensen, 1952). If the same situation holds for normal blood, we should be able to predict its absorption through a linear combination of the red cell and plasma components in it. The dotted line shows the absorption expected on the basis of protein concentration. It appears now that there is another, non-protein, process. This contributes a small but significant amount to the absorption of sound in normal blood which decreases as frequency increases.

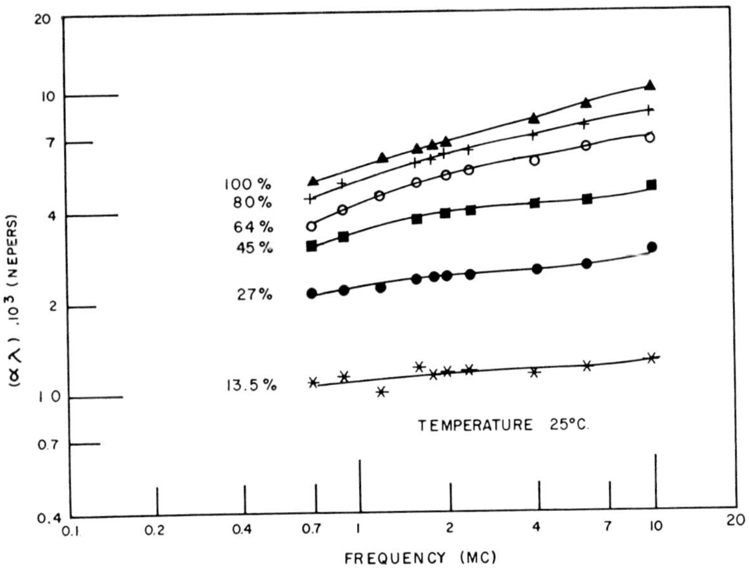

FIG. 6. Absorption of Sound in Solutions of Beef Red Cells in 0.9 gm./100 cc. NaCl Solution. Relative concentration of red cells is indicated in the figure. The absorption of water has been subtracted from the observed absorption to show the influence of the protein. Temperature 25° C.

A somewhat more detailed picture is shown in Fig. 6. Here concentrated red cells have been diluted to various degrees with isotonic saline. Note the change in the slope of the curves as the dilution proceeds, which is not anticipated on a linear basis and, therefore, indicative of the non-protein component of the absorption. The 2 Mc. data from this curve are plotted as a function of concentration in Fig. 7. Here the ordinate is in terms of absorption per gram of hemoglobin. The dotted line represents the absorption which would be expected on a molecular basis for dilution of red cells with isotonic saline (0.9 gm./100 cc.). Note that instead the absorption per cell continues to increase down to about 30 percent cells by volume. Normal packed cells were also diluted with 0.6 percent saline which is hypotonic and will cause the cells to swell and reduce the local concentration and the absorption per gram of hemoglobin. In spite of this, the cells gave a somewhat higher absorption than could be accounted for by protein content alone. At first for dilution with 0.3 percent saline the absorption decreases as dilution increases. Fig. 8 represents similar data, but for 10 Mc. At this frequency the absorption can be accounted for on the basis of protein content and the change in local hemoglobin concentration caused by the cellular volume changes.

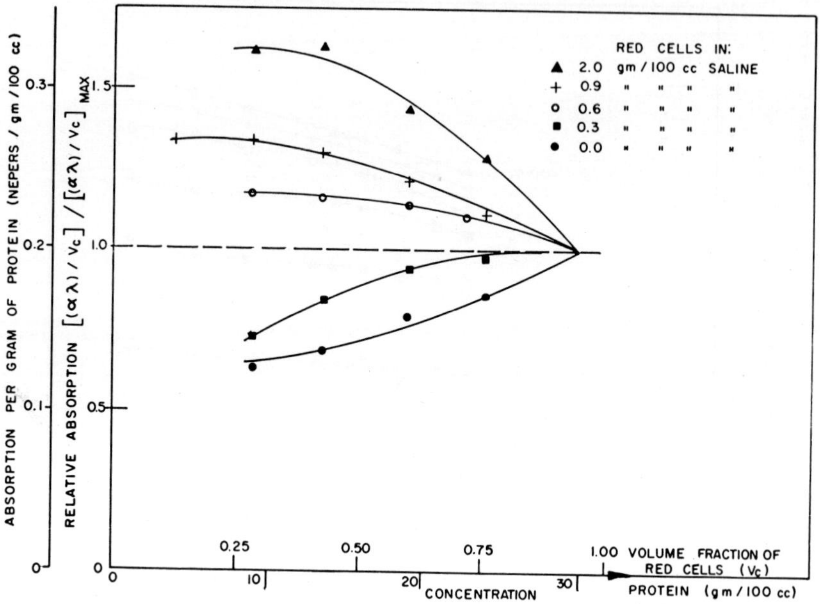

FIG. 7. Absorption of Sound by Beef Red Cells in Sodium Chloride Solutions (2 Mc.). Absorption per wavelength per cc. of cells relative to that observed at maximum concentration is plotted against volume fraction of cells. Beef red cells were diluted with solutions containing from 0 to 2.0 gm./100 cc. NaCl. The outer abscissa and ordinate give the equivalent quantities in terms of protein concentration.

The dramatic effect of the presence of intact cells on the absorption of sound is illustrated by Fig. 9. Here two solutions of identical Hb. concentration were prepared: One consisted of a mixture of equal parts of red cells and isotonic saline; the other, equal parts of red cells and distilled water. In the distilled water preparation the Hb. distribution was uniform because of hemolysis. In the saline preparation the cells were intact. The absorption of the saline preparation was nearly double that of the distilled water preparation. This was true, first, because the local concentration of Hb. was greater in the cells and, second, because of the non-protein absorption which is associated with the presence of intact cells in dilute solution. After measurement both samples were permitted to stand at room temperature while bacterial action caused hemolysis in the saline preparation. By the second day there was no apparent difference in the absorption. This illustrates that the effects observed in the dilution experiments arise simply from the presence of intact cells and do not depend upon a direct action of the salts on the protein.

The non-protein absorption increases with dilution and decreases with frequency, as shown in Figs. 7 and 8. This eliminates scattering as a possi-

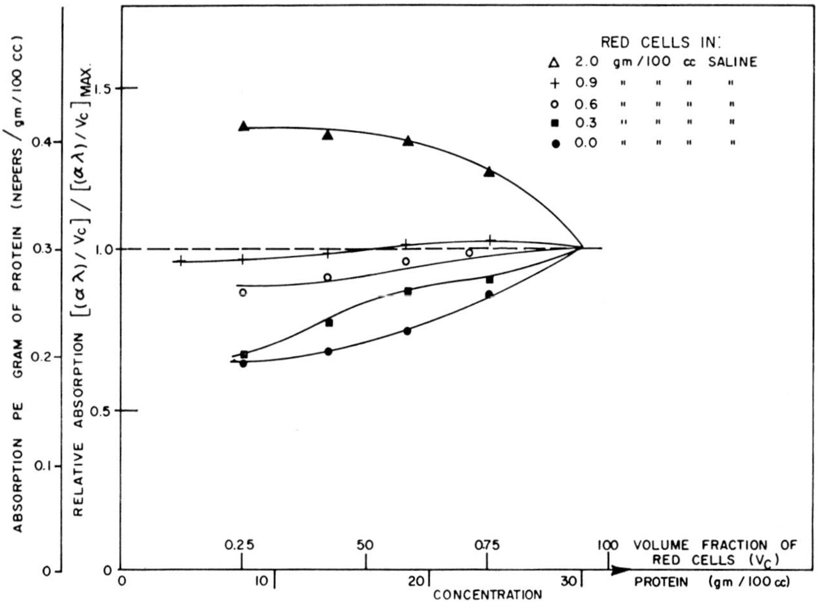

FIG. 8. Absorption of Sound by Beef Red Cells in Sodium Chloride Solutions (10 Mc.). Absorption per wavelength per cc. of cells relative to that observed at maximum concentration is plotted against volume fraction of cells. Beef red cells were diluted with solutions containing from 0 to 2.0 gm./100 cc. NaCl. The outer abscissa and ordinate give the equivalent quantities in terms of protein concentration.

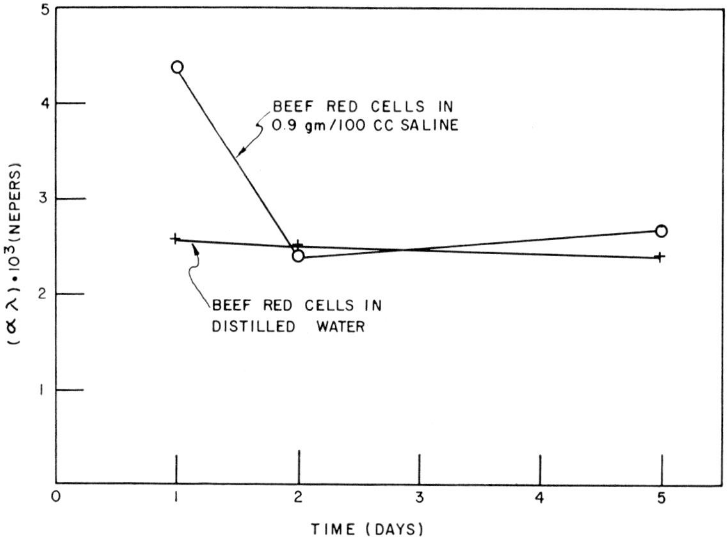

FIG. 9. Aging Effects in Beef Cell Solutions. A single sample of concentrated beef red cells was diluted (1) with an equal volume 0.9 gm./100 cc. NaCl solution, and (2) with an equal volume of distilled water. The absorption was measured immediately after dilution, and after standing at room temperature for five days.

ble mechanism for the observed effects. On the other hand, this behavior can be predicted considering the relative motion between the cells and the surrounding fluid. This relative motion is a consequence of the fact that the cells have higher density than the surrounding fluid and, therefore, tend to lag behind the water as frequency increases.

The absorption per wavelength for relative motion between suspended spherical particles and the surrounding liquid can be shown to be

$$\alpha\lambda = \frac{nR_w}{2\rho f} \frac{(m_e - M_e)^2}{M_e^2} \frac{(\omega/\omega_0)^2}{1 + (\omega/\omega_0)^2}, \tag{5}$$

where

$$\omega_0 = R_w/M_e, \tag{6}$$

$$M_e = M + m\left[1 + \frac{g}{4}\frac{1}{j\omega^{1/2}}\right], \tag{7}$$

$$m_e = m + m\left[\frac{1}{2} + \frac{g}{4}\frac{1}{j\omega^{1/2}}\right],$$

$$R_w = G\pi a\eta\,[1 + j\omega^{1/2}], \tag{8}$$

$$j^2 = a^2\rho/2\eta, \tag{9}$$

and

ω: frequency of observation,

ω_0: "Relaxation frequency",

R_w: Resistance,

M_e: Effective mass of particle,

M: Actual mass of particle,

m: Mass of a quantity of fluid equal in volume to that of the particle,

α: Radius of particle,

ρ: Density of the fluid,

η: Viscosity of the fluid.

Absorption of Sound in Tissue

It is interesting to speculate briefly on the applicability of protein and relative motion absorption to the case as found in the "solid" tissues of the body. Values of the absorption of sound per wavelength in tissues reported by Hueter range from 14×10^{-3} to 45×10^{-3} nepers. (He finds that values

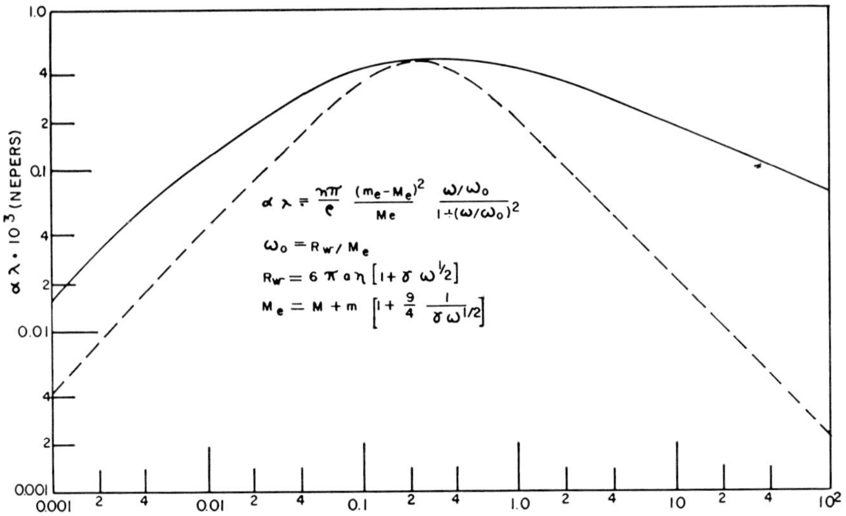

FIG. 10. Relative Motion Absorption. The absorption of sound has been computed (solid line) for a suspension of spheres of radius 2.4 microns, density 1.084 gm./cc., at a volume concentration of 13 percent, in a medium of viscosity $\beta = 0.01$ poise and density $\rho = 1$. The dashed curve shows the shape of the absorption vs. frequency curve which is obtained when the frequency dependence of the mass and resistance are neglected.

of $(a\lambda)$ are independent of frequency.) The protein content of these tissues is less than that found in the concentrated cell preparation of Fig. 3. Yet, the absorption in the tissues is higher by factors of 3 to 9. The other molecular components of tissue, water, salts, and fats, when taken separately all have comparatively low absorption. It appears, therefore, that the structure of the tissue at some level of organization is responsible for its high absorption.

It is rather unlikely that relative motion on a cellular level occurs in tissue, where the cells have a very tight organization. This follows from the fact that a pertinent discussion of the blood measurements reported above shows that no, or only minor, relative motion occurs with the packed erythrocytes. (For example, Fig. 11 demonstrates that the non-protein contribution is proportional to the cell concentration only up to about 25 volume percent. At a concentration of 43 percent the non-protein absorption per cell is already significantly reduced.) Relative motion of different parts of the cell, such as the nucleus and cytoplasm cannot be ruled out on the basis of information from the study of blood, since the erythrocytes are not nucleated. But, it is unlikely that such a process can account for the very high absorption of tissue.

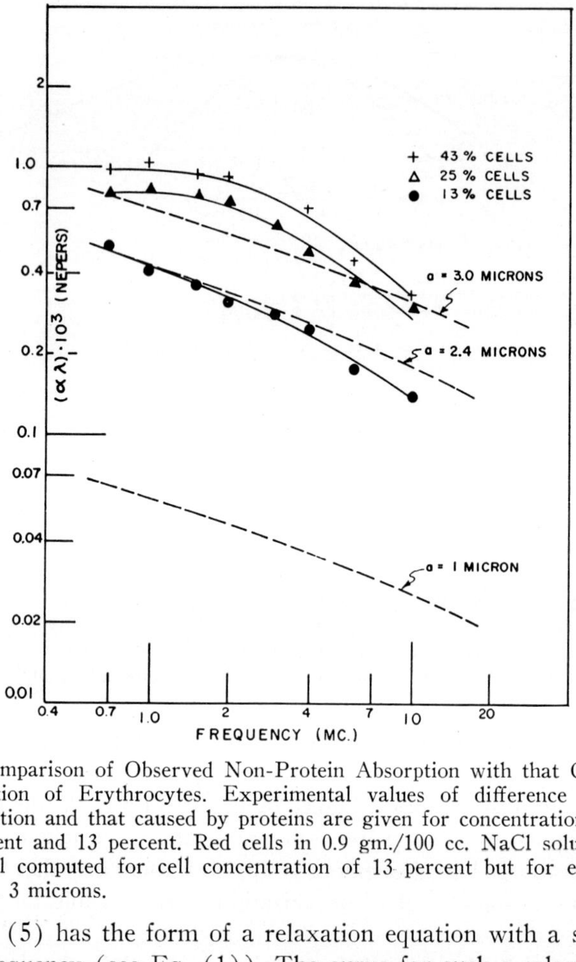

FIG. 11. Comparison of Observed Non-Protein Absorption with that Computed for Relative Motion of Erythrocytes. Experimental values of difference between observed absorption and that caused by proteins are given for concentrations of 43 percent, 25 percent and 13 percent. Red cells in 0.9 gm./100 cc. NaCl solution. Dashed curves are all computed for cell concentration of 13 percent but for effective radii a = 1, 2.4, and 3 microns.

Equation (5) has the form of a relaxation equation with a single characteristic frequency (see Eq. (1)). The curve for such a relaxation process is characterized by one single relaxation time and is given by the dotted line in Fig. 11. However, it is important to note that the parameters M_e, m_e, and R_w in Eq. (5) are frequency dependent and hence even the "relaxation frequency" $f_0 = \omega_0/2\pi$ itself becomes a function of frequency. As a result, the correct curve, which gives $(\alpha\lambda)$ as function of frequency has been found to extend over a somewhat wider frequency range than occurs in the case of simple relaxation processes, where the parameters are frequency independent.

The frequency range in which our measurements have been conducted is above the "relaxation frequency" for relative motion of red cells in blood if the relaxation frequency is defined as the frequency where $(\alpha\lambda)$ reaches its maximum. The experimentally observed "non-protein" absorption for several cell concentrations is shown in Fig. 11. In calculating the absorption by Eq. (5) it is necessary to estimate the radius of the sphere which would have the same effect as the red cell. The maximum and minimum half dimensions of the beef red cell are 3 and 1 microns, respectively. Curves using these values for the radius of the equivalent sphere are shown by dotted lines in the same figure for the 13 percent case. The value of the radius giving best fit to the 13 volume percent experimental data is 2.4 microns. The radius of a sphere having a value equal to that of the red cell is 2.3 microns. The agreement between experiment and theory is strong evidence that the non-protein absorption in blood arises from the relative motion between the cell and the surrounding fluid.

On the other hand, inhomogeneities in tissue are comparable to or in some cases larger than the wavelength of sound in the ultrasonic region. It seems more likely that the high absorption found for tissue may be caused by scattering at these interfaces. Scattering or reflection is a particularly effective mechanism for increasing absorption in a medium like tissue, because both transverse and longitudinal waves are generated by an irregular scatterer and the transverse wave is damped out completely after traveling only a few wavelengths.

There can be little question that a significant part of the absorption in tissue occurs at a molecular level through action of the sound on the proteins. However, it is very likely that we must look for a kind of absorption not found in blood to account for a large part of the non-protein absorption in tissue.

References

Carstensen, E. L. 1954a. Measurement of the dispersion of velocity of sound in liquids. J. Acoust. Soc. Amer. *26:* 858–861.

Carstensen, E. L. 1954b. Relaxation processes in aqueous solutions of $MnSO_4$ and $CoSO_4$. J. Acoust. Soc. Amer. *26:* 862–864.

Carstensen, E. L., K. Li and H. P. Schwan. 1953. Determination of acoustic properties of the blood and its components. J. Acoust. Soc. Amer. *25:* 286–289.

Piersol, G. M., H. P. Schwan, R. B. Pennell and E. L. Carstensen. 1952. Mechanism of absorption of ultrasonic energy in blood. Arch. Phys. Med. *33:* 327–332.

DR. HERRICK: Do you have any information on the leukocytes and other components of the blood?

DR. CARSTENSEN: This was not investigated but my reaction to this question is that all these components are present in comparatively minor quantities and it would be rather surprising if they contributed a large part to the total absorption. Certainly, however, before we say that we know exactly what the absorption of sound in normal blood is, we will have to take these factors into account.

Dr. Rosenberg: I believe—in a paper awhile back—you mentioned that in the case of the cell membrane because of its structure, its absorption would be two times greater than would be expected otherwise. I believe you used that as an explanation for the difference between the absorption in regular blood, compared to hemolyzed blood.

Dr. Carstensen: In the paper to which you refer, our conclusion was that the stromata contributed only an extremely small fraction of the total protein absorption. A measurement on the stromata alone suggested that the absorption per gram for the components of these structures might be as high as two times that of the abundant proteins hemoglobin and albumin. But, because of their relatively small quantity, these structural proteins would cause only perhaps 10 percent of the total absorption for a solution of red cells whether hemolyzed or intact.

The so-called non-protein absorption of our discussion today has been measured in such a way that protein absorption regardless of its source has been eliminated. The absorption of concentrated red cells of blood was measured. This value presumably included the small contribution of the stromata. When the cells were diluted, the absorption per gram of the protein did not change. This protein absorption, as determined from the measurements on the concentrated cells, was subtracted from the absorption observed at lower concentrations. The difference then is truly a non-protein absorption.

Dr. Busnel: Have you observed any differences between the warm blood from mammalians and cold blood from amphibians?

Dr. Carstensen: Unfortunately, we have no source of amphibian blood. For this work we have used beef, sheep and horse blood from the slaughter house.

Physical Aspects of High Amplitude Sound Phenomena

W. L. Nyborg

Department of Physics, Brown University, Providence, Rhode Island

In this paper I should like to review briefly some facts about recently discovered physical phenomena in which you may be interested. These phenomena are such that they might be important causes for the irradiation effects of high amplitude sound.

In considering the various aspects of a sound field, those that first occur to one are the oscillating characteristics: (1) the alternating pressures, which vary above and below atmospheric pressure, and (2) the alternating motions of the particles, described as "to and fro" in the usual acoustic textbooks. One might ask if there is any one of these alternating or AC characteristics which is the important one for effects of sound as an agent. This question would arise if we wished to know what distribution of irradiation effects to expect in a typical sound field, where the AC quantities are by no means uniformly distributed.

There is evidence (Goldman and Lepeschkin, 1952) that under some conditions pressure amplitude is the most important of the oscillating quantities. Fig. 1 shows typical distributions of pressure amplitude in a commercial exposure unit used by many people (Raytheon 10 kc. Oscillator DF101). The container indicated is a stainless steel cup furnished by the manufacturers; the bottom of the cup is a diaphragm, which is set into vibration during irradiation experiments. In obtaining the data of Fig. 1 the unit was operated at low amplitude so that cavitation effects were not important. (In the presence of cavitation it is nearly impossible to know what the pressure amplitudes are.) Measurements were made along the axis of the cup by S. A. Elder. A 1/16-in. barium titanate probe was used. The several curves are for different levels of filling in the cup.

It is clear that the distribution of pressure amplitude is far from uniform. The patterns are approximately describable in terms of simple standing waves. However, a really satisfactory theory for them must take into account the nature of the walls and of the diaphragm velocity distribution. We shall not discuss theoretical details here; suffice it to say that the experimental data in Fig. 1 can be explained rather well on the basis of conventional normal mode theory.

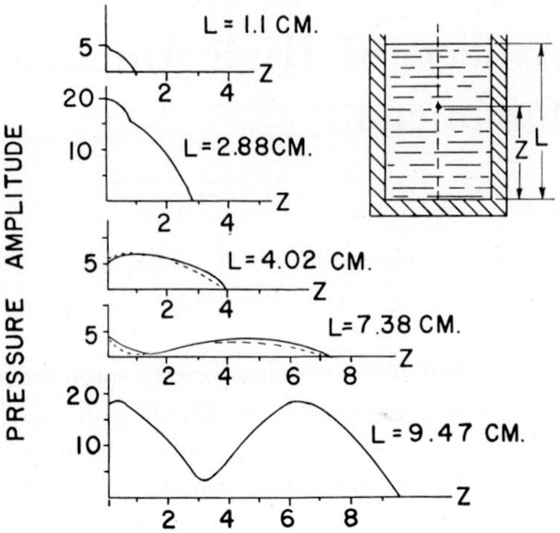

FIG. 1. Plots of Pressure Amplitude *versus* Height along the Axis of a Commercial Irradiation Vessel. Solid curves are experimental, dashed curves theoretical.

Using the ordinary acoustics dynamical equation it is possible to proceed from these data for the pressure amplitude p and obtain distributions of velocity amplitude u. Except near regions where p is minimum the amplitude u of velocity along any axis x is given approximately by

$$2\pi\rho f\, u = \delta p/\delta x, \tag{1}$$

where ρ is the liquid density and f the frequency. It is clear that the velocity distributions for the situation of Fig. 1, like the corresponding pressure patterns, would be nonuniform, exhibiting maxima and minima, and would be dependent on frequency and the height of liquid column.

Since the findings just discussed are probably representative for sonic and ultrasonic irradiation experiments (speaking here of non-focussed sound), it is likely that neither the AC pressure nor the AC velocity is distributed uniformly in a typical exposure chamber. Hence, if irradiation effects are associated with AC quantities, one must conclude that the "exposure conditions," or the "applied acoustic stimuli," are by no means the same in all parts of a container.

It is clearly important to know where one may expect maximum effects in a nonuniform field. Do they, for example, occur at maxima of either the pressure or velocity? Although interesting experiments have been carried out to answer this question, further detailed investigations are needed. For many conditions biological effects appear to be greatest at pressure maxima, but in some cases velocity seems to be the important parameter.

Closely associated with the practical question relative to conditions for maximum irradiation effects is the fundamental one concerning the basic mechanisms involved. Upon reflection one quickly realizes that a complete description of how a biological change is brought about by sound *cannot be given in terms of any AC quantity alone.* This conclusion is important to keep in mind, although it is immediately seen to be more a result of definition than of natural law. Thus AC motions (or AC pressures, whose existence is always due to AC motions) are *by definition* sinusoidal motions of particles about equilibrium positions. The motions of the surfaces of sound sources, such as vibrating diaphragms and piezoelectric crystals, are probably of this type to a fair degree of accuracy; as is to be emphasized, however, the particles of a medium irradiated by high amplitude sound will usually execute a motion of which the AC motion is only a part. The observed biological changes due to the sound are of the nature of increased or inhibited bio-chemical activity, coagulation of particles, and structure disintegration. These changes are, of course, nonoscillatory in character and are, in fact, observed only after a large number of sound cycles. They are evidently the result of processes which *proceed steadily in a given direction,* in spite of the oscillatory nature of the sound source motion to which they are due.

Although such processes may seem mysterious, they are familiar in physical acoustics and are coming to be fairly well understood in terms of mathematical theory. For example, it has been known since the time of Rayleigh that a steady rate of heating occurs at any point P in a steady state sound field, and also that shifts in the average pressure and velocity at P are caused by the sound. Mathematical techniques have been, and continue to be, developed for dealing with these phenomena. Some of the terminology employed will be useful for us here. Thus the AC or alternating components of pressure, velocity, etc., are called *first order* quantities, while the steady or steadily increasing components due to the sound are of second or higher order. The magnitude of a *second order* quantity is characteristically proportional to the square of the sound amplitude.

An example of a second order effect is the *heating* which always occurs in a steady state sound field, causing the temperature to rise continuously until an equilibrium temperature distribution is established. The initial rate of temperature rise is typically proportional to the square of the sound amplitude. The conversion of sound energy into heat, i.e., sound absorption, is discussed in detail elsewhere in this symposium.

Also in the second order category are *radiation* pressures or stresses; these are steady forces exerted on elements of a medium (or on obstacles in the medium) in a sound field. That these forces may be important in sonic irradiation effects seems evident. This subject has received much attention in physical acoustics, but more work is needed in order to deal with such situations as may arise in biology.

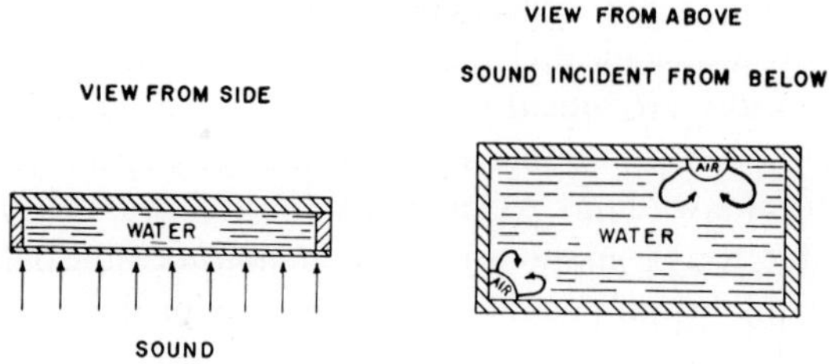

FIG. 2. Arrangement used in Experiments with Air-generated Sound.

Another second-order effect is one which has come to be called *acoustic streaming* or, sometimes, (rather ambiguously) hydrodynamic flow. By this is meant a steady vortex pattern of flow set up by sound in a fluid medium. Such motions may well be very important in contributing to sonic irradiation effects, not only by redistributing matter through convection, but also by exerting viscous forces on boundaries.

Still another important phenomenon, which might be regarded as an effect of second or higher order is the steady production of gas in a sound field. When one has a typical fluid exposed to sound of rather high amplitude, visible gas bubbles are produced. According to theories of Blake (1949), Rosenberg (1953) and others, these grow from small nuclei which are always present in liquids. The appearance of visible bubbles is ordinarily called *cavitation.* (Note: From such a definition it obviously follows that "cavitation" does not occur if the nuclei remain at their original submicroscopic size. It should not be assumed, however, that such nuclei, or invisible cavities, are not significant.) Bubble production is important, not only because dissolved gas is removed thereby, but especially because the generated bubbles are the sites for a great amount of activity. (Even the invisible "nuclei" may be active at high frequencies.) The precise nature of that activity is not known, but its existence is well established from the experiments of many people.

The special topic of this paper is one that has to do with DC flow, i.e., acoustic streaming, and also with the activity near bubbles. It turns out that when one has bubbles present in a sound field, one may observe characteristic micro-streaming patterns set up in the vicinity of these bubbles; such motions may be very important in sonic irradiation. The results to be described have been established only for visible bubbles, but may well have their counterpart also for invisible ones.

As far as the author is concerned, such motions were first observed in experiments done at the Pennsylvania State University in the course of interdepartmental research sponsored by the Air Force (Nyborg, Nertney and Spencer, 1950; Nyborg, 1954). One of the physicists' tasks was to design containers for exposing biological suspensions to air-generated sound from sirens and/or whistles. An experimental arrangement is shown schematically in Fig. 2. The container consisted of an optically transparent shallow cell. It enclosed a thin layer of water or suspension, a few millimeters deep; the latter was supported by a thin film transparent to the sound, which came from below. A transparent lucite cover plate kept the liquid from blowing away.

For our purposes, the main advantage of this arrangement was that here we could make direct visual observations of events taking place during sonic irradiation. Using indicating particles and low power microscopy, we found that if air pockets were present, characteristic steady vortex motions were set up near those air pockets. We also found that this kind of cell is not very practical for an interesting reason. It is difficult to fill the container without including air pockets; when these are present a great deal of the streaming motion takes place and an excessive amount of heating occurs.

Other aspects of the effects of such streaming showed up in an experiment done by a student of Frings and Boyd (Ackerman, Reid, Kinsloe and Frings, 1953). A small cell of the kind depicted in Fig. 2 was filled with a suspension of paramecia. Upon exposure to sound the latter were found to be killed quickly if the bubble-induced streaming was present, but only very slowly otherwise. The effect was evidently due to the bombardment of the little creatures against walls of the container. The kind of container shown in Fig. 2 is a rather special one and the conditions under which it was used were certainly special. The question naturally arose as to whether the same effects might occur under more general circumstances in other kinds of containers and with other frequencies. Since that time experiments have been carried out at Brown University which indicate that microstreaming phenomena near gas bubbles are indeed the rule, rather

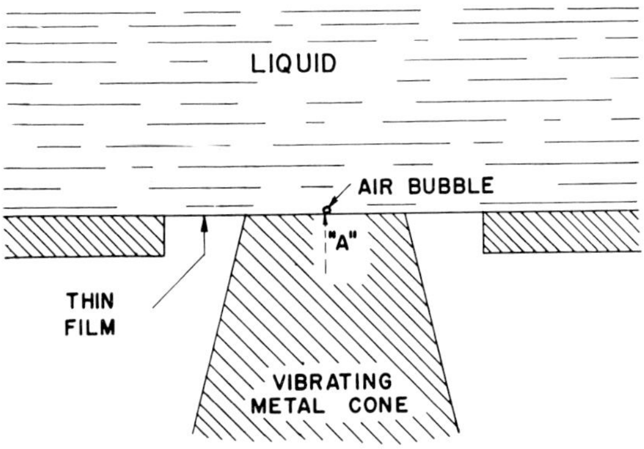

FIG. 3. Arrangement used in Experiments with Vibrating Metal Cone.

than the exception. Also, it appears that such motions may be of great importance in irradiation effects.

Fig. 3 shows a setup used by J. Kolb in certain experiments carried out by him. Again a layer of liquid is supported by film transparent to sound. This time the sound is generated by a vibrating metal cone, placed below the film as indicated. With this arrangement an interesting set of phenomena were observed.

As an illustration of typical findings let us suppose that one starts, in the absence of sound, with a medium which contains dissolved gas but is free of visible bubbles. The cone is then caused to vibrate, thereby setting up a sound field of moderate amplitude in the liquid. Observing with a low power microscope one soon finds tiny bubbles appearing and growing here and there on the upper surface of the film. After these reach a certain size they jerk loose and go towards the center of the cone tip, i.e., to the point "A" indicated by the tip of the arrow in Fig. 3. A few there combine to form a larger bubble. Once the larger bubble is present the smaller bubbles are even more strongly attracted to the point "A"; the migration of little bubbles towards the center and the consequent growth of the large bubble through combination is then greatly speeded up.

This process continues until the bubble at "A" grows to resonant size (about 0.6 mm. diameter) for the 10 kc. frequency. It then becomes very unstable and darts about in many directions. In a rather short time it comes to rest at the edge of the container. A new bubble then appears and begins to grow at "A," etc.

It is possible to give a simple picture of this, following, in a general way, a discussion given by Rosenberg (1953). Let p^* be the instantaneous pressure in the neighborhood of a small bubble and let v^* be the instantaneous volume of the latter. In a sound field p^* will have two major parts. The first is a constant P_0, the hydrostatic pressure, independent of time and also of space, except for a small variation with height. The second part varies sinusoidally in time with an amplitude $p(x)$ which varies in space; for simplicity we here assume the space variation is only along the direction of an arbitrary coordinate x. Hence we have

$$p^* = P_0 + p(x) \cos \omega t. \tag{2}$$

The bubble volume also has two parts: a constant part v_0, giving the equilibrium volume corresponding to the pressure P_0; and a sinusoidally varying part whose amplitude is proportional to the alternating component of pressure and whose phase may differ from that of the pressure by an angle α. Thus

$$v^* = v_0 + b\, p(x) \cos (wt + \alpha), \tag{3}$$

where b is a constant. The fact that the pressure varies across the surface of the bubble causes a net force (analogous to buoyant force) to be exerted on it. The instantaneous value of this force F_x, directed along x, is

$$F_x = -v^* \, (\delta p^*/\delta x) \tag{4}$$

Substituting values for p^* and v^* from Eqs. (2) and (3) into Eq. (4), we obtain a result for F_x whose time-average is not zero. This means that a *steady* force acts on the bubble, its value is given by

$$\langle F_x \rangle = -\tfrac{1}{2}\, b\, p \frac{\partial p}{\partial x} \cos \alpha = -\frac{b}{4} \frac{\partial (p^2)}{\partial x} \cos \alpha \tag{5}$$

For bubbles well below resonant size $\cos \alpha = -1$ and the steady force is in the direction of increasing pressure amplitude. The physical significance of this situation may be easily seen. During the compression part of a sound cycle the bubble is of reduced size and, because of the way v^* enters in Eq. (4), the magnitude of F_x is therefore less than during the expansion part of the cycle. (The magnitude of $(\delta p^*/\delta x)$ is, of course, the same in a given part of the compression half of the cycle as in the corresponding part of the expansion half.) But during compression the force is in the direction of decreasing pressure amplitude and during expansion, in the opposite direction. Hence during a sound cycle a net force exists, in the direction of increasing pressure amplitude.

Conversely, for bubbles well above resonant size $\cos \alpha = 1$ and the steady force is in the direction of decreasing pressure amplitude.

With these ideas in mind the facts previously described are readily explained. We expect the sound field in the liquid to be such that the pressure amplitude is maximum at the point "A" and falls off with distance from this point. Hence small bubbles will move toward "A." As a larger bubble forms at "A" and grows to approach resonant size it will radiate a scattered field of its own of higher and higher amplitude. Since this scattered field consists approximately of a spherical wave the growing center bubble will itself be the site of a pressure maximum and the acceleration of small bubbles toward "A" will be enhanced. When the center bubble becomes of resonant size $\cos \alpha$ becomes zero and this bubble is no longer attracted to "A." Finally, when the bubble becomes a little greater than resonant size it is repelled from "A" and seeks a region where the pressure amplitude is minimum.

The arrangement of Fig. 3 is favorable for observations of the kind described above because lighting conditions are good, and because a pressure maximum keeps the center bubble fixed in the field of view. Nevertheless, the same phenomena very likely occur under rather general conditions. This suggests a special reason why the pressure maxima are often found to be the important regions for irradiation effects: active bubbles tend to form there and these exert effects of their own.

The initial purpose of the experiments just described was to study streaming effects near bubbles. Kolb found that the arrangement of Fig. 3 is well suited for observation of such effects. He used a fairly viscous liquid like glycerin, in which small bronze particles were suspended. In the presence of sound, after a bubble has formed at "A," circulatory motions may be observed in the fluid adjacent to the bubble. When the bubble is small, or the sound amplitude low, the motions appear as a slow churning in a vortex pattern; the latter has symmetry about the vertical axis through "A." As the bubble grows, or the sound amplitude increases, the streaming velocities increase. When the bubble is near resonant size the motion is usually very vigorous and chaotic, even for only moderate sound amplitudes.

Elder has recently made further study of these events. He has investigated the streaming patterns as a function of bubble size, sound amplitude and liquid viscosity. His arrangement is similar to that depicted in Fig. 3, but differs in that the lower boundary of the container was formed, not by a plastic film, but by a vibrating steel diaphram; the frequency was about 10 kc. Elder found that the most general type of streaming pattern consists mainly of two oppositely directed vortex rings, a lower one and an upper one. (see Fig. 4) The sense of the latter is such that the direction of flow is downward, i.e., towards the bubble, at points on the vertical axis through the bubble. At the frequency of 10 kc. in a liquid of low viscosity and at low amplitudes the height of the lower layer is very small; only the upper streaming is then observed, except under close scrutiny. As viscosity increases, the height of the lower layer increases, and for liquids of high viscosity may predominate.

The streaming pattern is dependent in a rather complicated way on the sound amplitude; the pattern also is a function of bubble size, perhaps mainly because the vibration amplitude of the bubble is dependent on its size. Details on these matters will be published elsewhere.

The photograph shown in Fig. 5, obtained by Elder and Jackson, shows

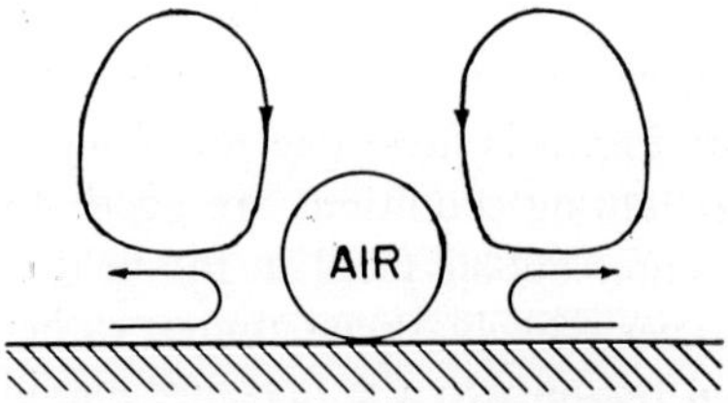

FIG. 4. Sketch of Acoustic Streaming near Vibrating Gas Bubble.

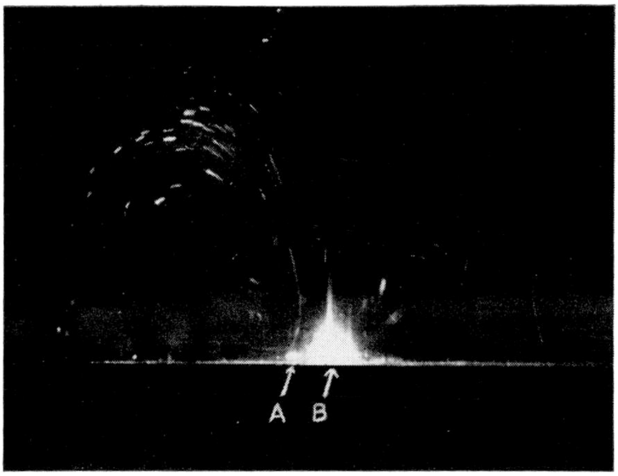

FIG. 5. Photograph of Acoustic Streaming near Bubble above Vibrating Diaphragm. Diaphragm indicated by horizontal bright line at bottom of picture. Bubble is at "B." Vertical bright line through center of B is an artifact. The vortex motion, seen especially well on the left, is that of the upper streaming (see Fig. 4); this streaming is symmetrical about a vertical axis through the bubble, though it does not appear so because indicating particles are scarce on the right. The lower streaming is confined to a small region "A."

the streamlines in a liquid of moderate viscosity at fairly low amplitude. Silver particles were used as indicators. The bubble which appears in the lower center is about 0.6 mm. in diameter, and thus is approximately of resonant size for the frequency, 10 kc., employed. The bubble rests on the plane boundary of a vibrating steel diaphragm; the portion below this boundary is simply an optical reflection. There are two directions of streaming present here. The obvious one is what was called the "outer layer" in the previous discussion; the streaming is downward, toward the bubble, along the vertical axis. The lower layer is barely visible, and appears only as a bright spot in the photograph.

There is good evidence that this bubble-associated streaming is the intermediate agent for laundering and degreasing effects of sound. A simple demonstration is to coat a film or plate with colored grease, then immerse it in a liquid bath and irradiate with sound (only moderate amplitude is required). Bubbles tend to form on the coated surface. By observation with a microscope one can see grease being removed from sites of the resonant-size bubbles. When the sound is turned off small clear areas are seen at the bubble positions.

Penn, Yeager and Hovorka (1954) have recently investigated a completely different kind of situation, where effects of this kind appear to be involved. By Schlieren optical methods they observed that concentration

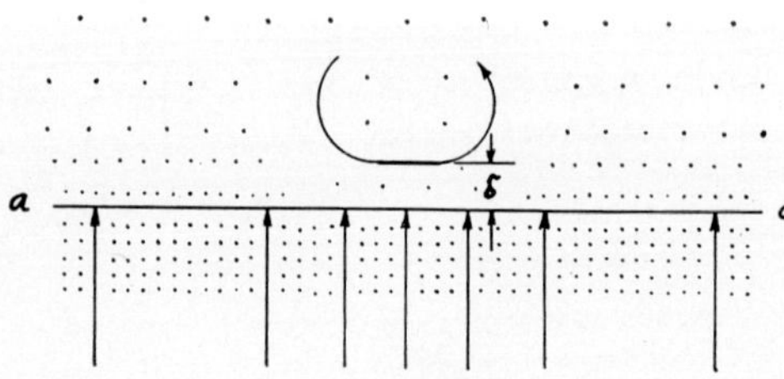

FIG. 6. Sketch showing the Effect of Acoustic Streaming on Transfer of Solute across a Boundary.

gradients near an electrode in a liquid are greatly affected by the presence of sound waves, and especially when bubbles are present. It is reasonable to suppose that bubble-induced streaming is playing an important role here.

In general one may expect rate processes of many kinds, with which living organisms abound, to be greatly affected by convection due to acoustic streaming. Such a possibility has been suggested previously by Lehmann (1953). Fig. 6 is a highly schematic sketch indicating the kind of effect to be expected. The line *aa* represents a real or fictitious boundary below which exists a kind of gaseous, liquid or solid solute material densely distributed throughout a solvent. The solute diffuses across the boundary *aa* at a rate which depends, among other things, on the vertical gradient $(d\rho/dy)$ of the solute density ρ, evaluated at the boundary. (If the boundary consists of a real membrane $(d\rho/dy)$ may be replaced by $(\Delta\rho/\Delta y)$, where $\Delta\rho$ is the difference in solute density on the two sides of the membrane and the membrane thickness is Δy.)

In the absence of convection, the density ρ may vary rather slowly with height and the rate of transfer across the boundary may be relatively slow. However, suppose a circulatory flow is present, as depicted in Fig. 6. Liquid of high solute density will then constantly be swept away from points near the boundary and replaced by liquid of low solute density. A high gradient of ρ will then develop in the vicinity of the sweeping action. The resulting high gradient $(d\rho/dy)$ at the boundary will cause a greatly increased transfer of matter across areas above which there is localized convection.

Arguments, similar in a general way to that just given, can be used to show how localized convection can accelerate diffusion from solid granules or liquid drops into the surrounding liquid, and also can accelerate certain kinds of chemical reactions. It is clear that any rate process that depends on concentration gradients in a liquid is likely to be affected.

It is natural to ask whether there is anything about these convection effects which is peculiar to acoustic streaming. Could not the same effects be produced by mechanical stirring?

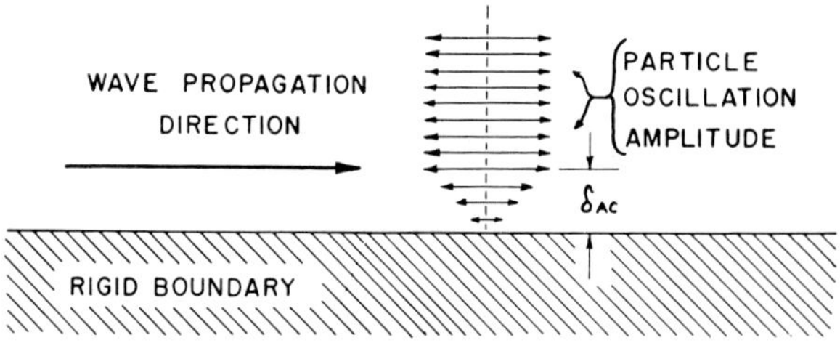

FIG. 7. The Acoustic Boundary Layer.

One difference which may be pertinent to biological problems is that acoustic streaming can take place in an enclosed space not accessible to a mechanical stirrer. Thus, as early as 1930, Harvey (1930) observed turbulent motion in plant cells being irradiated with ultrasonics, and was convinced of its significance.

Another difference is that with acoustic streaming high velocity gradients are to be expected, hardly attainable with a mechanical stirrer. In order to understand why this should be, it is well to consider very briefly a few characteristic features of basic situations where streaming occurs, and for which physical theory exists. These features also very likely apply to bubble-associated acoustic streaming, for which theory has been only partially developed.

Suppose a sound wave travels along a rigid boundary, as indicated in Fig. 7. If the frequency is high and the viscosity of the fluid above the boundary not too great, the amplitude of particle oscillation in the wave will drop rather abruptly from its free space value to zero at points near the boundary. The region very near the boundary, where the particle amplitude is changing rapidly, is often called the *acoustic boundary layer.* An index of the boundary layer thickness is δ_{ac}, the distance from the boundary where the amplitude is $(1 - e^{-1})$ or 0.63 times its free field value. Specifically δ_{ac} is given by

$$\delta_{ac} = (\mu/2\pi\rho f)^{1/2} \tag{6}$$

where μ is the shear viscosity coeffiicent of the liquid, ρ the liquid density and f the frequency. Taking 1.0 poise as a representative viscosity and 1.0 gm./cc. as a representative density for liquids of biological interest we obtain $\delta_{ac} = (0.4/f^{1/2})$. For the frequencies 10^4, 10^6 and 10^8 cps we obtain 4×10^{-3}, 4×10^{-4} and 4×10^{-5} cm., respectively, for δ_{ac}. At ultrasonic frequencies the boundary layer is thus microscopically thin.

It is this boundary layer which is responsible for acoustic streaming in many instances. Mathematically, a solution of basic hydrodynamical equations in which the acoustic boundary layer appears is used to calculate the streaming solution. It was Lord Rayleigh (1884) who developed this theo-

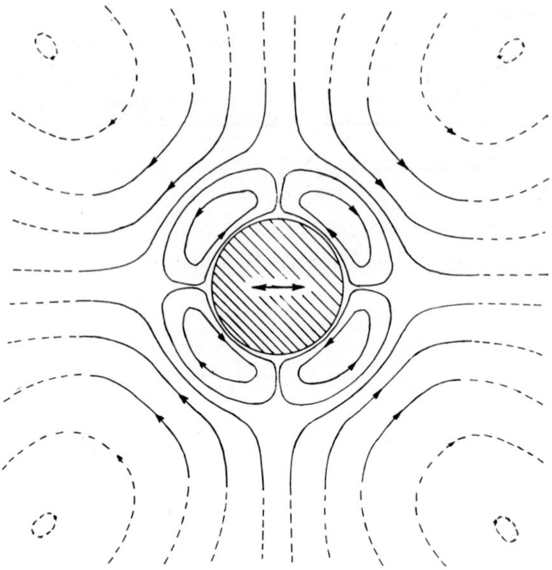

FIG. 8. Acoustic Streaming near an Oscillating Cylinder. The arrow in the cylinder gives the direction of oscillation. (After Holtzmark et al., 1954.)

retical technique; one of the first problems to which he applied it was that of the vortex motion responsible for the well known dust piles in a Kundt's tube experiment.

A satisfactory solution for the streaming near a small cylinder in an oscillating fluid was given recently by Holtsmark, Johnsen, Sikkeland and Skavlem (1954) and shown by them to agree well with experiment. Improvements were made by Raney, Corelli and Westervelt (1954); the latter authors also give a critical analysis of theory and experiment bearing on this problem. In general an eight-fold array of vortices is found, as indicated in Fig. 8. As one starts at the surface of the cylinder and proceeds outward along a radius in any direction the tangential component of velocity increases from zero to a maximum, decreases to zero, reverses sign, increases to a smaller maximum then steadily decreases. The radial distance from the surface of the cylinder out to the point of reversal has been called the DC boundary layer thickness δ_{dc}. Raney et al. present a curve relating experimental results for δ_{dc} to those for δ_{ac}; the fact that data for both air and water fall on this curve suggests that the latter may be generally valid. From this curve one finds that for frequencies high enough so that (δ_{ac}/a) is less than 0.02, where a is the cylinder radius, the ratio $(\delta_{dc}/\delta_{ac})$ always lies between 2.0 and 3.0; for lower frequencies $(\delta_{dc}/\delta_{ac})$ rises above this range of values.

Let ϵ be the radial distance from the surface of the cylinder out to the point of maximum tangential velocity. Then ϵ is always less than δ_{dc}; hence, in the high frequency range, ϵ is of the same order of magnitude as δ_{ac}. Referring to Eq. (6) we have that

$$\epsilon \sim (\mu/2\pi\rho f)^{1/2};$$

typical values of this constant were given previously. This result strongly suggests the difference to be expected between results of mechanical and ultrasonic "stirring." A mechanical rotator or shaker is typically of very low frequency; the generated "boundary layers," if they may be said to exist, are of much greater thickness than those produced ultrasonically. Ultrasonic waves therefore have a unique ability to cause localized high gradients of velocity and hence high viscous stresses.

Results similar to those for the cylinder have recently been found by Lane (1955) for streaming near an oscillating sphere.

For the case of streaming near a vibrating gas bubble there is as yet no adequate theory; the problem is complicated by a number of different features. A major cause of the streaming is believed to be the acoustic boundary layer associated with the (approximately spherical) wave scattered from the bubble as it interacts with the lower boundary. Elder has found that the maximum velocity occurs at a height above the boundary roughly comparable to δ_{ac}; this result is similar to those discussed previously for the cylinder. This bubble-associated acoustic streaming appears to offer a particularly effective way of causing localized high gradients of velocity, and the possible importance of this phenomenon in causing irradiation effects should not be ignored.

References

Ackerman, E., J. J. Reid, H. Kinsloe and H. W. Frings. 1953. Biological effects of high-intensity sound waves. WADC Tech. Report 53-82. 51 pp.

Blake, F. G., Jr. 1949. The onset of cavitation in liquids. Technical Memorandum No. 12. ONR Contract N5ori-76. Acoust. Res. Lab. Harvard Univ. Cambridge, Mass.

Elder, S. A. Work done in partial fulfillment of the requirements for the Ph.D. degree in physics at Brown University. (Pub. pending.)

Goldman, D. E. and W. W. Lepeschkin. 1952. Injury to living cells in standing sound waves. J. Cell. and Comp. Phys. *40:* 255–268.

Harvey, E. N. 1930. Biological aspects of ultrasonic waves, a general survey. Biol. Bull. *59:* 306–325.

Holtsmark, J., I. Johnsen, T. Sikkeland, and S. Skavlem. 1954. Boundary layer flow near a cylindrical obstacle in an oscillating, incompressible fluid. J. Acoust. Soc. Amer. *26:* 26–39.

Kolb, J. Fulbright fellow at Brown University for the year 1952–53. (Pub. pending.)

Lane, C. A. 1955. Acoustical streaming in the vicinity of a sphere. J. Acoust. Soc. Amer. *27:* 1082–1086.

Nyborg, W. L., R. J. Nertney and J. W. Spencer. 1950. Techniques for exposing biological suspensions to air-generated sound. J. Acoust. Soc. Amer. *22:* 683. Abstract.

Nyborg, W. L. 1954. Controlled sonic irradiation of living organisms. WADC Tech. Report 53-128. 40 pp.

Penn, R., E. Yeager and F. Hovorka. 1954. The interaction of acoustical waves with concentration gradients. J. Acoust. Soc. Amer. *26:* 950. Abstract.

Raney, W. P., J. C. Corelli and P. J. Westervelt. 1954. Acoustical streaming in the vicinity of a cylinder. J. Acoust. Soc. Amer. *26:* 1006–1014.

Rayleigh, P. 1884. Trans. 175.

Rosenberg, M. D. 1953. Gaseous-type cavitation in liquids. Technical Memorandum No. 26. ORN Contract N5ori-76. Acoust. Res. Lab. Harvard Univ. Cambridge, Mass.

DR. WEISSLER: An alternate explanation for killing of paramecia, removal of grease, is mechanical impulse at the collapse of cavitation bubbles. Is it possible by careful observation of the removal of colored grease from the vicinity of the attached bubble to determine whether the removal appears to be greater right at the point of attachment of the bubble or in those areas where there seems to be a great deal of streaming towards the bubble?

DR. NYBORG: From observations made with low-powered microscopes, the indication seems very strong that it is streaming. We know about where the streaming is greatest, and we can see about where the removal of the material is greatest. However, I will admit that more detailed study should be made to nail that down for sure.

A point that should be made here is that this was pretty low amplitude sound. It is probably not what you would call cavitating sound at all. These effects can be noticeable even for sound pressure of tenths of an atmosphere or even as small as hundredths of an atmosphere.

DR. WEISSLER: Did you inject the bubble?

DR. NYBORG: Yes.

DR. WEISSLER: This was not a bubble that appeared spontaneous?

DR. NYBORG: No. In the experiments done at Penn State the bubbles were a millimeter or two in diameter; these can easily be put in artifically.

DR. BALDES: Could you state the approximate intensities used in your work?

DR. NYBORG: I do not think that I can give you a meaningful value for the intensity in these experiments. The pressure amplitudes were in order of 0.1 of an atmosphere or less. I think that the smallness of the amplitudes is an important thing to keep in mind. Actually, we had to go to pains to get sufficiently small amplitudes. Motions could be observed for sound pressure amplitudes of about 0.01 atmospheres; in terms of decibels the level would be about 150 db (referred to 2×10^{-4} dynes/cm.^{2}).

DR. HERRICK: We have been making an interesting study of the degassing of the cornea of the eye, which makes a nice test object because of its structure. We find that if we use oil as an accompanying medium we get a degassing effect that we do not get if we use boiled water. I was wondering if this might not be an excellent test object for coupling mediums. What did you use for your diaphragm, and was there any heat developed because of the coupling effect? Was your medium kept temperature-controlled?

DR. NYBORG: These amplitudes were low enough so that not very much heat was generated, and the temperature did not rise to an appreciable extent. In the experiment at Penn State a rubber dam was used and a plastic plate. A great deal of heat was generated when exposed to a field of something like 160 or 155 db. The amount of heat generated was so great that the experiment was just not acceptable in that form.

Progress in the Techniques of Soft Tissue Examination by 15MC Pulsed Ultrasound

J. J. Wild and J. M. Reid

Medico-Technological Research Department, St. Barnabas Hospital, Minneapolis, Minnesota

SINCE THE LAST Symposium, our efforts have become concentrated more and more, as experience grew, on improving instrumentation aimed at the diagnosis and detection of cancer; an exciting business. For the benefit of those members of the audience who were not present at the last Symposium (1952) it is proposed briefly to review the early background of our work before going on to developments.

Early in 1949 the senior author decided to investigate the possibility of applying technological developments of the recent world conflict to the direct study of bowel function. In this simple manner biology inherited a tremendous technical effort, the Naval Ultrasonic Radar Trainer AN/APS-15-Z-1 resting at the Naval Air Station at Wold-Chamberlain Field, Minneapolis. A fruitful partnership was formed between Dr. Finn J. Larsen, now director of the Minneapolis-Honeywell Research Department, who had had a considerable amount to do with the design of the Radar Trainer, and a bio-medical man, the senior author. With the encouragement and help of Dr. Larsen, access was obtained to the Naval Trainer.

The Navy machine worked as follows (Fig. 1): A source of timing pulses initiates each cycle; a transmitter generates each pulse as an electrical voltage. A transducer of quartz is used to convert this pulse to a short train of ultrasonic waves. A receiver is coupled to the same transducer to pick up and amplify voltage produced in the transducer by echoes returning from the system. The display units show the results continuously on a cathode ray tube. The attenuation at 15 mc. is within the range predictable from Hueter's data (1948), of the order of 17 to 25 decibels per cm. in the breast.

Some simple experiments were designed to determine whether the theoretical resolution of about 1–1½ mm. in depth—1 microsecond pulse—could be realized at 15 mc.

A piece of dog bowel was removed and opened at the mesenteric attachment to form a sheet of tissue (Fig. 2). It soon became apparent that the

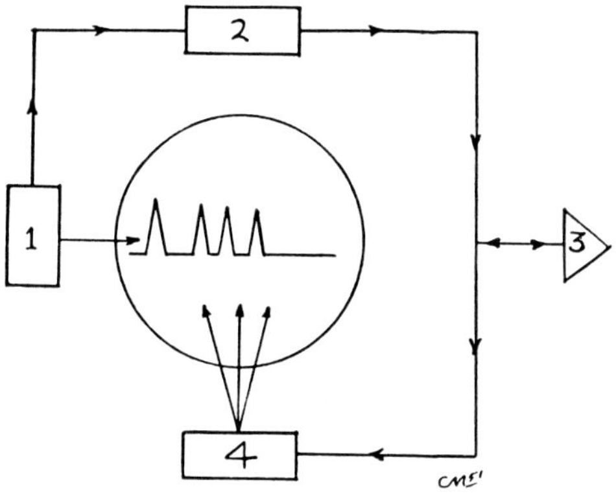

FIG. 1. A Schematic Diagram of the Apparatus. The pulse timer (1) starts the trace on the oscilloscope and times the bursts of sound energy produced by (2) into the piezo-electric crystal (3). Returning signals pass to amplifier (4) and are recorded continuously on the oscilloscope as shown.

small difference in thickness of the bowel specimen, between the middle and the ends, could be observed with certainty.

A small chamber was then constructed, set up on a table and filled with boiled distilled water. One, two, and three layers of fresh dog bowel could be identified when set upon the instrument (Wild, 1950). Since the proposed bowel studies would require a collapsed instrument for insertion into

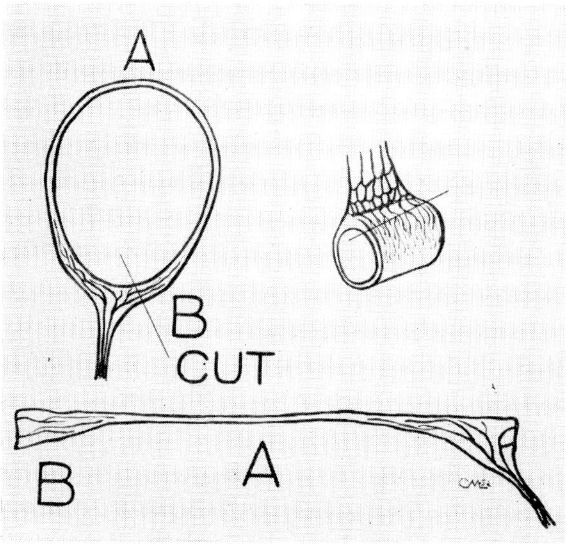

FIG. 2. Method of Obtaining a Sheet of Biological Tissue with Slight Variations in Thickness between A and B.

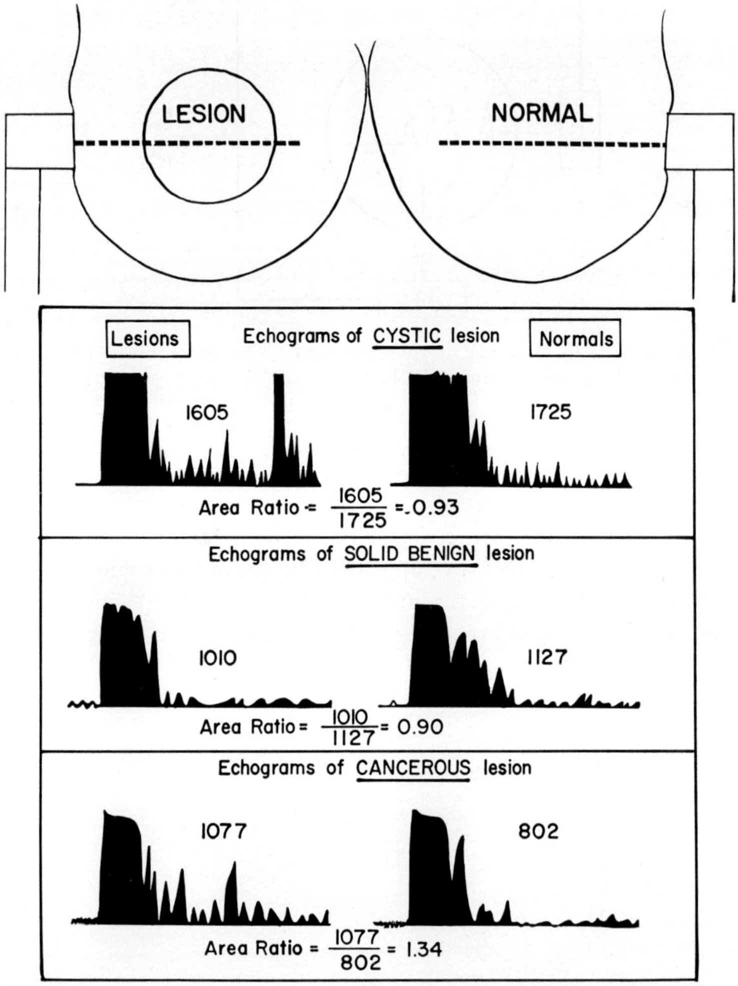

FIG. 3. The Area Ratio Discovery. Uni-dimensional echograms of the lesion and of normal tissue in the same subject at the same setting of the machine were recorded. The trace was projected on to paper ruled to form squares and the area under the trace computed. The conclusion reached was that more sound was returned from cancer tissue than from normal tissue and less sound was returned from benign lesions than from normal tissue. This result gave encouragement to proceed to two-dimensional presentation.

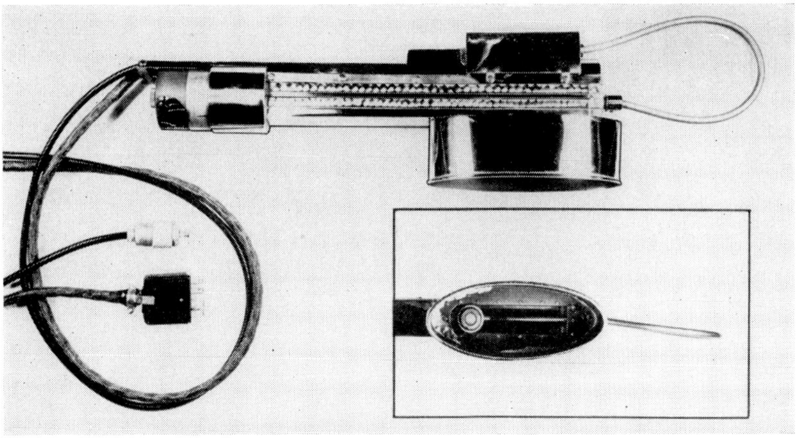

FIG. 4. Two-dimensional Body Surface Scanning Instrument.

the bowel, a water-filled balloon seemed a logical development. The problem posed was whether a useful amount of sound could be driven through the containing rubber membrane. The quickest way to find out was to close the chamber with a rubber membrane and repeat the experiments (Wild, 1950). Thus, the first "Echoscope" (Wild and Reid, 1952) came into being.

It was found that echoes could be obtained, even with the closed echoscope, from the interface between dissimilar tissues such as fat and muscle

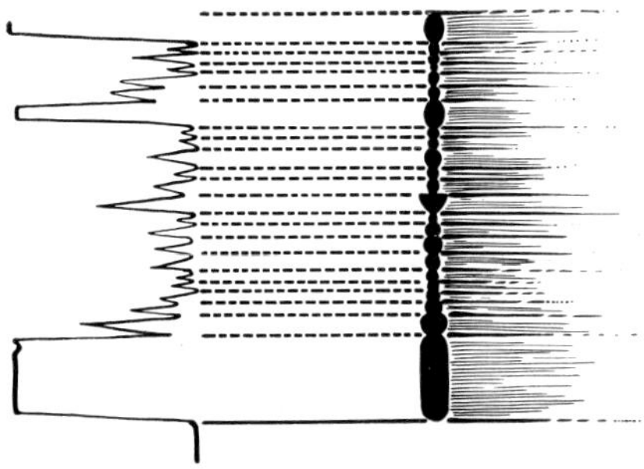

FIG. 5. Two Types of Uni-dimensional Cathode Ray Traces Obtained From Tissues are Shown. The time base is from below up in both types. The graphic trace shows the echoes expressed in terms of strength as deflections of the base line. To the right is an exaggerated equivalent intensity modulated trace. The echo strength is expressed as areas of differing brightness in the trace. The intensity modulated trace can be used to produce echographic tissue patterns in two dimensions; up and down and side to side.

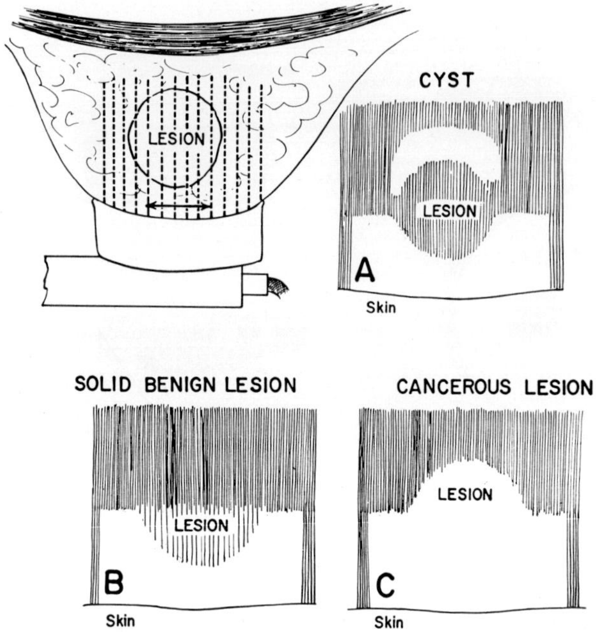

FIG. 6. Direct Visualization of Lesions of the Breast. Direct visualization of lesions of the breast was anticipated from the area ratio discovery. The lesions would be revealed by contrast in the "normal" background. A benign lesion returning less sound than normal tissue, would appear as a "hole" or less dense area of echoes (A and B). Cancer, returning more sound than normal tissue, would appear as an area of denser echoes at a range where normal tissue echoes were less dense (C).

(Report to U. S. Navy, 1949). It was also found that the echoscope could be held in the hand and applied to the specimen. A fresh operative specimen of a nonmalignant tumor of the intestine was taken (Wild and Reid, 1953). Three blocks of tissue were cut, a piece of lobulated intestinal fat, a piece of the tumor, and a block containing a piece of tumor and naturally attached lobulated fat. Without altering the controls, a series of echograms were recorded from the specimens. It was found that a number of echoes were returned from the fatty tissue and none from the tumor. In the naturally composite specimen a transposition of the recognizable fatty tissue echo complex was observed, according to which type of tissue was first traversed by the sound beam.

Further proof of echo production from within tissues was obtained by directing the sound beam across the fibers in a cube of beef muscle. Reid subsequently demonstrated the anisotrophy of striated muscle by observing almost no echoes when the sound beam was directed along the muscle bundles (Wild and Reid, 1953).

A fresh operative specimen of the human stomach containing a cancer

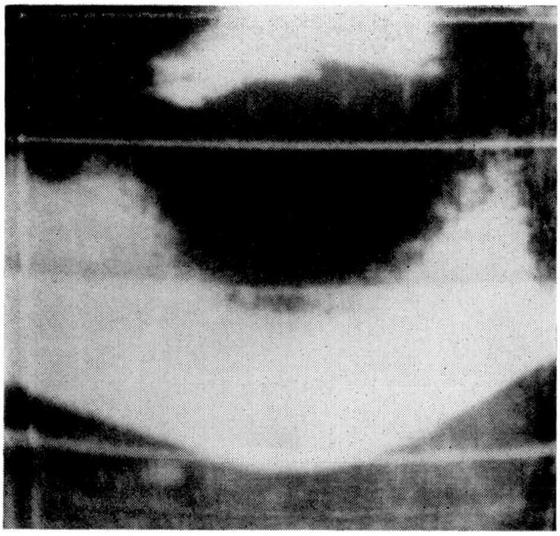

FIG. 7. A Liquid Filled Cyst of the Living Breast. A liquid filled cyst 1½ cm. in diameter is revealed by a circular area of no echo returns (black) outlined almost completely by the contrasting high echo density normal tissue (white). The horizontal lines are 1 centimeter range marks.

(carcinomatous ulcer) was examined, and the echograms of the normal stomach were found to differ considerably from those of the infiltrated stomach of the same thickness (Wild, 1950). This experiment introduces a concept of control widely used in biology. All variables were held constant except one, the structure of the stomach wall. Various cancer specimens were examined in the same way, as well as freshly removed whole brains (French, Wild and Neal, 1950; Ibid., 1951a). By this time it was felt that living intact tissues should be tried instead of fresh specimen.

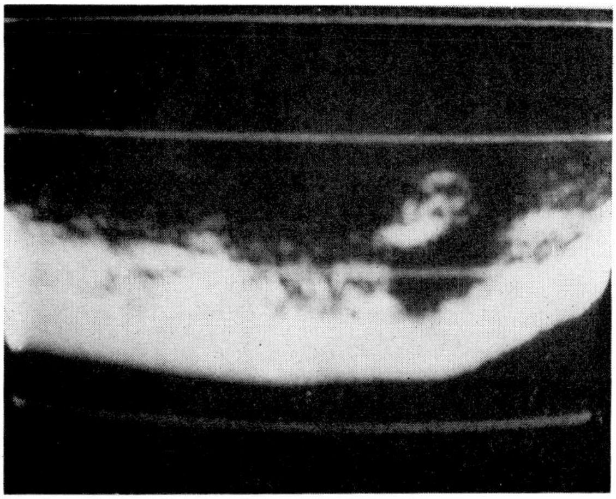

FIG. 8. A Small Cyst of About 7 mm. Diameter is Shown.

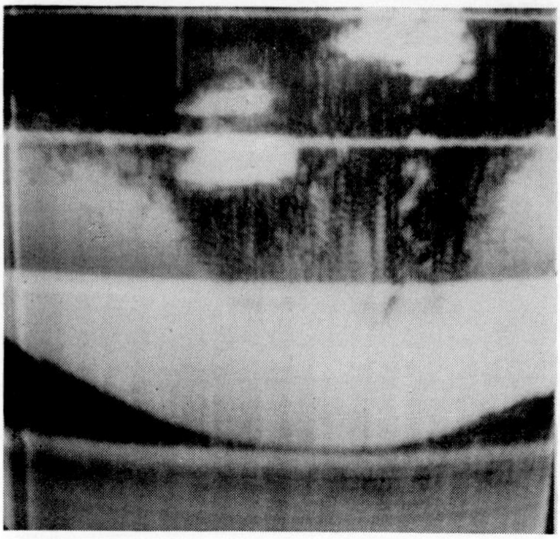

Fig. 9. Two Cysts in One Clinical Lump. Echoes from cellular debris within the cyst liquid can be seen.

The question of damage was answered directly by animal experimentation on living intact brain tissue (French, Wild and Neal, 1951b). No damage was demonstrated up to 8 weeks after exposure. The average intensity of our present transducers has been determined by absorption in a water bath calorimeter to be less than 70 mw. per square centimeter at a repetition rate of 1 kc. At the duty factor of 10^{-3}, this corresponds to a peak intensity of less than 70 watts/cm.^{2}

Before leaving the Naval establishment we were able to examine lumps in the breasts of two women. A difference was observed in the records of the two cases, one cancerous, the other non-cancerous (Wild and Neal,

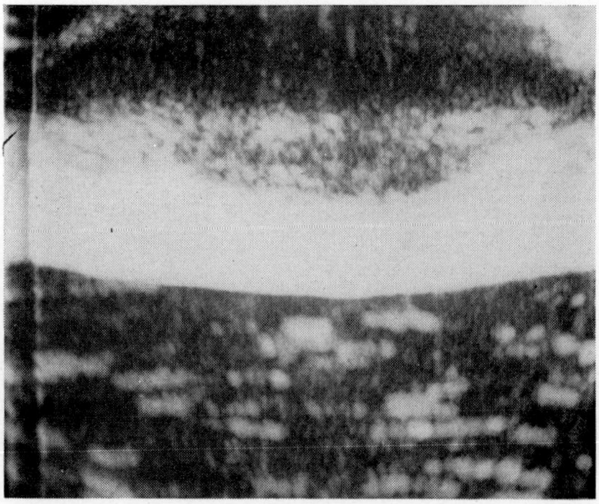

Fig. 10. Echogram of a Solid Non-malignant Tumor (Fibro-adenoma).

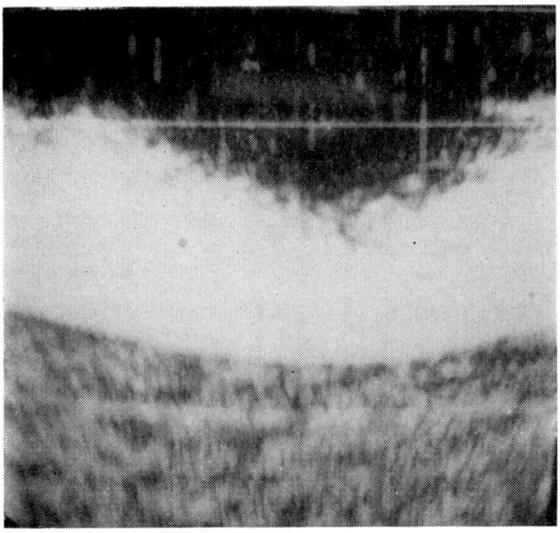

FIG. 11. Echogram of a Solid Non-malignant Tumor (Fibro-adenoma). Here the tumor returns almost no echoes and is revealed as a deficiency in the normal tissue pattern.

1951). We had by now accumulated enough data to interest the U. S. Public Health Service, who have supported this work almost entirely up to the present.

The basic units of the Echograph which Reid built follow conventional sonar and radar principles. The high frequency of 15 mc. allowed an apparently adequate definition with straightforward techniques. The use of commercially available crystals and non-critical circuits gave us a working machine for clinical use as quickly as possible. The pilot experimental evidence that the fresh cancer specimens from the stomach, rectum, and brain differed from the normal tissues of origin pointed the way to a clinical series with biological control. Abnormalities in the human breast discovered clinically were known to be a convenient source of material, since such abnormalities are almost always removed for microscopic diagnosis.

Nineteen consecutive cases (Wild and Reid, 1951) were examined by the graphical method of displaying results, unidimensional echography, comparable to a needle biopsy. Echograms of the abnormal tissue were compared with echograms of comparable normal tissue (Fig. 3).

The records were examined statistically and a possibly significant entity, the area on the echogram between the trace and the base line, was revealed. In all of the eleven tumors subsequently diagnosed malignant, the ratio of the tumor-record area to control-tissue-record area was found to be greater than unity. Six of the eight non-malignant abnormalities were found to have an area ratio less than unity.

At this time, we examined a tumor in the living brain at operation with the skull removed. The records showed a cancer when examined in the light of our experimental evidence, in spite of the pre-operative diagnosis

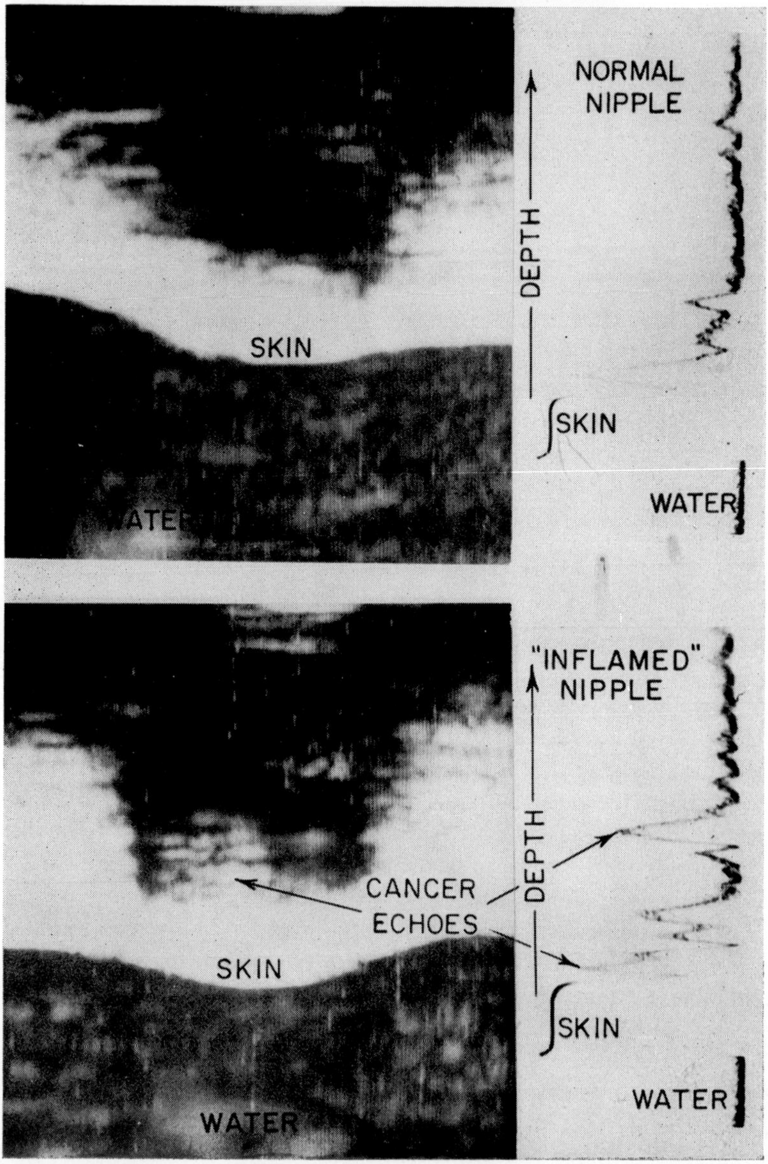

FIG. 12. A Composite of Uni-dimensional (Right) and Two-dimensional (Left) Echograms of the Same Lesion. The time base (depth) from below upwards is the same in both types of record.

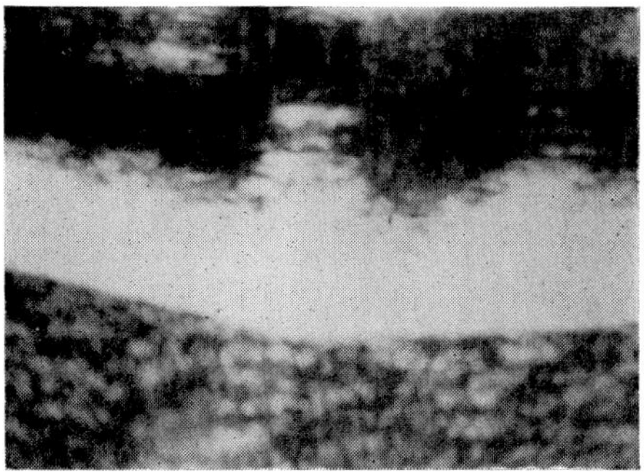

Fig. 13. Echogram of a Cancerous Nodule of the Breast (Adeno-carcinoma).

of non-cancer (meningioma). Cancer was diagnosed by the microscope (Wild and Reid, 1953).

The work up to this point tended to show that echoes were coming from many small tissue elements, such as concentrations of elastic and connective tissue, ducts, arterioles and capillaries, and fat lobulations.

The geometry of tissues such as the breast is very complicated, even over a few centimeters. Accordingly, scanning techniques were investigated to see if recognizable signal patterns arising from small tissue abnormalities could be distinguished from the normal background patterns.

Some pilot two-dimensional echograms obtained with a quickly constructed compromise apparatus were shown at the last Symposium (Wild and Reid, 1952; Ibid., 1953).

With this scanning instrument, we were able to obtain some confirmation of the validity of the area ratio discovery. We succeeded also in obtaining an encouraging set of echograms of a tumor in the thigh muscle (Wild and Reid, 1952).

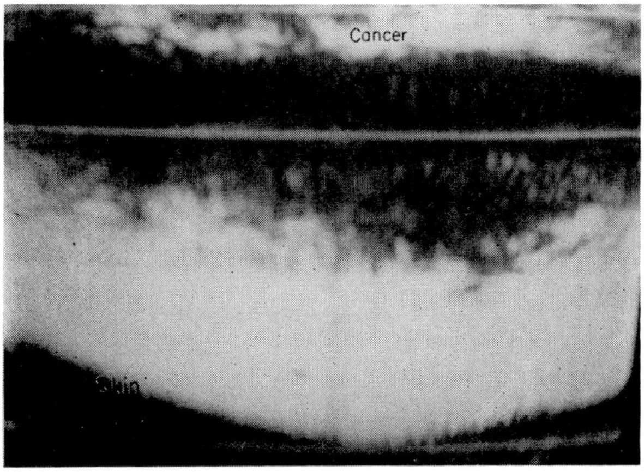

Fig. 14. A Layer of Cancer is Shown at a Depth of 3 Centimeters from the Skin.

This work prompted the construction of a two-dimensional instrument (Fig. 4) in which the transducer moves along a straight line at right angles to the sound beam (Wild and Reid, 1954). The instrument had a skin coverage of 6.5 cm., which was considered adequate for small lumps.

The relationship between the graphical and intensity-modulated display methods is shown in Fig. 5.

On the basis of our previous work, we expected to obtain the types of two-dimensional pictures shown in Fig. 6.

Fig. 7 shows a living, intact, liquid-filled cyst typical of those found in 15 of our recent clinical series with the instrument. The circular region of no signals from within the cyst liquid, the absence of signals from generally smooth side walls, and the relatively strong echoes from the tissue on the far side of the cyst (indicating a low attenuation for the cyst liquid) can be seen.

Our definition appeared good enough to visualize a 7 mm. diameter cyst (Fig. 8).

Cellular debris within a double cyst is shown in Fig. 9.

In the case of a solid, non-malignant tumor, since less sound is returned from the tumor than from surrounding normal tissue (Figs. 3 and 6), we shall expect a defect in the normal background of the two-dimensional echogram.

The mottled area of lower intensity signals in the center of Fig. 10 can be compared with the normal tissue pattern at each side.

CLINICAL RESULTS OF THE EXAMINATION OF 77 PALPABLE ABNORMALITIES IN THE HUMAN BREAST

Of 27 malignant lesions,	we correctly diagnosed	26
	we did not diagnose	1
Of 50 non-malignant lesions,	we correctly diagnosed	43
	we did not diagnose	7

To give an idea of the confidence to be placed in the results <u>before</u> operation with our present apparatus

Of the 33 lesions <u>we</u> <u>called</u> malignant:	we correctly diagnosed	26
	we incorrectly diagnosed	7
Of the 44 lesions <u>we</u> <u>called</u> non-malignant:	we correctly diagnosed	43 (98 %)
	we incorrectly diagnosed	1

Thus, at present, a woman has a 98% chance that we are right if we tell her she does not have cancer in the "lump" in her breast.

FIG. 15. Results of 77 Lesions of the Breast Confirmed by Microscopical Diagnosis are Shown in Tabular Form. The figures are arranged in two forms as explained.

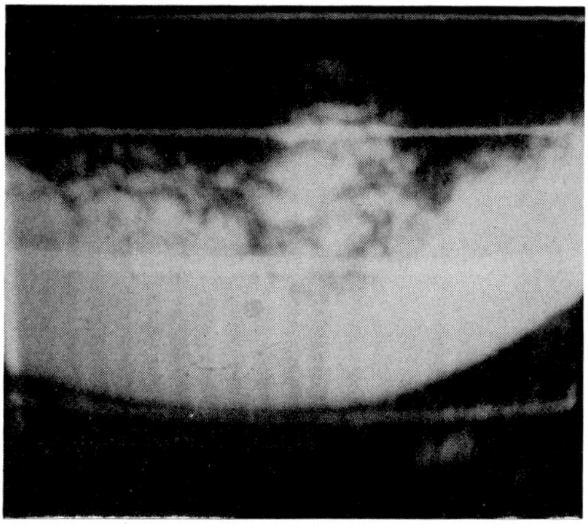

FIG. 16. An Echogram of a Dense Fibrous Lesion is Shown Which Was Incorrectly Diagnosed as Malignant (Compare with Fig. 13).

Fig. 11 shows a condition typical of 13 lesions which we called non-malignant correctly. The low signal intensity from the tumor compared to that of the normal tissue on either side gives the impression of a "hole" in the section.

One type of non-malignant, two dimensional echogram which we have seen shows no demonstrable difference from the normal picture taken from the other breast over an area comparable to the size of the lesion.

What will a deposit of cancer tissue look like? The tumor returns more sound than does the comparable normal tissue (Figs. 3 and 6).

A cancer, 7 mm across, shown in Fig. 12, was successfully revealed as a group of high intensity signals within a clinically "inflamed" nipple. The tumor could not be felt by the attending physician even after he was told of its presence by us. The area ratio was 1.34. We believe that this was the first unequivocable visualization of a cancer in the living subject. It was declared publicly at the Centennial meeting of the Minnesota State Medical Association as a malignant tumor, *before* the biopsy was performed.

Some of the malignant lesions in the series showed up as a "mountain" of greater signal intensity arising in a normal background of low intensity (Fig. 13). Other malignant lesions showed greater signal intensity over the entire scanned area than from a comparable area of normal tissue. Fig. 14 shows a plaque of cancer tissue near the pectoral muscles at the far limit of our present range.

Second Clinical Series

We have now examined with satisfactory biological control a total of 77 lesions of the human breast which were biopsied and diagnosed by the

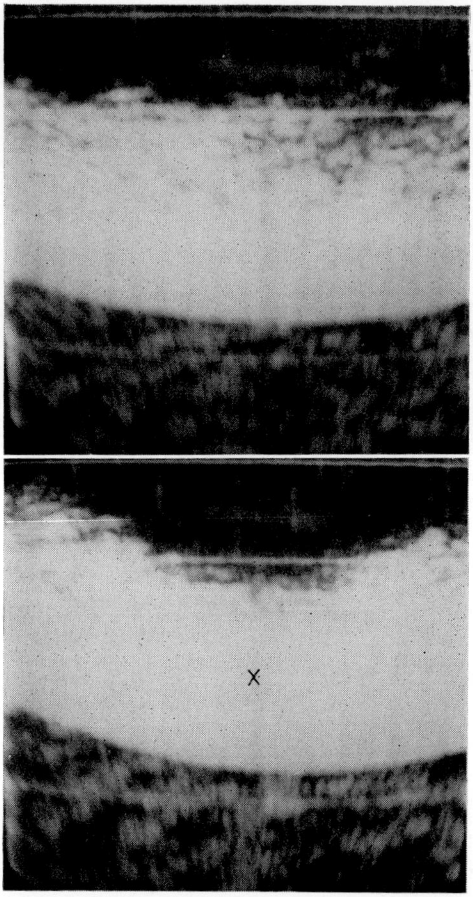

FIG. 17. Necrotic Lesion. The lower echogram was obtained from a lesion that was found to be internally degenerated (necrotic) when removed surgically. Comparison with the upper echogram of normal tissue at the same setting of the apparatus revealed the denser echo pattern in front of the "hole" at "X".

pathologist. The results are tabulated in Fig. 15. Of these 77, 27 lesions were diagnosed malignant and 50 were diagnosed non-malignant by the pathologist. Of the 27 malignant lesions, we correctly diagnosed 26, and of the 50 non-malignant lesions, we correctly diagnosed 43. These figures may be expressed differently to give a better idea of the confidence to be placed in the results. Since our diagnoses are reported to the referring doctor before biopsy, no one knows into which category the patient will fall. Taking the lesions in the classifications into which we placed them:

Of the 33 lesions that we called malignant, we correctly diagnosed 26 or 79 percent.

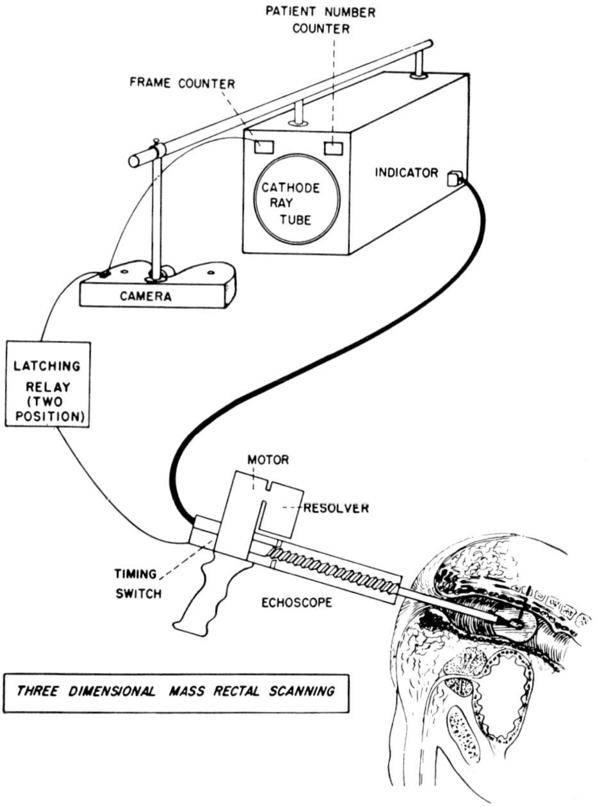

FIG. 18. Arrangement of Equipment for Obtaining the Three Dimensional Information from the Lower Bowel.

Of the 44 lesions that we called non-malignant, we correctly diagnosed 43 or 98 percent.

Thus, with our present undeveloped apparatus, there is a two-percent chance of our making the more serious mistake of calling a malignant lesion non-malignant.

Fig. 16 is typical of 5 benign lesions which appeared malignant.

Some of the malignant echograms proved deceptive until examined carefully. At the first glance, the lesions in Fig. 17 (lower) appeared as a "hole" similar to some of the non-malignant solid tumors (see Fig. 11). However, an important difference is that the "hole" is surrounded or at least partially fronted by a region of greater signal strength than the normal echogram (Fig. 17 upper) at the same range. These lesions were reported to have internal degeneration.

In conclusion, we would like to show some serial echograms obtained

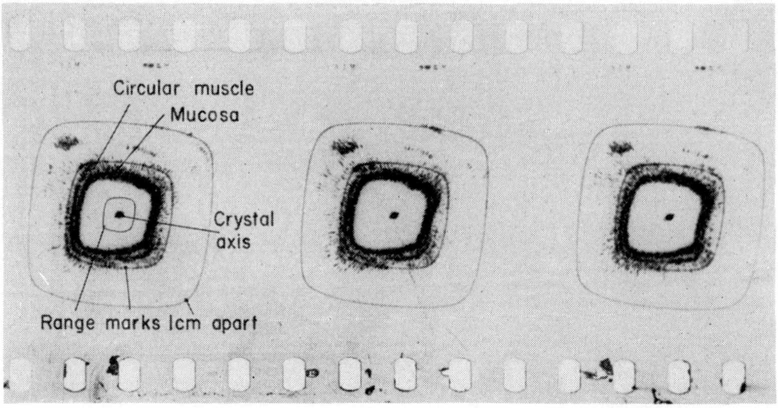

FIG. 19. Three Consecutive Two Dimensional Echograms of Normal Human Lower Bowel are Shown. The concentric structure of the lower bowel wall is defined.

from the lower nine inches of the bowel of a human volunteer. The general arrangement of the equipment is shown in Fig. 18. A scanning head attached to a rod was inserted into the bowel through a sigmoidoscope. Degassed water was injected into the rubber balloon surrounding the scanning head and the whole assembly was driven in a circular motion so that the sound beam swept through the bowel wall. Upon engaging a half-nut, the balloon began to screw its way out of the body and an automatic camera took pictures of the bowel echo patterns on the display cathode ray tube. Thus, a strip of film was produced with a series of circumferential scans of the bowel wall (Fig. 19).

Three consecutive frames are shown at the most distant point reached by the sound beam. The circular group of dense signals next to the rubber membrane could have been returned by the mucosa, followed by a ring of signals which could have been returned by the circular muscle coat of the bowel. The discontinuous groups of signals further out could have been returned by the teniae coli. The range marks are 10 millimeters apart so that the thickness of the bowel and the rubber membrane at this point was about 3–4 millimeters. The square pattern of the clear space in the middle representing the water-filled balloon is not a peculiarity of the subject's bowel but an artifact due to a technical imperfection.

References

French, L. A., J. J. Wild, and D. Neal. 1950. Detection of cerebral tumors by ultrasonic pulses; pilot studies on post-mortem material. Cancer *3:* 705–708.

French, L. A., J. J. Wild and D. Neal. 1951a. Attempts to determine harmful effects of pulsed ultrasonic vibrations. Cancer *4:* 342–344.

French, L. A., J. J. Wild and D. Neal. 1951b. The experimental application of ultrasonics to the localization of brain tumors. Preliminary report. J. Neurosurg. *8:* 198–203.

Hueter, T. 1948. Messung der Ultraschallabsorption in tierischen Geweben und ihre Abhangigkeit von der Grequenz. Naturwiss. *35:* 285–287.

Report to U. S. Navy, 1949.

Wild, J. J. 1950. The use of ultrasonic pulses for the measurement of biological tissues and the detection of tissue density changes. Surgery *27:* 183–188.

Wild, J. J. and D. Neal. 1951. The use of high frequency ultrasonic waves for detecting changes of texture in living tissues. Lancet *1:* 655–657.

Wild, J. J. and J. M. Reid. 1952a. Further pilot echographic studies on the histological structure of tumors of living intact human greast. Am. J. Path. *28:* 839–861.

Wild, J. J. and J. M. Reid. 1952b. The application of echo-ranging techniques to the determination of structure of biological tissues. Science *115:* 226–230.

Wild, J. J. and J. M. Reid. 1953. The effects of biological tissues on 15 megacycle pulsed ultrasound. J. Acoust. Soc. Amer. *25:* 270–280.

Wild, J. J. and J. M. Reid. 1954. Echographic visualization of lesions of the living intact human breast. Cancer Research *14:* 227–282.

DR. HOWRY: What is the frontal area or diameter of the crystal driver you are now using?

DR. REID: The crystals themselves are about 1 cm. across. They are the same crystals that were used in the ultrasonic trainer.

DR. HUETER: Would you put on Slide No. 17 again please (Ed. note: Figs. 3, 5 and 6), which seemed to be sort of a summarizing slide, and indicate how the information relates to the several diagrams?

DR. WILD: This was a composite to show the transfer of the information from the uni-dimensional method to the two-dimensional scanning.

DR. HUETER: Have you ever planted any artificial lesions in tissues? Would you consider that as a valuable procedure in such work?

DR. WILD: We were thinking about it.

DR. HUETER: Could you explain in terms of this slide your term of area ratio?

DR. WILD: The area ratio is computed by projecting the trace on to paper ruled in squares. The magnification is quite high, and we count squares to determine the area between the trace and the baseline, discounting with the usual conservatism anything that looks like it is not more than half a square. We arrive at the units or number of squares between the trace and the baseline.

We don't take out the skin signal because we don't know where it stops on the record. Some cancer starts at the skin, so we would not know where to cut the record. With an electronic integrator, we can give you some idea of how valuable that area ratio is. The area ratio work has done its job from my point of view, because it showed we could visualize some of the lesions, if not all of them, so, right or wrong, we used it as a stepping stone to the next stage, in biology. We will have to go back and verify the value of the area ratio and stand up to criticism, no doubt.

DR. HUETER: I noticed from your scans of the bowels that apparently gain is a very important factor. In one case you obtained a considerable detail as you scanned and in another case practically none so you evidently had changes in gain.

If you make a comparison between a lesion and a control, the coupling of the transducer to the body in both the control and experimental case would have to be done with extreme care in order that the area ratio have significance. Do you think this is very critical or that it can be readily accomplished?

DR. WILD: Failure of coupling can be seen at once. The way we normally operate is to put the transducer on the area and examine the lump for a little while, and then by instinct Dr. Reid knows where to put the controls. Usually with about two applications we are showing the maximum difference.

DR. HUETER: Isn't this twiddling of the controls?

DR. WILD: Nothing is twiddled. When we take the records, nothing is twiddled between the taking of the normal and the taking of the lesion. That is one of the important things. If the machine drifts significantly I want to know about it, because the whole thing falls down, but I have been assured it does not drift in between a given setting and the taking of records.

DR. REID: I should also like to point out all our pictures are taken before the lesion is removed by the doctor, before it is biopsied and on the smaller lesions we have no idea what they are, so all the records we have are taken under identical conditions before we have the faintest idea as to the outcome.

DR. BALLANTINE: I wonder if Dr. Wild would go over the statistics again.

DR. REID: What we did here was to express them as percentages of the way we had diagnosed them. There are four categories.

Thirty-three we declared malignant, and 44 we declared non-malignant. Of the 33 we called malignant, 26 of them were malignant, therefore a certain number that we called malignant were not malignant. However, all the lesions that we worked on, i.e. that are reported here, were biopsied; so we are far less conservative than present surgical practice in this experimental diagnostic work. Of the 44 we called non-malignant, 43 actually were non-malignant. This includes the one we called non-malignant that was malignant, which is a mistake in the more serious direction. I did it this way, because the previous method of determining the number of times we were right and the number of times wrong would not give too good an idea of the confidence to be placed in the results at the time we diagnosed it.

DR. BALLANTINE: How about the breast tumors that were solid rather than cystic? Could you separate those into malignant and non-malignant categories?

DR. WILD: Except for those highly dense fibrotic tumors. The last slide (Fig. 16) looked like one type of tumor.

DR. REID: Out of the entire group of non-malignant lesions four were in this category, of which three were in the same patient.

DR. BALLANTINE: That did not account for all of them? You had one malignant tumor of this type—did you not?

DR. WILD: Yes, we did.

DR. BALLANTINE: There were seven that you thought were malignant. How many of those were solid in contrast to cystic tumors?

DR. REID: They were all solid tumors in that there was not a large single cyst such as the one we showed. Some of them had small cysts within them on a microscopic scale.

DR. BALLANTINE: So that misses were in the solid benign tumors?

DR. REID: That is right.

DR. BALLANTINE: The point I am trying to clarify in my own mind is that you cannot tell the histology of the tumor by this method, but you can tell whether it is cystic.

DR. WILD: We can recognize the cysts immediately in the clinic.

DR. BALLANTINE: You mean by this method?

DR. WILD: We can visualize them directly.

DR. REID: We have not attempted to break it down any more than that into the histological classes. We have been trying to find a correlation index in degrees of malignancies, but this is rather difficult to tie down.

DR. NYBORG: Is there a possible explanation for the extra reflection from the tumors?

DR. WILD: I was listening to Dr. Carstensen this morning. He was talking about packed red cells, and I did not quite get the whole gist of the thing, but I am going to look into it more. At present we feel it may be either the high cell concentration of the cancer occurring in a disorganized manner as packed red cells. Let us call it that—as packed cells, with very little connective tissue occurring in a background of normal properly organized tissue, and that may be the difference. We do not know yet.

DR. HOWRY: There is one thing we observed which would explain that to some extent. After all, fat has a different impedance than does tumor tissues, and this is particularly important for malignant masses that have extended out into the breast structure. It is then surrounded by a high contrast medium, so you would expect a somewhat higher reflection coefficient or diffused reflection coming back from a malignant, rather than benign. It is largely conjectural, although we have inspected that idea to some extent.

Techniques Used in Ultrasonic Visualization of Soft Tissues

D. H. Howry

Ultrasonic Research Unit, University of Colorado School of Medicine, Denver, Colorado

THE GENERAL METHOD by which pulsed ultra-high frequency sound is used to produce a cross sectional picture of body structures is now fairly well known in the field of acoustics. In method of operation our equipment is similar to that used by Wild and Reid. Several essential differences exist, however, which make the operation of our equipment different from theirs: 1. Our instruments operate at a central frequency of two megacycles and use a special converging lens system. The use of the lower frequency allows us greater penetration of the sound beam into the tissues, while the focusing action improves the horizontal resolving power. 2. A gain compensator circuit is incorporated in the amplifier which serves to make echoes produced by a given size and type structure near the surface appear to be identical to those produced by the same structure when lying deep within the tissue. This compensator in effect corrects for the loss of signal intensity produced by absorption and dispersion of the sound in tissue. 3. A gain equalizer is used which makes all portions of the beam appear to be of equal intensity even though the absolute intensity, as measured in water, varies considerably because of the focusing effect of the lens. 4. A long time constant automatic volume control is incorporated in the equipment since it was found from initial studies that the average gain of the receiver needed to be somewhat different in areas such as the back of the neck as compared with the front, for accurate and correct visualization.

Automatic preset correction systems of this type are believed to be essential to the successful operation of this equipment to produce picture standardization, as it was previously found that by turning the numerous controls on our earlier equipment the operator was able to influence the picture according to his preconceived idea of how the picture should look (by emphasis or de-emphasis of various picture elements).

Fig. 1 shows a rather typical example of the type of anatomic differentiation that could be achieved by our earlier instrument under optimum conditions. This figure is a view through the right upper arm. There is a fair anatomic correlation between the various nerves, arteries and veins, and a

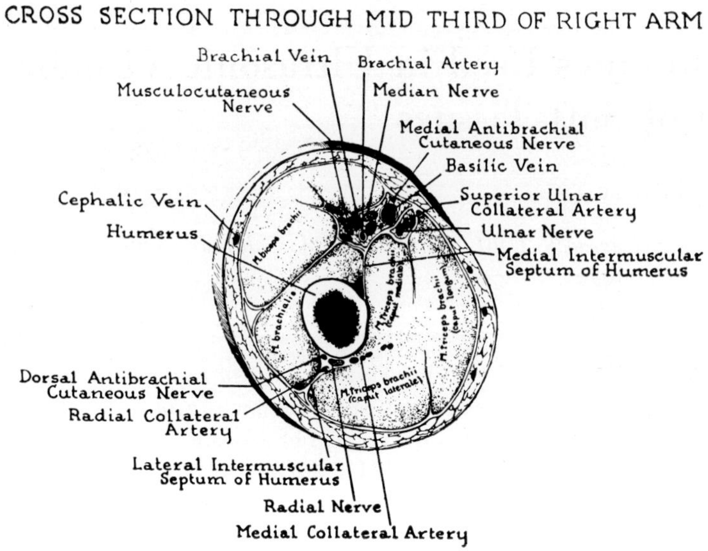

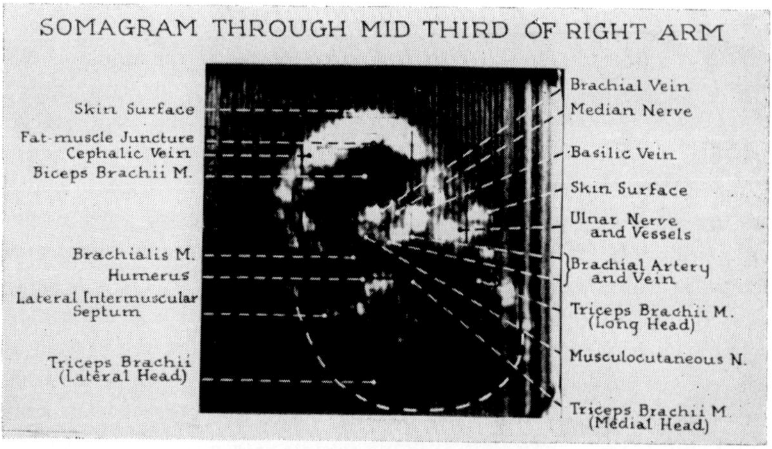

FIG. 1.

few of the fascial planes, as seen in the sound picture (somagram) and the cross section anatomy diagram shown above. However, many tissue structures in this area do not show well. The definition achieved in this study was of the order of 1/16 of an inch resolution in both axial and horizontal directions.

There are several methods by which sound pictures of this type can be used to make a diagnosis. They all have their parallelism in radiology. Di-

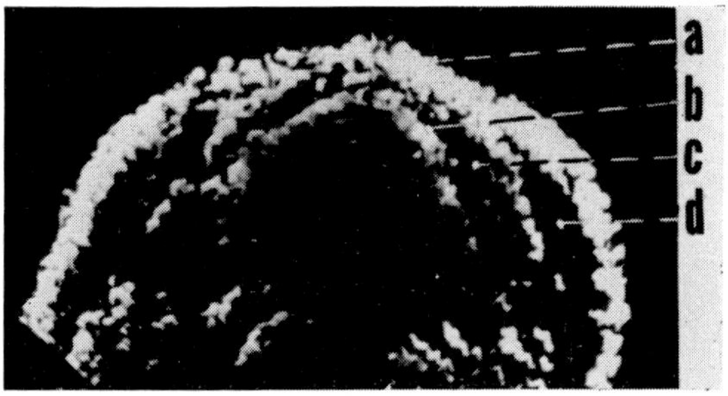

FIG. 2. Somagram of Colloid Goiter: (a) Skin surface. (b) Trachea. (c) Thyroid. (d) Sternocleidomastoid muscle. The somagram cross section of the anterior neck shows displacement of the sternocleiodmastoid muscle away from the trachea by an enlarged thyroid. The enlargement is principally on the right.

rect visualization of the abnormality can be applied, as is done in tuberculosis of the chest, or the displacement of a normal structure can be used as the significant point. Fig. 2 shows, for example, a very large thyroid which has pressed the skin and sternocleidomastoid muscle out of the way to give a very abnormal picture. For this view it was necessary to make two separate somagrams and later paste them together, as a simple B scan type presentation does not allow one to see around curved structures.

Fig. 3 is a cross-sectional somagram of the neck of one of our engineers. It was possible in this study to outline the trachea, internal jugular vein, carotid artery, portions of the anterior strap muscles, and some segments of the vertebral column. To produce this picture it was necessary to make four separate ultrasonic pictures—each from a different 90° oblique quadrant of the neck—as it is not possible to get accurate picture detail when a structure lies at any substantial angle, other than perpendicular to the beam. Neither is it possible to get pictures when the structures are shadowed or hidden behind air-filled or bony tissues. Despite the fact that we were able to identify many of the structures in the normal neck, the visualization was far from complete and very difficult to reproduce.

Also illustrated in Fig. 3 is a method of visualizing the motion of structures within the body such as pulsating blood vessels. This is achieved by stopping the mechanical scan and using a slow electronic horizontal sweep on the oscilloscope. Motion of the blood vessels can be seen as a shift in the corresponding echo positions on the oscilloscope in a graphic form. It was possible in this study to identify the pulsating wave form of the artery, and the alpha, beta and gamma waves of a deep neck vein. It is felt that moving target indicator techniques could very well be applied to this aspect of the work and may be of value in both physiology and clinical medicine. We are currently investigating such a system for studying the heart's wall thickness and amplitude of motion.

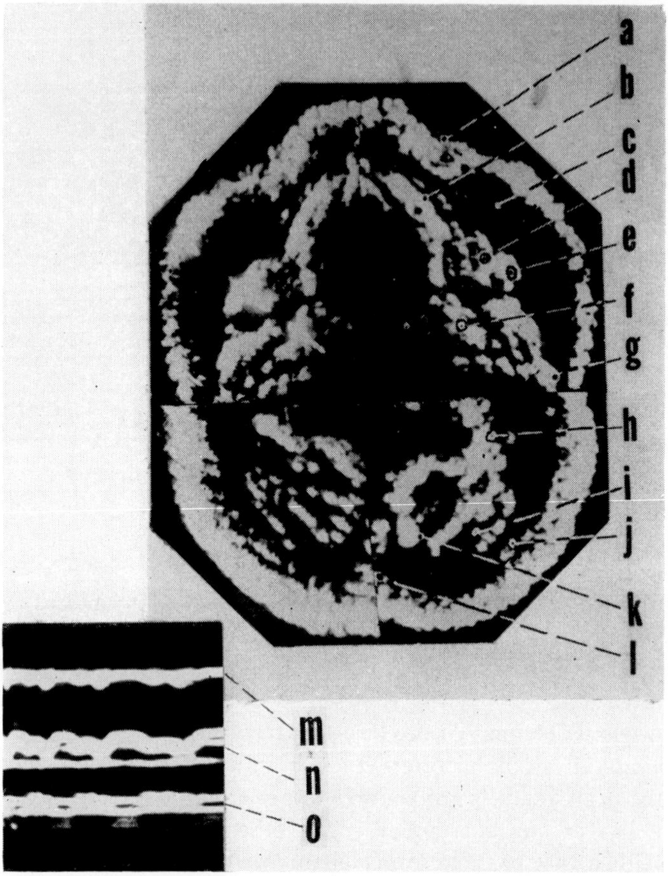

FIG. 3. Cross Section Somagram of the Normal Neck at the Level of the Fifth Cervical Vertebra. (a) Skin surface. (b) Trachea. (c) Sternocleidomastoid muscle. (d) Carotid artery. (e) Internal jugular vein. (f) Vertebral vessels. (g) Fascia colli lateralis. (h) Transverse process of fifth cervical vertebra. (i) Splenius capitis muscle. (j) Trapezius muscle. (k) Spinous process. (l) Ligamentum nuchae. Below: A graphic, time amplitude, visualization of the wave motions of the skin over the carotid artery (m), the carotid artery (n), and one of the deep neck veins (o).

Additional studies were made on breast tumors, liver disease, tumors of the salivary glands, metastatic carcinoma, etc. (Howry and Bliss, 1952; Howry, Stott and Bliss, 1954; Howry, Holmes and Cushman, 1955; Holmes, Howry, Posakony and Cushman, 1955; Howry, 1955; Howry, Holmes, Lanier and Posakony, 1954; and Howry, Posakony, Cushman and Holmes, 1956). Although we did demonstrate some of the changes produced by these diseases, it was recognized that the visualization was neither reliable nor accurate, and therefore no really useful information could be obtained by an extended period of clinical investigation with the equipment available.

It was initially believed by this group, and apparently by others, that adequate echo information would be received regardless of the angular position of the reflecting structure. Reason for this belief is to be found in the fact that materials testing devices which use the pulsed ultra-high frequency sound have operated adequately, despite the fact that a flaw or crack may lie at a substantial angle to the penetrating sound beam and still be adequately seen. Careful evaluation of numerous preliminary studies made upon ourselves and clinical cases demonstrated that this concept was grossly in error. Instead of the sound being reflected in a non-specular fashion (in all directions), sound is reflected from body structures as if it had struck a mirror-like surface. Evaluation of this phenomenon on test objects of various sizes and shapes demonstrated that a change in direction (from normal) of the reflecting structure by 6° produced a decrease in the amplitude of the echo received by over 10 to 1. When the same structure was rotated so that it was 12° off normal, the amplitude of reflection fell to $\frac{1}{100}$ of that obtained when the same structure was flat on toward the beam. The seriousness of this problem can be more easily recognized when it is recalled that the actual power received from a structure so turned at 12° is $\frac{1}{10{,}000}$ of that received when the identical structure was in a perpendicular direction. This effect is the principal cause for the loss of visualization of curved structures in such areas as in the neck. In Fig. 3, which was our best previous result, the majority of the muscle planes are seen only in short horizontal segments where these muscles presented a surface nearly perpendicular to the sound beam.

Very small structures (small with respect to a wave length) will reflect substantially in all directions. Studies were made, therefore, to establish how small objects would have to be before we could be sure that their sound echoes would be reflected back to the receiving crystal regardless of their angular position. We found that such objects would have to be less than $\frac{1}{32}$ of an inch or spherical in shape before we could depend upon the fact that they would be received regardless of their position. Unfortunately when objects are of such small size, they intercept only a small portion of the energy of the beam and reflect it in all directions; therefore, the amplitude of these echoes is then decreased to approximately $\frac{1}{100}$ of the amplitude to be expected from the identical object, were it of larger size and had it a surface perpendicular to the beam. Some carcinomas, and a few other pathologic processes, do probably represent the non-specular type of reflectors, as small filaments of carcinoma tissue invade through normal tissue and serve as a very diffuse type of reflector.

It has been suggested that since Wild and Reid use a substantially

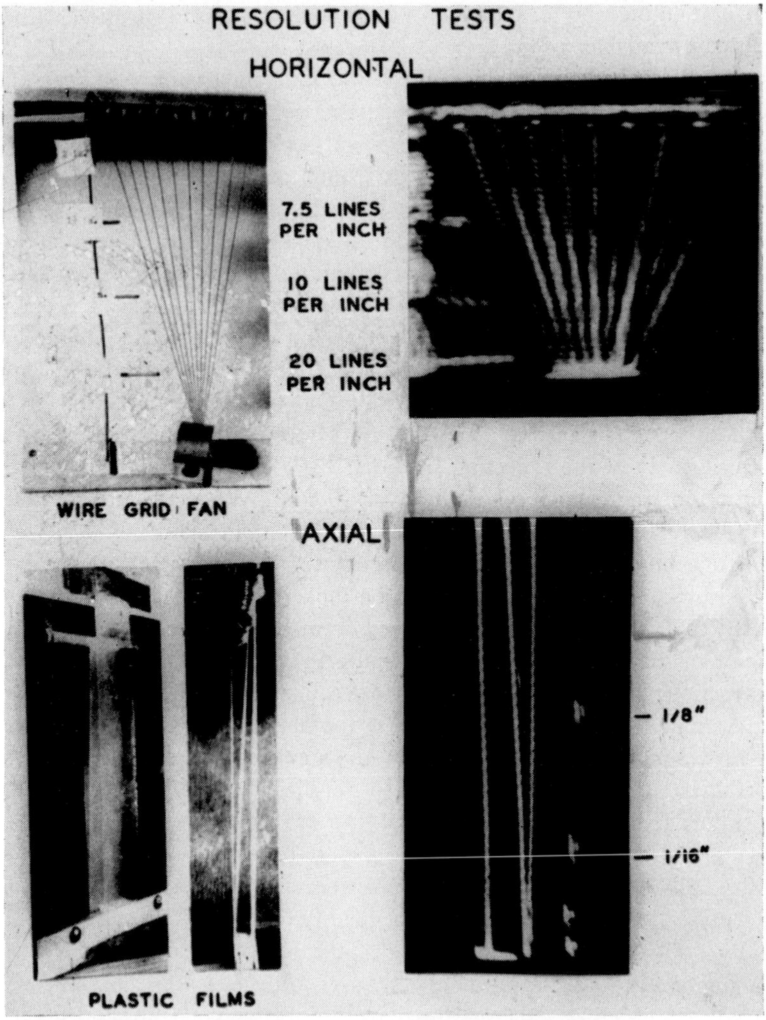

FIG. 4. Test Objects and Somascope Resolving Power Tests. Above: Horizontal resolving power test. On the left is a fan-like wire grid test object. On the right, a somagram horizontal resolving power test, as seen on the image screen. Below: Range resolving power test. On the left are two views of a wedge-shaped plastic film test object. On the right is the range resolving power test as seen on the image screen. (The bright spots are markers which are placed where the films are separated by $\frac{1}{8}$, $\frac{1}{16}$, $\frac{1}{32}$, and $\frac{1}{64}$ of an inch.)

higher frequency, they may realize an advantage in their present studies. Our objective, however, has been to produce an instrument of wide clinical use which will accurately portray the location of tumors, and their relationship to normal structures, and show changes in anatomic structures,

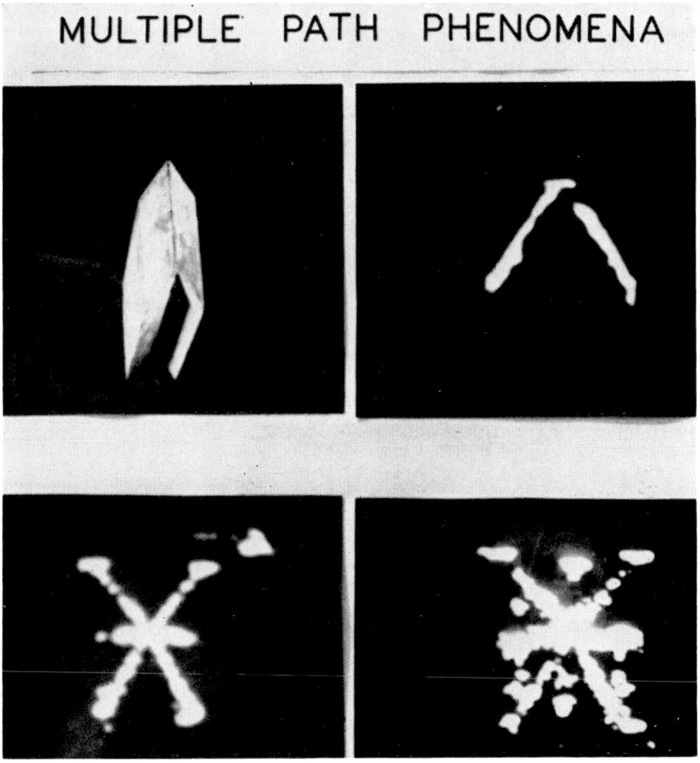

FIG. 5. Somagrams Illustrating Serious Picture Distortions Produced by Multiple Path Reflections From a Simple Wedge and a V Block Test Object. (Test object above left.)

such as the liver, kidney, etc. It is not believed that raising the frequency greatly helps this situation.

Investigation was undertaken to see whether we could operate our equipment at the higher power levels required to see around large curved structures, and at the same time see small structures. Earlier studies (see Fig. 4) demonstrated that we were able to obtain a resolving power in the horizontal direction of approximately 20 objects to the inch, and, in the range direction, 32 objects to the inch. When one attempts to duplicate such resolving power studies with the equipment increased in sensitivity approximately 100 times, he finds that the azimuth resolution falls to approximately 3 or 4 objects to the inch and completely destroys any picture detail, as the beam has for all practical purposes become wide and paintbrush-like. In the axial, or range dimension, resolving power does remain somewhat better than in the azimuth direction; however, it is grossly inadequate for the clinical evaluation of delicate soft tissue structures.

In addition to the above described problems, an even more serious problem was identified. When structures of fairly simple geometry present surfaces with steep angular sides, numerous false echoes or picture artifacts are produced. As an example, it was found that although at high power a pointed or inverted V-shaped object would produce a satisfactory picture, a V-shaped object produced serious distortions because of picture artifacts which caused it to look like an X with a bar through its center. The additional artifact structures (ghost echoes) were caused by multiple reflections of the sound beam (Fig. 5). From these studies, and others, made with more complex objects, we felt that accurate definition could not be achieved by the methods which we had previously employed, and that in all probability some of the structures seen in our previous illustrations did not represent true tissue processes, but rather were false echoes derived from the sound ricocheting around inside the body much like a ball on a billiard table.

The seriousness of these combined problems can be best demonstrated by making a picture of a complex object by ultrasound as is shown in Fig. 6. In Fig. 6 a lead brick with a multiangular surface is illustrated. Applied to it are two layers of curved plastic sheets, and a small wire is placed vertically in a notch in the brick. This construction results in the maximum opportunity for (1) failure of visualization of the structures because of angular and curved surfaces, (2) the maximum opportunity for the production of false echoes or ghosts, (3) the loss of range and azimuth resolution at the lead surfaces, when the wire and plastic are detectable (due to the latter's small reflection coefficients), and (4) the maximum opportunity for the sound shadows produced by the lead to obscure picture detail. At the top left (Part I) is a diagram of the cross section of the structure studied. Parts II through VI of this illustration demonstrate the inadequate and inaccurate picture information obtained regardless of the direction from which the sound beam approached the test object.

Our recent work, therefore, has primarily been the development of an instrument which allows the sound head to scan horizontally back and forth, and simultaneously travel around the structure under study which corrects for the above deficiencies. This type of complex picture registration we choose to call a "compound circular scanning system." The desired improvement in the final sound picture is seen in Part VI, where all details of the test object are seen in their entirety, along with an improvement in both the range and azimuth resolving power, and a suppression of the picture artifacts. A more detailed explanation of how these improvements are achieved is as follows.

By operation of our equipment so that it will see echoes which extend over a practical amplitude range (100 to 1) we are able to see only a 12° segment of the front of any curved structure, such as the plastic films illus-

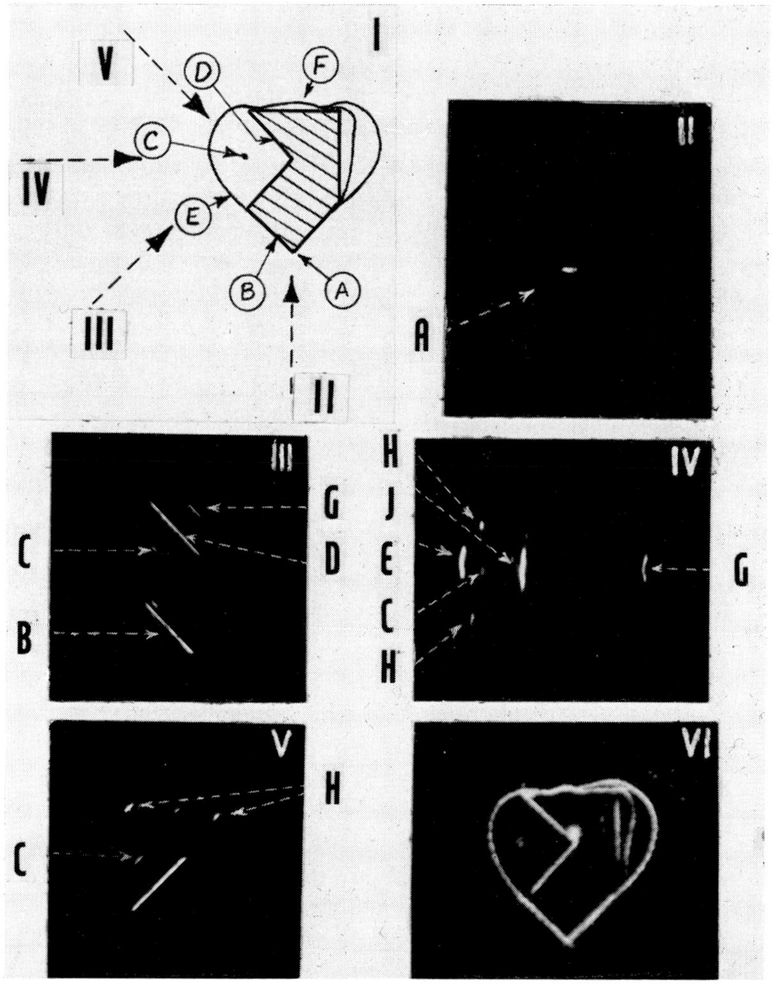

FIG. 6. Somascope Studies of a Complex Test Object. Part I (upper left) A lead brick is diagrammed by the cross hatched area in the central portion of this illustration: (A) point of lead brick, (B, D, and F) flat surfaces of the lead, (H) corners of the brick, (J) base of the notch. The brick is covered by two layers of thin sheet plastic which are combined on the left side (E). In the central portion of the "V" shaped notch on the left side of the brick a small wire is placed (C). Sound pictures were made from the directions II, III, IV and V as indicated by the accompanying arrows, and illustrations. "Ghost," or multiple path reflection echoes, are shown on the somagrams III through V by (G). Part VI (lower right) shows the improved results obtained by "compound circular scanning," achieved by allowing the sound head to travel completely around the structure illustrated while short picture segments were produced as shown in the previous four illustrations. The composite picture is only slightly distorted, and shows few picture artifacts. (Compare with Part I).

trated (Part IV). Yet the base of the notch is grossly blunted due to the inherent breadth of the beam at this amplitude level. The notch thus assumes a line-like projection horizontal to the direction of scan. The small wire in the notch of the V is likewise shown as a line, (Parts III through V); as is the point of the brick (Part II). Despite such loss of resolution, the angular surfaces of the brick are demonstrated only when the beam is perpendicular to them (Parts III and V). However, by allowing a horizontal back and forth scan, as the transducer is slowly moved in a circle completely about the object, one is able to pick up superimposing consecutive segments of all portions of the lead brick, plastic sheets and metal rod, and consequently print the test object in its true outline form, regardless of the angle at which any segment lay during a particular horizontal scan. Similarly, compound circular scanning results in the partial elimination of the sound shadows, since at some time during the circular scan nearly all structures present an unshadowed surface to the transducer.

The improved resolving power is achieved since the straight line segments obtained from each horizontal scan of the brick and the metal rod intersect to form a figure similar to an asterisk (*). The center of this asterisk is a spot. Consequently, by properly aperturing the camera so that only structures which are seen repeatedly on different scans produce enough total light to be registered on the film image, one is able to largely rid himself of the line segments, leaving only their points of intersection in the picture.

The troublesome artifacts produced on any single horizontal scan, due to multiple reflections, are caused to largely disappear since they shift their position on the screen at a rate which is twice as fast as the unit is rotating. Thus, true structures can be made to form superimposing patterns, and to register several times, while false echoes ("spooks") will usually not superimpose and are thus eliminated on the final picture.

Fig. 7 illustrates more clearly how one is able to achieve a range for azimuth exchange of information and thereby an improved definition. The test object in this case is a series of 1/16 of an inch wires which look much like the rungs on a ladder. They are spaced ½ inch apart. If one scans these wires lengthwise down the test object, line-like segments are produced whose variation in width is a graphic illustration of the focal pattern of the transducer (Fig. 7, Part I). Turning the wire grid sideways so that each of the wires is at the same distance, one finds each wire forming a line which is approximately ¼ inch in width (Part II). By allowing the sound head to scan back and forth while traveling completely around the grid, a series of bright spots are produced which are approximately ¼ inch in diameter (Part III). However, the central portion of each of these spots is actually of much higher average light intensity than are the surrounding

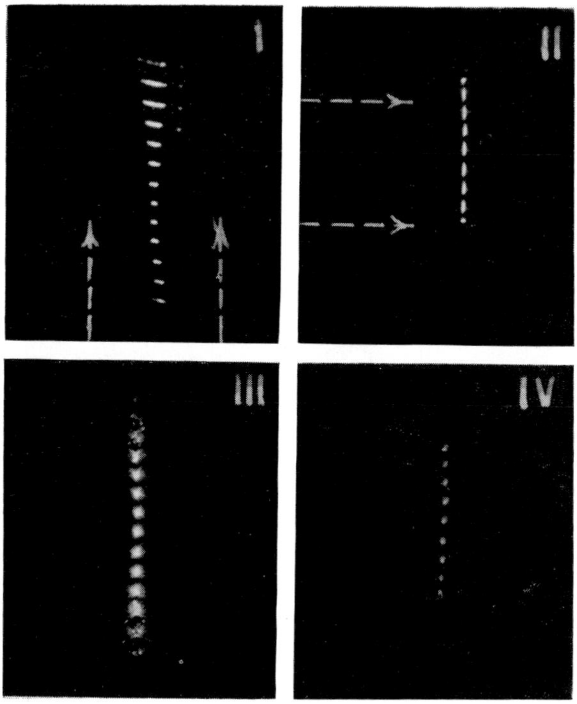

FIG. 7. Compound Circular Scanning of a Wire Grid Test Object. Part I shows the sonic picture obtained when the sound beam travels only down the long axis of the test object in the direction indicated by the arrow. Part II illustrates the sound picture obtained by scanning the test object at 90° from the previous picture (see arrow). In both of these illustrations the apparent width of the wires greatly exceeds their true diameters. Part III illustrates the picture obtained by allowing "compound circular scanning." In this picture the sound head was allowed to scan horizontally back and forth while travelling completely around the test object. The intensity of the light is much the highest at the center of the circular spots, thus, by decreasing the light intensity at the film by aperturing the camera, as compared with Part III, the true size and shape of the wire grid is shown (Part IV).

outer portions. Therefore, by aperturing the camera down several stops and making a picture of the identical type as is shown in Part IV, one is able to pull the spot size down to nearly the true dimension of the wires themselves without sacrificing other technical factors (such as operating the receiver at a lower gain setting) to achieve the picture.

Compound circular scanning then represents a new system of acoustic information processing which appears to offer many advantages from the practical standpoint of accuracy of picture details regardless of the amplitude of the echo signals produced. It achieves four advantages over the simple B scan system which we had previously employed: (1) it allows us to see structures which do not have a plane presented perpendicular to the

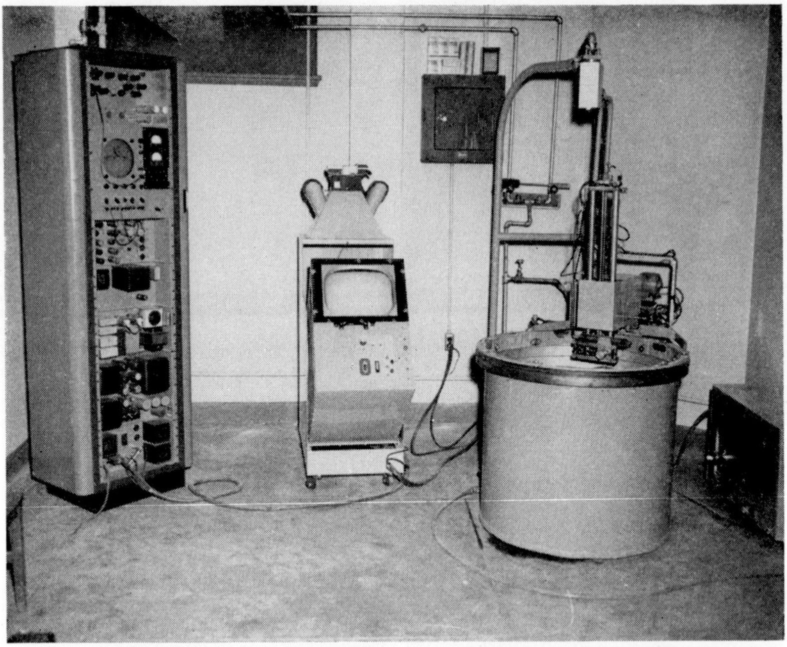

FIG. 8. Experimental Somascope at the University of Colorado. On the left is seen: the pulse generator, receiver amplifier, gain compensators and monitor oscilloscope. At the center is shown: the main viewing unit with associated photographic equipment and viewing hood. On the right is shown: the tank in which the patient is immersed, the transducer, the horizontal, vertical, and circular scanning mechanisms. On the far right is a constant temperature circulation pump.

sound beam; (2) we see structures which at times lie in the sound shadow of some sonically opaque object; (3) we are able to improve our resolution by an exchange of range for azimuth resolving power from strong reflectors, while showing the small and weakly reflecting structures accurately; and (4) we nearly rid ourselves of "spooks" or picture artifacts which were highly troublesome in previous studies.

Fig. 8 illustrates the equipment that is currently being used, and shows the water tank in which the patient sits, the screen of the oscilloscope and associated equipment.

Since the basic research studies had demonstrated that one must expect to receive signals which would differ in amplitude by over a 100 to 1 amplitude range (despite the use of compound circular scanning), it was found necessary to further improve the range resolving power of the system. Several methods were investigated in an effort to shorten the wave train of the echo signals. One method of reducing the echo length is by use of a system of plugging, that is, following an initial excitation pulse by a

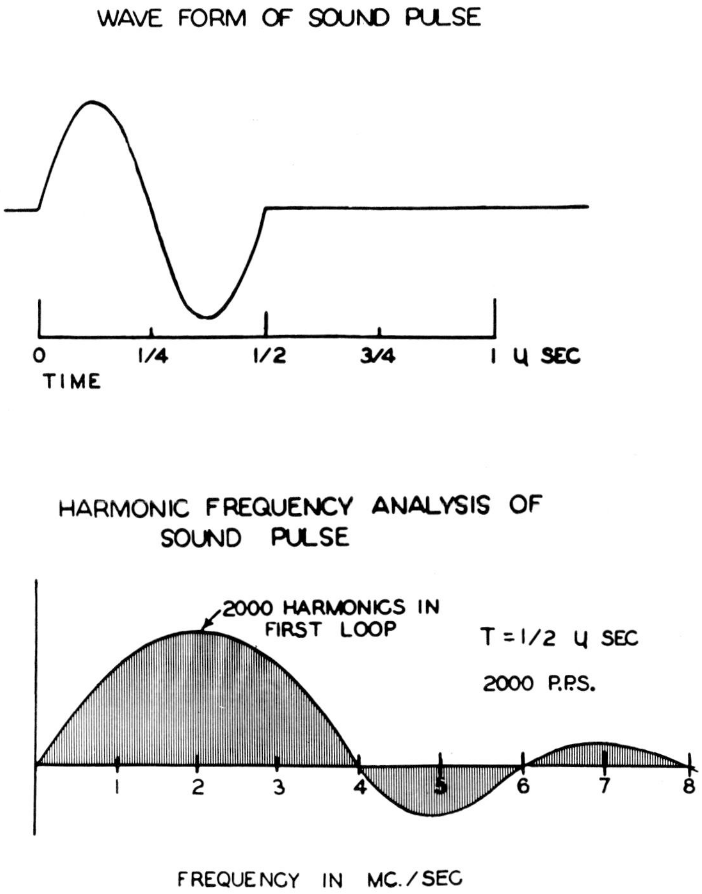

FIG. 9.

second pulse phase to stop the oscillation. By such a method one can realize a single cycle of oscillation in the water; however, the ringing of the crystal on receiving the echo still remains. By the use of two double pulses phased properly in time, the echo will be composed of two oscillatory cycles out of phase with each other and it is possible to reduce the ringing so that the echo becomes approximately one cycle long. Investigation of this method showed that we could expect to obtain resolving power of approximately 1/32 of an inch in tissue over a 40 to 1 db range.

The complex echoes contained in one long-ringing echo complex can also be processed by a phase detection system so that the individual echoes can be seen clearly, regardless of their original amplitude-phase relationship. (A new system of echo ranging based on this method has been designed,

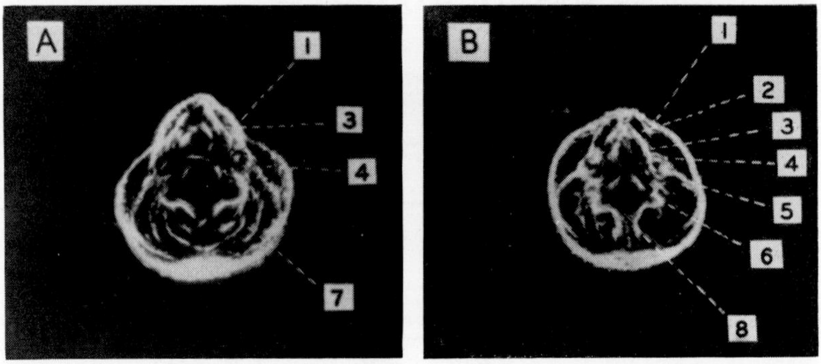

FIG. 10. Somascope Studies of the Normal Neck. Compound circular scanning of the two normal necks, and the resultant improvement in picture detail is shown above. (1) Skin surface. (2) Thyroid. (3) Trachea. (4) Sternocleidomastoid muscle. (5) Fascia colli lateralis. (6) Transverse process. C.4. (7) Fascial planes between posterior neck muscles. (8) Spinous process. C.4.

which is best called a phase modulation system, as compared with pulse echo and frequency modulation systems.)

The best solution of this problem was simpler than either of the above methods. A mechanical impedance matching transformer was designed that transformed the high impedance crystal vibration down to the low impedance of water. This is done through multiple thin layers which slowly bring the mechanical impedance down to that of water, thus preserving both wide band width and power efficiency.[1]

The question of the frequency spectrum in these echo pulses is difficult to answer without actually measuring the spectrum. However, if the wave form is just a single cycle long (which is closely approximated by all the above methods), a very wide spectrum is present. The fact that the crystal is cut to a two megacycle thickness is of no particular significance under these conditions. Fig. 9 shows the Fourier analysis of a one cycle sinusoidal wave with a pulse length similar to ours. This figure illustrates the approximate frequency spectrum present under our experimental conditions.

The azimuth resolving power of our equipment has also been the subject of extensive study. One method of achieving a narrow beam is to use a high frequency crystal of small driver area as is done in the equipment of Wild and Reid. In such a system a beam of approximately one centimeter diameter is obtained. Some time ago we applied focusing techniques and found it possible to achieve beams which were about half-way between the optical type of focusing and that achieved with a plane wave radiator, so that in

[1] The methods devised to shorten the echo pulses were reported in detail at the Symposium; however, since they have been published elsewhere, they are only summarized in this paper (Howry, 1955).

the linear dimension the beam is several inches long and yet remains under ⅛ of an inch in diameter. Several methods of further improving azimuth resolving power are under study.

Not all of our difficulties have been eliminated by the previously described methods; however, a considerable improvement has been achieved in the quality of the picture produced by our new equipment, as is shown in Fig. 10.[2] The most serious deficiency that still exists is that echoes pass above and below the receiver crystal, but a multiple array of receivers placed in a vertical dimension will reduce this difficulty. It is believed that by the application of the methods described in this paper, an instrument of general clinical usefulness will result.

Acknowledgments

The author gratefully acknowledges the contributions made to this project by J. H. Holmes, M.D., D.Med.Sc.; R. R. Lanier, M.D., Ph.D.; G. J. Posakony, C. R. Cushman, and the many engineers who have made this research possible.

References

Holmes, J. H., D. H. Howry, G. J. Posakony and C. R. Cushman. 1955. The ultrasonic visualization of soft tissue structures in the human body. Trans. Am. Clin. Climat. Assn. *67:* (in press).

Howry, D. H. 1955. Techniques used in ultrasonic visualization of soft tissue structures of the body. Convention Record I. R. E. Part *9:* 75–88.

Howry, D. H., and W. R. Bliss. 1952. Ultrasonic visualization of soft tissue structures of the body. J. Lab. and Clin. Med. *40:* 579–592.

Howry, D. H., J. H. Holmes, C. R. Cushman, and G. J. Posakony. 1955. Ultrasonic visualization of living organs and tissues; with observations on some disease processes. Geriatrics *10:* 123–128.

Howry, D. H., J. H. Holmes, R. R. Lanier and G. J. Posakony. 1954. Use of ultrasonic pulse echo techniques for the visualization of soft tissue structures and disease processes. Third Annual Conference on Ultrasonic Therapy. Washington, D. C.

Howry, D. H., G. J. Posakony, C. R. Cushman and J. H. Holmes. 1956. Three dimensional and stereoscopic observations of body structures by ultrasound. J. App. Physiol. (In press.)

Howry, D. H., D. A. Stott and W. R. Bliss. 1954. The ultrasonic visualization of carcinoma of the breast and other soft-tissue structures. Cancer *7:* 354–358.

Dr. Howry: One thing I neglected to say. I have not in any way contradicted Dr. Wild's and Dr. Reid's work, because we have not investigated the same problems as they have. They are most assuredly operating

[2] This figure was described but not illustrated during the Symposium.

over a full 60 db range. They are not trying, apparently, to get the last ounce out of definition which is what we are trying to do.

DR. WILD: I would like to add that we are attacking the known sites of cancer and holding the cancer up, so to speak, on the end of a rubber membrane. There are certain known sites of cancer of high incidence in the body, and by balancing it on the end of this rubber balloon, we have the tissue for examination fixed.

DR. HOWRY: You are comparing the picture of one type against another which is being called standard, and from that arriving at the information—without making any definite statement that, it is the true picture of the tumor. I think from that standpoint it is quite clear. You are certainly getting significant results.

DR. WILD: In answer to one of Dr. Hueter's former questions, we have gone to the brain of a child through the foramen and picked up a metal tube which was in there for the surgical therapy of hydroencephalocele.

DR. HUETER: I was not only thinking of putting such foreign objects in there, but perhaps of coagulating the tissue or changing the tissue in some way and thus making it pathological, and then observing the progression of changes in the echoscope.

DR. WEISSLER: Did all of your work take place at 2 megacycles or have you explored a range of frequencies?

DR. HOWRY: We have been working from 180 kc. up to about 20 megacycles. I think there are some advantages in raising the frequency somewhat. I do not plan to go as high as Dr. Wild and Dr. Reid have. If we want to double our resolving power in the azimuth, we must go to 6 megacycles and I think that is where we are going.

DR. HUETER: You actually do not use one frequency as you said. You use a band, and you may want to shift the band up. However, I would like to ask another question of both speakers. Dr. Wild specified his range as being about 4 cm. and yours as probably a little larger, but how do you specifiy range? What defines your 4 cm.?

DR. WILD: By identifying the tumor when we can see it, and observing the range markers which are plugged in on the basis of the average velocity of sound in tissue.

DR. HUETER: If you put a small scattering object in the tissue and move it further back, you would continue to see it until it is ground in noise. It is sort of a gradual limit. You have to increase your gain, probably.

DR. REID: The depth which you can perceive reflecting objects depends on the sound reflected, obviously.

DR. HUETER: That depends on the kind of tissue penetrated.

DR. REID: Quite often we have picked up the pectoralis muscle which underlies the breast.

DR. HUETER: What is your range?

DR. HOWRY: I do not know. We have gone clear through the body several times; unintentionally. The thing I was going to say, however is apparently, Dr. Reid and I have substantially the same circuits. The transducer is placed at some distance from the tissue and is coupled to it by a water standoff.

If you are operating over some kind of a circuit device you cannot have a simple time varied gain as used in radar. You must have a keyed-time gain so in essence the gain curve of the receiver must start when the first echo comes back. You allow the first major echo to trigger the gain compensator and then you allow the gain of the amplifier to increase in a quasi log fashion, so you are able to receive echoes of identical intensities regardless of where they are.

DR. HUETER: I notice, too, one difference between the pictures shown. You had in some pictures, Dr. Wild, double reflections, and Dr. Howry did not have them. Apparently you used a rather large water delay or a larger one. Now would you consider using a larger water delay and what are your reasons?

DR. WILD: Yes. Our range is a matter of convenience. The range of our crystals in water as designed by the Navy was 18 inches in water. We did some reflection studies, multiple reflections on distilled water versus blood. We got a ratio of 5 to 1. We have 20 reflections.

DR. REID: Dr. Hueter's point is that the multiple reflection we get is the skin signal which is rereflected off the crystal face, and then off the skin again occurring much further along the linear time base. In fact, it is twice the distance from the transmitted pulse to the first skin signal to the second one, and that is as far as we dare to go. On some specimens that acted as a new transmitter pulse and reduplicated the first set of signals, so any signal that occurs after that time cannot be absolutely identified as to the spatial position of the structure that caused it, so we look no further than that second reflection that comes back. Most of the pictures had it chopped off. You did see the similar thing inside that double cyst picture, the left-hand cyst had a rereflection between the near and the far walls. This is as much of a spook as we have been able to readily identify.

Indications and Contraindications for Ultrasonic Therapy in Medicine

J. H. Aldes

Department of Rehabilitation, Cedars of Lebanon Hospital, Los Angeles, California

INCREASED EXPERIENCE with ultrasonic therapy has resulted in a better understanding of its various methods and techniques, and their specific indications and contraindications.

Ultrasonic Instruments

Numerous types of ultrasonic instruments are available, with frequencies varying in range from 800,000 to 4,000,000 cycles per second, and a total energy output of 10 to 60 watts. Recommended ultrasonic modalities should have a frequency between 800,000 and 1,000,000 cycles per second with a maximum intensity of 3 watts/cm.^{2} with a total output of 15 watts. Some units produce more than one frequency, are equipped with more than one applicator or transducer, and the frequency can be adjusted to the requirements of any specific treatment. Applicators or transducers come in different sizes and shapes and the area of contact, or the radiating surface, ranges from 4.5 to 12.5 square centimeters.

For general use a transducer with a contact surface of about five square centimeters is recommended; with the output limit of 3 watts/cm.^{2} the total power administered will not exceed 15 watts. This range minimizes the damage of excessive dosage. Whatever type of unit is used, calibration of the output must be checked at least once daily. In our work a Siemens Dosimeter has been employed for this purpose. Many of the more recent ultrasonic instruments are equipped with a correctly calibrated gauge which indicates throughout the treatment whether the contact is good or faulty, as well as the amount of acoustic power transmitted to the affected area. Nevertheless, we have found it advisable to continue using the Dosimeter in order to double check the calibration of the gauge.

Methods and Techniques of Application

In the use of ultrasound an impeccable method and technique of application are of vital importance. This includes correct selection of frequency, intensity and duration of each application. A faulty technique leads to poor results and could be injurious to the patient. Two methods of application are distinguished: the direct and the indirect method. Ultrasound does not pass through air. Therefore, a suitable contact medium, known as the coupling agent, is introduced between the soundhead or transducer, and the skin area to be treated. For direct application we have experimented with mineral oil, soap emulsions, paraffin, lanolin, and liquid petrolatum, and have found that the latter is the most satisfactory coupling agent. In the indirect method best results are obtained by use of degassed water as a coupling agent. The indirect method is used whenever the area to be treated is irregular, precluding direct contact with the entire surface of the soundhead, as with elbows, hands, knees, ankles and feet.

Dosage

The dosage used in the direct method is determined prior to application. The head of the transducer is moved slowly over the oiled skin surface, and the wattage regulator set to the proper dosage. Any discomfort felt by the patient indicates either undue intensity of the sound waves or an insufficient amount of coupling agent. The sensory reactions of the patient must be determined by neurologic examination prior to start of therapy, in order to make sure that he is able to detect pain. During the entire course of sonations the Dosimeter is continuously checked to ascertain whether the selected dose is actually administered, and at the same time fluctuations of the wattage are kept to a minimum.

In our experience frequencies of from 800,000 to 1,000,000 cycles per second have proved most satisfactory in the majority of cases. With frequency of this range the half value layer amounts to between 3.5 and 4.5 centimeters. It is thus possible to reach any of the sites to be sonated, provided the approach is not abnormally impaired by intervening interfaces, such as air spaces, adipose tissue, periosteum or bone. As to intensity, best results were obtained with a low dosage varying from 0.2 to 2.0 watts/$cm.^2$ Ordinarily the range between 0.2 and 1.5 watts/$cm.^2$ was selected, but a higher dose—up to 2.5 watts/$cm.^2$—is required in obese or muscular individuals.

The site to be sonated must be carefully considered in selecting the optimal dose, as the depth of the target point below the skin surface varies in different parts of the body. For example, the overlying tissue is thicker in the gluteal area than in the forearm, and therefore the dose for the gluteal area must be higher than that for the forearm. The dose is adjusted to the specific disease and the severity of the pathologic condition, refractory cases calling for a greater amount of sonation. Furthermore, each time a treatment is given the physician should take into consideration the subjective and objective findings, and fit the dose to the prevailing circumstances.

Ultrasonic radiations are administered in a sequence of series, each series usually consisting of 12 sonations. In acute cases sonations are given every day, in mild or chronic cases every other day. Application periods vary from 3 to 20 minutes. Whenever further treatments are required after completion of the first series, sonations are resumed following a rest period of two weeks. In some cases a third or even a fourth series becomes necessary, but after the second series, the interval between ultrasonic applications is extended. Continuation of sonations over more than four to six weeks without rest periods in between is ill-advised and definitely contraindicated. Best results were obtained by applying the radicular and neurotrophic therapy of Tschannen and Stuhlfauth, in which sonations are administered not only to the local area, but also the respective nerve root areas (Head's zones).

Contraindications for Ultrasound

The areas of the body for which ultrasonic therapy is contraindicated are: brain, eyes, thyroid, stellate ganglion, cardiac area, parenchymal organs (such as spleen and liver), spinal column, and reproductive organs. Special precautions are required in sonating certain other parts of the body, especially the sternum, scapula, bony prominences and epiphyses of juvenile bone. Ultrasonic therapy is also contraindicated in pregnancy, certain gynecological conditions, in the presence of benign and malignant tumors, in patients with tuberculosis, bronchiectasis, and other types of lung involvement, fractures, and thrombophlebitis. In elderly patients ultrasonic therapy should be administered with great caution, and only small doses are used. The number of contraindications is steadily being reduced through development of better ultrasonic equipment, the use of minimal doses, and research on improvement of techniques (Fig. 1).

The application of ultrasonic therapy calls for a thorough understanding of the theories, methods and techniques of medical ultrasonics, and can be regarded as safe only in the hands of physicians who are willing to take the necessary time required to supervise and apply ultrasonic therapy. Further progress of ultrasonic therapy in medicine depends on continued laboratory and clinical research. It is necessary to investigate more precisely the absorption of ultrasonic radiation and its effect on specific normal and diseased tissues. On this basis we hope to be able to determine the usefulness of selective dosages, and to determine more precisely the indications and contraindications of ultrasonic therapy.

We have been doing some intensive experimental research using pigs as our laboratory animal. Our main project is to determine whether the therapeutic dosages can disturb growth. In addition, we are utilizing ultrasonic radiation to determine whether there is a cessation of function of the female and male organs when therapeutic dosages of ultrasonic radiation are given in those areas where the glands are located. We have also done a great deal of work on the healing of skin ulcers. We are producing skin ulcers by ultrasonic radiation of high dosage and then therapeutically healing them.

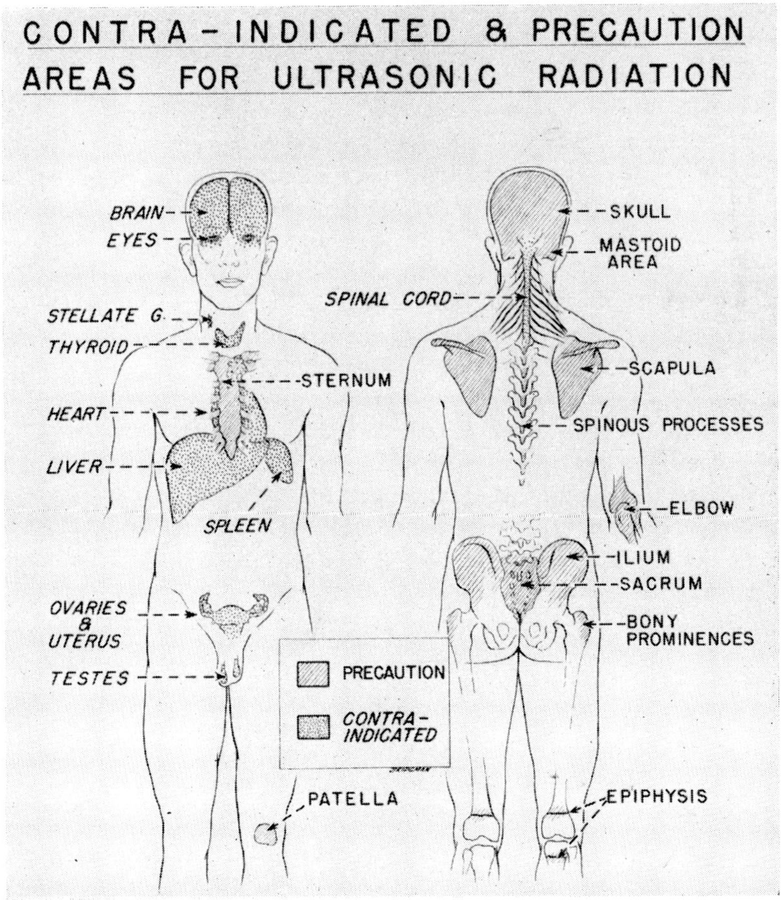

FIG. 1. Contraindicated and precaution areas for ultrasonic radiation.

We have found that therapeutic dosage is more beneficial than some of the other preparations, medicinal as well as plastic.

Since 1939 when Pohlman and his co-workers demonstrated favorable therapeutic results from ultrasonic radiation in the treatment of sciatica and brachial plexus neuralgia, countless articles have been published reporting beneficial as well as damaging results from this type of therapy.

Indications

The findings of the earlier investigators in the use of ultrasonic therapy in medicine were so impressive that it was decided five years ago, in 1950, to start a clinical research project for the study of ultrasonic therapy at Cedars of Lebanon Hospital, Los Angeles, California. In view of the fact that the literature had shown that the best results were reported with spinal arthritis both in the cervical and lumbosacral areas with and without radiculitis, we felt it best to try out this new type of therapy on these conditions. We also felt that it would be more beneficial in evaluating this type of therapy to utilize patients having cervical or lumbar arthritis, with and without radiculitis, who had previously failed to benefit from any other type of conservative therapy such as diathermy, microtherm, infra-red, hot-packing, massage, roentgen therapy, and various types of immobilization. We did not include any patients in these series who had surgery to the spine for these conditions and continued to have symptoms. The first group of patients in the above category totalled 121, of which 29 had cervical arthritis, 42 cervical arthritis with radiculitis, 19 lumbar sacral arthritis, and 31 lumbar sacral arthritis with radiculitis.

Ultrasonic radiation was administered in a series of eight to twelve treatments at intervals of 48 hours. These sonations were administered paravertebrally in the region of the cervical spine and trapezius areas bilaterally, for the condition of cervical arthritis. When there was radiculitis accompanying cervical arthritis, the sonations were continued to the shoulder joint and included the deltoid area. In addition, indirect therapy was given to the hand and lower third of the forearm, following the course of the radiculitis in the nerve and body. Each patient received one full series of treatment. If the responses were favorable but improvement only transient, another series was given, after a therapeutic holiday of ten days prevailed. Whenever it appeared advantageous a third series was administered. In this group of patients 40 percent of them had one series and 50 percent, two series; ten percent had three series. Most satisfactory results were obtained by increasing both intensity of radiation and duration of treatment from one series to the next. In the first series the intensity averaged from 0.5 to 1 watt/$cm.^2$, and the duration of the treatment, three to five minutes. The intensity of the second series ranged from 0.75 to 1.2 watt/$cm.^2$ The duration for each side is approximately five minutes. The third series intensities ranged from 1.2 to 1.5 watt/$cm.^2$ In this series the duration of time ranged from 8 to 10 minutes on each side. The intensity for the indirect method when the patient had radiculitis, where we sonated the lower forearm and the hands, ranged from 0.5 to 1 watt/$cm.^2$ with a duration of five minutes to each extremity.

We have noticed, not only in our first group of patients in which ultrasonic radiations were used but also throughout the entire program, that if adequate intensities of ultrasonic radiations were given, the patient usually had the reaction of marked discomfort which came on approximately three hours after radiation. This discomfort was relieved by mild sedation such as aspirin or Pabirin. Only in the more apprehensive patients did we have to use codeine or the derivatives of codeine. We noticed that with those patients who showed this reaction of discomfort, the final results were better. This reaction was noted only during the first few radiations and then subsided completely. When an inadequate intensity was used, that is, a low wattage, this reaction did not occur; and if we kept on with the same low intensity, the results were not as good as if we had increased the intensity. The bases of this reaction, according to our experience, are probably due to the local biochemical and physiological effects in the area that is being sonated. There is no doubt of the increase of vascularization in that area as well as loosening up of the fibrous and spasmodic tissues, and when this occurs, there is an irritation to the nerve endings in that area, setting up this pain syndrome. Under no circumstances, however, should the patient suffer pain at the time of radiation. If this occurs, then the intensity is too high and it must be cut down immediately.

Prior to ultrasonic therapy, patients were completely evaluated, including blood and urine examinations as well as roentgen studies of the involved area. Fourteen days after the final series the patient was rechecked. Thereafter every patient, that we were able to follow was re-evaluated at monthly intervals for the next five years. At the present time we have followed 3,485 cases.

As temporary favorable response might be due to the psychological lift of a new type of treatment, 25 patients of the same age level with similar complaints of corresponding durations were selected as a control group. The first series of treatments was given in the usual manner, but with the current turned off; none showed any improvement. After an interval of ten days another series of treatments was administered, this time with the current on. The results in the control group compared favorably with those in the original group of 121 patients.

Results of Clinical Study

The following table shows our general results in our preliminary study, with an eight-month evaluation in the use of ultrasonic radiation in spinal arthritis, and a thirty-six-month evaluation, in our five-year study. In evaluating the results of ultrasonic radiation in this study, as well as in others, we are reporting, the following is the classification we used:

Apparent permanent improvement	(+3)
Apparent good improvement	(+2)
Partial improvement	(+1)
No improvement	(+0)

The evaluation of our results necessarily contains a subjective element, since we depended largely upon the statements of our patients. One objective criterion used, however, was the increase in range of motion in the affected area (Table 1).

Repeated roentgen, blood and urine examinations revealed no abnormal

TABLE 1

Results in the use of ultrasonic radiation for spinal arthritis
Preliminary group 1950–1951—8 month evaluation

Pathology	No. of patients	Frequency of ultrasound in C.P.S.	Intensity of ultrasound in w/cm²	Duration of sonation in minutes (total)	Other therapy applied	Results (total)
Arthritis, Osteo Cervical (with & without radiculitis)	71	800,000 to 1 megacycle	0.5 to 1.5	6 to 10	none	
Arthritis, Osteo Hypertrophic (with and without radiculitis)	50	800,000 to 1 megacycle	0.5 to 1.5	6 to 15	none	
TOTAL	121					42% (+2 & +3) 57.8% (+0 & +1)
Five year study—36 month evaluation						
Arthritis, Osteo Cervical (with & without radiculitis)	320	800,000 to 1 megacycle	0.5 to 1.5	6 to 20	Hydrotherapy & hot packs	
Arthritis, Osteo Dorsal (with and without radiculitis)	83	800,000 to 1 megacycle	0.5 to 1.5	6 to 20	Hydrotherapy & hot packs	
Arthritis, Osteo Lumbar (with & without radiculitis)	400	800,000 to 1 megacycle	0.5 to 1.5	6 to 20	Hydrotherapy & hot packs	
TOTAL	803					78% (+2 & +3) 22% (+0 & +1)

changes, and no ill effects were noted. The response of male and female patients was not significantly different, but younger patients responded more readily. Patients with cervical hypertrophic arthritis and radiculitis showed better, more rapid, and more constant results than those with arthritis of the lumbosacral area. Patients showing questionable or no improvement following the first or second series responded encouragingly when in the third series ultrasonic therapy was combined with other forms of conservative therapy, particularly infra-red irradiation, hot packs, and hydrotherapy. Since this original group of patients on which ultrasonic therapy was initiated five years ago, we have treated 923 patients having spinal arthritis. This included not only the cervical and lumbar spines but also the dorsal spine. We were able to follow 803 of these over a period of three years. There were 320 cases of cervical, 83 cases of dorsal, and 400 of lumbar. Approximately one-third of these cases had radiculitis symptoms associated with their osteoarthritis.

In our last evaluation of the entire series, as of April 1, 1955, the overall percentage of relief of symptoms was 78 percent. The remaining 22 percent, although showing some improvement, were not completely free of symptoms and had to have another series or two, on an average of every six months, to obtain relief.

Bursitis

In early 1951, following the encouraging results we were getting in ultrasonic therapy in spinal arthritis, we decided to institute ultrasonic radiation to a small controlled group of patients with subdeltoid bursitis, in order to compare this new type of therapy for this condition with the more conventional form of treatment. In treating subdeltoid bursitis with ultrasonic radiation we find that it produces a powerful and deep micromassage, exerts localized thermal action, and increases intracellular metabolism; it causes exudates and precipitates to be absorbed and tissue deposits to be broken up; it loosens tissues, relieves edema, decreases hypertonicity of the muscles, and produces a local analgesia causing an immediate relief of pain.

Treatment Procedures

Prior to the application of ultrasonic radiation, it is important that in addition to the physical and laboratory examinations, x-rays should be taken of the cervical spine and shoulder joint to rule out any contraindicated pathology and confirm the possibility of a calcareous deposit in the subdeltoid bursa. In our application we followed the radicular and neurotrophic techniques of Tschannen and Stuhlfauth in which we sonate not only the local area of the subdeltoid bursa, but also the nerve roots of the

TABLE 2

Results in the use of ultrasonic radiation for subdeltoid bursitis

Preliminary studies 1951—11 month evaluation

Pathology	No. of patients	Frequency of ultrasound in C.P.S.	Intensity of ultrasound in w/cm²	Duration of sonation in minutes (total)	Other therapy applied	Results (total)
Subdeltoid Bursitis	157	800,000 to 1 megacycle	0.4 to 1.5	6 to 10	none	73.8% (+2 & +3) 26.2% (+0 & +1)

Preliminary study two series of ultrasonic radiation, 1951—12 month evaluation

Pathology	No. of patients	Frequency of ultrasound in C.P.S.	Intensity of ultrasound in w/cm²	Duration of sonation in minutes (total)	Other therapy applied	Results (total)
Subdeltoid Bursitis	35	800,000 to 1 megacycle	0.4 to 1.5	10 to 20	infra-red and hot packs	28.6% (+2 & +3) 71.4% (+0 & +1)

Preliminary study—36 month evaluation

Pathology	No. of patients	Frequency of ultrasound in C.P.S.	Intensity of ultrasound in w/cm²	Duration of sonation in minutes (total)	Other therapy applied	Results (total)
Subdeltoid Bursitis	672	800,000 to 1	0.4 to 1.5	10 to 20	Hot packs	83.8% (+2 & +3) 16.2% (+0 & +1)

cervical plexus. However, we cannot go into the detailed treatment procedure here and therefore we shall just mention a few important items.

In the acute cases sonation was given daily; in the chronic every other day. It has been our experience that a minimum of six sonations is required before beneficial results can be expected, but a full course generally consisted of nine to twelve treatments. A rest period of two weeks followed the first series of sonations, and if symptoms persisted, which was rare, a second series of six sonations was given. If necessary, a third and even fourth series was administered after rest periods between each series. In the treatment of subdeltoid bursitis with calcareous deposit, stationary sonation was applied in addition to the gliding technique directly over the area where the deposit occurred. For the stationary application both intensity and duration were greatly reduced, and only 0.1 to 0.25 watt/cm.^{2} was administered for a period of one to three minutes.

In evaluating these results we used the same classification, except that we took into consideration the pain syndrome as well as the range of motion of the affected shoulder. Our evaluation in this particular study is classified as follows (Table 2):

Apparent permanent improvement—no pain, full range of motion	(+3)
Apparent good improvement—no pain, 80 percent of motion	(+2)
Slight improvement—no pain, 50 percent of motion	(+1)
No improvement	(+0)

Of the 41 patients who obtained little or no improvement from either ultrasonic or conventional therapy, 35 were given another series of ultrasonic treatments, starting and terminating the treatment this time with infra-red heat, or hot packs when muscle spasms were present. These patients, who had reacted poorly to conventional or ultrasonic therapy, when either one of these forms of treatment was given independently, showed that good results could be achieved by a combination of these treatments.

In a group of 210 patients there were 36 who had subdeltoid bursitis with calcareous deposit. Of this group 48 percent showed either complete disappearance or decrease of the calcareous deposit following ultrasonic therapy. Our findings indicate that no constant relationship exists between the decrease or disappearance of calcareous deposit and improvement of symptoms of bursitis. Most patients experienced relief after the deposit had been reduced, but we found that ultrasonic radiation may be effective even when the deposit failed to show any response.

During this five-year period we have treated 672 cases of subdeltoid bursitis of which 108 had calcareous deposits. Their overall percentage of relief of symptoms with full range of motion, loss of pain and discomfort, averaged 83.2 percent. The remaining 16.8 percent had partial to good im-

TABLE 3

Results in the use of ultrasonic radiation in rheumatoid arthritis
Three year study—24 month evaluation

Pathology	No. of patients	Frequency of ultrasound in C.P.S.	Intensity of ultrasound in w/cm²	Method of sonation	Duration of sonation in minutes (total)	Other therapy applied	Results
Arthritis, rheumatoid Upper extremities	37	800,000 to 1 megacycle	1.0 to 1.5	Subaqueous	5 to 10	Hydrotherapy	63% (+2 & +3)
Arthritis, rheumatoid Lower extremities	21	800,000 to 1 megacycle	1.0 to 1.5	Subaqueous	5 to 10	Hydrotherapy	37% (+0 & +1)
Arthritis, rheumatoid Marie-Strumpell's	53	800,000 to 1 megacycle	1.0 to 2.5	Direct	5 to 20	Hot packs	53% (+2 & +3) 47% (+0 & +1)
TOTAL	111						58% (+2 & +3) 42% (+1 & +0)

provement and range of motion, which averaged at least 60 percent. In the entire series all patients benefited but the group in the 16.8 percent bracket were those who had bursitis of a chronic nature for an average duration of time prior to treatment by ultrasonic therapy of eight and a half months.

Rheumatoid Arthritis

In the treatment of rheumatoid arthritis we had 111 cases, 53 of which were Marie-Strumpells. As you know, in this condition there is a soft tissue calcification which involves the anterior and posterior ligaments of the entire spinal column with a calcification of the intervertebral ligaments. These patients show by x-ray a characteristic bamboo-type of an ankylosis. The results with conventional types of therapy have not been too encouraging. However, ultrasonic treatments in this condition have shown positive results.

The frequency used in the Marie-Strumpell's cases remains the same as in other cases, but the intensities must be higher in order to get beneficial results. In our series the intensities vary between 1.0 and 2.5 watts/cm.^{2}, and were determined by the amount of pathology, as well as by the symptoms. In our first group of patients when using lower intensities, the results were very poor but as we stepped up the intensities as well as the duration, our results became more encouraging. We have also found that the combination of ultrasonic therapy, followed by hot packing to the area, gives the best results. We feel that further investigation must be done in this specific pathology.

Rheumatoid arthritis affects the upper and lower extremities with marked deformities. The results have not been as spectacular as in other types of arthritis. We have had 37 cases involving the upper and 21 involving the lower extremities. The method of treatment on these cases was indirect. The intensities ranged from 1.0 to 1.5 watts/cm.^{2} and the duration again depended on the amount of pathology present.

In this group of 111 cases, we have seen our poorest results in our continuous rechecks, and noted percentage for overall relief of symptoms was 58 percent. (See Table 3.)

Arthritis, Hypertrophic, Joint Involvement

This group embraces arthritis changes, both osteo and hypertrophic, of not only the major joints of the body but also small joints of the hands and feet. In this group we were able to study 807 joint involvements which comprised 603 cases.

The shoulder, hip and knee joints sonations were applied by the direct method. The elbow, wrist, hand, knee, ankle and foot were usually treated by the indirect method. In this group the overall percentage of relief of

TABLE 4

Results in the use of ultrasonic radiation in hypertrophic arthritis

Five year study—36 month evaluation

Pathology	No. of patients	Frequency of ultrasound in C.P.S.	Intensity of ultrasound in w/cm^2	Method of sonation	Duration of sonation in minutes (total)	Other therapy applied	Results
Arthritis, Hypertrophic	603 (807 joints)	800,000 to 1 Megacycle	0.7 to 1.5	Direct or subaqueous depending on area to be sonated	5 to 15	Hydrotherapy and hot packs	79% (+2 & +3) 21% (+0 & +1)

symptoms with increase of motion of the various joints averaged 79 percent. (See Table 4.)

Orthopedic Intra-Articular Conditions

In this type of pathology we have compared the results of using the oral medications which have been isolated from the adrenal cortex, Cortisone and Hydrocortone, and then Cortisone followed by ultrasonic therapy. We have also used intra-articular injections of Hydrocortone Acetate in the common articular arthritic conditions.

Approximately three years ago we began an investigation into the use of Hydrocortone Acetate followed by ultrasonic therapy, and in this study we used the same approach as in previous research, where we compared not only the reported results on the use of Hydrocortone alone, but also when administered along with ultrasonic therapy. In this dual approach to the traumatic articular arthritic conditions, we took into consideration the dispersion power of ultrasound.

Prior to clinical use of ultrasound along with Hydrocortone Acetate, we conducted animal investigations, to indicate the value of this mechanical property of ultrasound. In this study we injected a mixture of opaque substance plus Hydrocortone into the knee joint of a pig. We found through direct observation, by means of arthrotomy and x-ray, that the drug was dispersed more completely throughout the entire synovia of the knee joint when ultrasound was used following the intra-articular injections.

Our initial series included 108 patients with 126 joint involvements and covered the following pathological conditions: Chronic periarthritis of the shoulder joint, chronic bursitis of the shoulder joint with calcareous deposit and capsulitis; osteo, hypertrophic, and degenerative arthritis; epicondylitis; synovitis secondary to chronic rheumatoid arthritis; traumatic synovitis; gouty arthritis with secondary bony changes.

Each injection of hydrocortone averaged 100 mg., or 4 cc. of the drug, which contains 25 mg. per cc. The direct method of ultrasonic irradiation was used for the shoulder, hip and knee; and the indirect method for the elbow, wrist and ankle. The neurotrophic radicular application was used in each case preceding the local direct or indirect sonation.

In our control series we used a group of patients having the pathological conditions mentioned. This group numbered 37 patients with 50 joint involvements. Intra-articular injections were given with the same technique as in our regular series, only hydrocortone acetate was used alone. We found in this study that our best results were obtained by injections of 100 mg. every 36 hours. A total of four 100-mg. injections were given. After receiving the large single doses, the patient showed improvement within two hours and had less regression between injections than with smaller doses. We also found that the objective signs of improvement, such as decreased swelling, tenderness, redness and warmth and increased range of motion without pain generally followed subjective signs of improvement more quickly with the larger single doses. In addition, by giving an injection every 36 hours until four had been administered, we noted that the objective signs were of longer duration. This control group averaged 16 days of marked improvement before any regression, subjective or objective, was apparent. In our regular series in which we used hydrocortone and ultrasonic therapy we had the best results in chronic bursitis of the shoulder joint with calcareous deposits and capsulitis. Here we found that 93 percent of the cases had persistent marked improvement which had continued 18 months, which was the time of our last checkups. The remaining 7 percent could be classified at that time as having moderate improvement since they have histories of slight regressions, though they never returned to the level of subjective or objective symptoms they had prior to therapy.

Our next best results occurred in those patients having hypertrophic or degenerative arthritis of the knee joint with synovitis. 91 percent of this group still showed a level of marked improvement at the 18-month follow-up. They all were fully ambulatory and had only mild and infrequent pain on motion. The remaining 9 percent of this group could be classified as obtaining 60 percent improvement. Their regression periods, although not frequent, revealed moderate pain and swelling of their affected joint on motion.

Our third best results were with epicondylitis. Though we had just six cases, five of them showed complete and continuous disappearance of symptoms. The one case which did not respond completely had only short periods of mild discomfort.

In the group with arthritic changes in the hip joint we found that we could classify 83 percent as having continued marked improvement. The average age of those showing improvement in this group was 59, while the 17 percent that could be classified as having only mild or moderate improvement averaged 71 years of age. In the patients having synovitis secondary to chronic rheumatoid arthritis we noted that 85 percent retained their level of marked improvement at their 18-month checkup. Of the remainder, 10 percent could be classified as having persistent mild improvement, and 5 percent as little or no improvement. In the 15 percent not showing marked improvement, the patients had frequent general flare-ups of the rheumatoid condition. Our most rapid results were in traumatic synovitis. The objective signs of swelling, redness, warmth and painful motion subsided on an average within two hours after the first injection and sonation. In these cases the majority needed only two injections and four ultrasonic treatments.

In both the control and the regular series our pretherapy examination always consisted of x-rays of the involved area, range of motion of the affected joint, complete blood count, sedimentation rate and urine. This examination was repeated at regular intervals. We found that if the individual had an elevated white count and sedimentation rate, it declined to normal levels more quickly when Hydrocortone plus ultrasonic radiation was used, then when Hydrocortone was used alone.

In comparing the control and regular series, we found our overall percentage of improvement in all cases showed that injections of Hydrocortone alone gave improvement that lasted an average of 16 days, and the improvement level could only be classified as moderate. When Hydrocortone plus ultrasonics was used there was marked improvement, and on an average this level was retained for 18 months, which was the last checkup. In the combination therapy method we found that regression was less marked after each treatment than when Hydrocortone was used alone. In statistically comparing the remission of symptoms in both the regular series and the control group, we found that when ultrasonics were used along with Hydrocortone injections, 89 percent of those cases retained a level of marked improvement for 18 months. The remaining 11 percent treated retained their marked improvement plateau for 6 months, and then regressed only to a level of 50 percent, or moderate improvement at the 18 month checkup.

In the control group which received Hydrocortone alone, 80 percent of the cases retained a level of moderate improvement for 16 days and the remaining 10 percent showed regression after 7 days. We also found that the subjective and objective signs were eliminated more rapidly when Hydrocortone was administered in combination with ultrasonics, and the range of motion of the joint then returned more quickly to normal levels.

This study has revealed to us that in severe chronic articular conditions, ultrasonic therapy plus intra-articular injections of Hydrocortone is the treatment of choice, but continued investigation into this procedure is necessary, not only to establish the amount of Hydrocortone to be injected, but also to determine the best level of ultrasonic radiation and the number of sonations required for these conditions.

In this 3-year study in the treatment of intra-articular arthritis we have used this approach on 301 cases, or 342 joints which comprised 93 shoulders, 31 elbows, 30 wrists, 52 hips, 79 knees, 37 ankles. Our total percentage of relief of symptoms with increased motion of the joints involved was 93 percent. (see Table 5.)

Epicondylitis

In 1953 we started our investigation of the clinical use of ultrasonic therapy for epicondylitis. Again in this pathology we found that, compared to our previous experience in the use of ultrasonic therapy, our results

TABLE 5

Results in the use of ultrasonic radiation in the treatment of orthopedic intra articular conditions

Preliminary report—18 month evaluation

Pathology	No. of patients	Frequency of ultrasound in C.P.S.	Intensity of ultrasound in w/cm²	Method of sonation	Duration of sonation in minutes (total)	Other therapy applied	Results
Arthritis, Osteo Inter-articular	108 (126 joints)	1 megacycle	0.8 to 1.5	Direct and subaqueous depending on area to be sonated	5 to 15	Hydrocortone inter-articular Hydrotherapy	89% (+2 & +3) 11% (+0 & +1)

36 month evaluation

Pathology	No. of patients	Frequency of ultrasound in C.P.S.	Intensity of ultrasound in w/cm²	Method of sonation	Duration of sonation in minutes (total)	Other therapy applied	Results
Arthritis, Osteo Inter-articular	301 (342 joints)	1 megacycle	0.8 to 1.5	Direct and subaqueous depending on area to be sonated	5 to 15	Hydrocortone inter-articular Hydrotherapy	93% (+2 & +3) 7% (+0 & +1)

were not as outstanding as we felt they should be. Therefore, we utilized the same procedure that we had with intra-articular arthritis by using Hydrocortone injections followed by ultrasonic therapy. To compare this new therapy with the previously accepted therapeutic practices, we first used ultrasonic radiation on the group of patients on whom all forms of conservative treatment had failed. This group was comprised of the two patients who had received Hydrocortone alone without beneficial results, and the 15 patients who had received other forms of conservative treatment and had shown little improvement. These patients all had a traumatic etiology for the epicondylitis, normal blood count, and except for a flick of calcium noted in the lateral epicondylar region in five cases, x-ray findings were negative.

Examination of these patients prior to ultrasonic therapy revealed tenderness about the lateral epicondyle on palpation. Tests for the extensor capri radialis brevis and extensor digitorium communis, and also the "door knob test" were positive. Three of these patients had pain over the radial-humeral joint on palpation. The average duration of symptoms in this group was 91 days.

The application of ultrasonic radiation to the lateral epicondylar area was by means of a cone-shaped applicator which was attached to a regular transducer having a piezo-electric quartz crystal surface of 12.5 cm. The tip of the cone had a radiating surface approximately 2.5 cm. in diameter. The cone-shaped transducer was necessary in order to obtain direct contact to the irregular surface about the lateral epicondylar area. The intensity used in this area ranged from 0.5 to 1.0 watt/cm.^{2}, and a very slow, gliding, rotating movement was made with the transducer over the lateral epicondylar area. The length of time of each sonation was approximately five minutes.

The second part of the ultrasonic therapy was performed under water, using water as the coupling agent. This sonation was given over the entire extensor area of the forearm, and was administered with a gliding, rotating movement covering 20 cm. of skin surface in one minute with the head of the transducer 1.3 cm. away from the forearm. This radiation was given with a regular transducer having no cone attachment but having a crystal surface of 4.5 cm.^{2} We feel that, in our experience, the smaller radiating surface in a regular transducer is better for sonation. The frequency used with this transducer remains the same, but the intensity varies from 1 to 1.5 watts/cm.^{2}

In a group of 19 cases in which no previous treatment of any kind had been given, ultrasonic therapy was administered in the same manner as in the first group. Complete relief was noted in 16 cases after two weeks. The average duration of symptoms of this group prior to treatment was four

TABLE 6

Results in the use of ultrasonic radiation in the treatment of epicondylitis

Two year study—18 month evaluation

Pathology	No. of patients	Frequency of ultrasound in C.P.S.	Intensity of ultrasound in w/cm²	Method of sonation	Duration of sonation in minutes (total)	Other therapy applied	Results
Epicondylitis	144	1 to 3 meg.	0.5 to 1.2	Direct and subaqueous	5 to 15	Hydrocortone interarticular	97% (+2 & +3)
						Hydrotherapy	3% (+0 & +1)

weeks. In the three cases which did not respond, in this group of 19, we infiltrated the lateral epicondyle with 25 mg. of Hydrocortone and followed the injections with ultrasonic radiation using the cone radiation technique to the lateral epicondyle. The rationale of using Hydrocortone followed by ultrasonic therapy is to utilize the dispersing power of ultrasonic radiation to spread the Hydrocortone throughout the pathologic tissue about the lateral epicondyle. In these three cases, six radiations plus Hydrocortone injections gave relief of all symptoms. In another group of 35 patients we used the same technique of ultrasonic radiations preceeded by injections of 25 mg. of Hydrocortone into the lateral epicondyle. The average duration of symptoms in this group was approximately four weeks. Thirty-four patients (97 percent) showed complete relief of all symptoms at the end of their third treatment, a treatment being given every other day. One case required two additional treatments before full relief was accomplished.

In the 71 cases which had ultrasonic therapy alone or with Hydrocortone the percentage of male and female, and the average age of the group were about the same as in the previous group. Etiologic factors were also similarly distributed. The follow-up period in this group has been two years. Symptoms have not recurred, and x-rays following ultrasonic radiation showed no deterioration of the bone.

The total group of patients with pathologic conditions known as epicondylitis numbered 144. In the overall percentage of complete cessation of symptoms in the full range of elbow joint and forearm was 97 percent. The 3 percent that did not show complete results were a group of patients who had a chronic condition of epicondylitis for an average length of time of 18 months. In all the cases showing good results the average number of maximum radiations was five, and the minimum three. (see Table 6.)

Acute Traumatic Miscellaneous Conditions

In this group of conditions in which we have found that ultrasonic radiation has been very beneficial we have included myositis, 200 cases; fibrositis, 210; sprains (ankle, knee and wrist), 180; with an overall total of 590. The length of convalescence has been shortened at least 75 percent with the use of ultrasonic therapy.

In about 50 percent of the fibrositis cases the condition occurred both in male and female and were of the chronic stage, the type that we see in the menopause age bracket. In these cases ultrasonic radiation has been more beneficial than any other type of physical therapy agent. The myositis and fibrositis cases were treated by the direct method, with a range of intensity of 0.5 to 1.5 watts/cm.^{2} and in sprains of the ankle and wrist the indirect method was used, with an intensity of 1.0 to 1.2 watts/cm.^{2} The overall percentage of relief and cessation of symptoms was 93 percent. We feel that in the previously mentioned cases in which ultrasonic therapy has been investigated, that we can definitely recommend this type of radiation, but we must stress that the individual who is applying ultrasonic therapy must have a thorough knowledge of the superficial anatomy, as well as the superficial neuroanatomy of the human body. He or she should have precise knowledge of the techniques of medical ultrasonics and should realize that the intensities and durations should be varied from day to day, depending on the objective and subjective symptoms of the patient. The approach to treatment is entirely different from that of other physical therapy agents, and the success of ultrasonic therapy is due only to the precautions and care given to the application of ultrasonic radiation.

There are several pathologic conditions that we feel are still in the experimental stage. There have been numerous articles on these various pathologies, but in our clinic, it is our opinion that even though the results are encouraging, we are not ready to recommend ultrasonic radiation as the treatment of choice. The pathologies still under investigation by our experimental group are the dermatological conditions of local dermatitis that are usually a contact type of dermatitis. We have 18 of these cases. Here we have used frequencies of 3,000,000 cycles per second with an intensity of 0.5 watt/cm.^{2} and treated these conditions as they occur on the extremities, by the indirect method. Our results in these types of cases have been encouraging. We have seen relief of symptoms such as itching and cessation of symptoms in about 60 percent of the cases.

In Herpes Zoster, especially of the thoracic area, we have had 27 cases. These we have treated with the direct method, using a frequency of 3,000,000 cycles per second and intensities of 0.5 to 1 watt/cm.^{2} and radiating over the area of the peripheral nerve involvement. Usually these cases occur in the mid-dorsal area and with the spread of dermatitis under the breast line. Care must be taken in radiating over the anterior chest area. We felt that in this area the lower intensities are best. In our group of cases, we have been able to decrease the severe itching sensations approximately 50 percent within the second radiation treatment and to effect a gradual cessation of this symptom in about 10 radiations. The dermatological condition seen in the skin does remain for a number of weeks following the radiation but gradually disappears. An overall percentage of relief in these cases is approximately 71 percent. The group that did not fall in this category are of a chronic nature. Our best results are with the group that we have seen in the first week of occurrence.

In Dupytrons Contractures, we have a pathological condition of fibrositis of the sub-cutaneous layers of the palms of the hands as well as the plantar surface of the feet. With this there is a contracture of the tissues in the hand. The recognized therapy has been surgery in which the contracting tissues are severed. The procedure is very radical, and the patient is incapacitated for many weeks. Ultrasonic therapy for this condition has been showing encouraging results. It must be combined with stretching and with a splint that will keep the fingers and hand extended following each radiation. In our group of 18 cases we have shown improvement in about 61 percent of the cases. The number of treatments must be determined by the results obtained. The radiation must be given under water. The best frequency is 3,000,000 cycles per second but we believe better results would be obtained if a frequency of 2,000,000 cycles per second would be used. Intensities should range from 0.2 to 0.7 watt/cm.^{2}

Circulatory Disturbances

In circulatory disturbances of a mild nature, such as seen in the geriatric group, especially of the lower extremities, we have found that radiation should be used in the neurotrophic approach, that is, radiating over the lumbar plexus. In these individuals we have found that it is best to use the indirect method, particularly for the lower extremities. The results that we have obtained are very encouraging, and we have been able to give relief to approximately 50 percent of our cases.

Ulcers

Dermatological ulcers, due to circulatory disturbances, have been benefited by ultrasonic therapy. These ulcers occur over the lower third of the leg and about the ankles. We have had 37 of these cases in our series. They have all had a duration of 3 to 10 years, with every type of conservative therapy as well as surgery performed on them, with no permanent results. We have found that the indirect method of ultrasonic therapy using a frequency of 800,000 to 1,000,000 cycles per second with an intensity of 0.5 to 1 watt are very beneficial. In this series of 37, we have 10 cases that we now have followed for three years which have been completely healed and have shown no recurrences. The overall percentage of improvement is 73 percent.

Keloids

In this series we have collected 33 cases. Two cases occurred in the ear lobes following puncturing of the lobe for cosmetic purposes. The other cases are post-wounds with keloid formation. With ultrasonic therapy in acute cases the "itching" sensation has been reduced with three radiations, and the thickness and width of the keloid formation dimensions reduced about 50 percent after the first series of ultrasonic radiation, the series totalling 12 radiations. We have been using frequencies of 1,000,000 cycles per second with intensities of 0.5 to 1 watt, depending on the location of the keloid and the extent of the pathology. The duration of treatment for each area extends from three to ten minutes. In our series we feel that we have seen improvement in about 50 percent of the cases.

Operative Scars

With the advances of surgery of the chest and the extensive post-operative wounds we have noted more painful scars than in previous surgery. A study of this is being made with the Department of Surgery. Ultrasonic radiation is being given within three days after surgery at the time the skin sutures are removed. The frequency used in these cases is 3,000,000 cycles per second, but we do feel that 2,000,000 cycles per second would be adequate. The intensities are very low, from 0.2 to 0.5 watt/cm.^{2}, the duration depending on the extent of the wounds. This research problem has just started. We are already encouraged by the results, and we feel that in this small group we have been able to help at least 75 percent of them.

Summary

Continuing laboratory and clinical investigations on ultrasonic radiation, as well as the exchange of ideas on the potentialities of ultrasonic radiation, at symposia such as this, and the presentation of scientific papers in this field at general medical meetings, will help to eliminate the fear and doubts on the value of ultrasonic therapy by our colleagues. Such efforts will increase the understanding of the importance of ultrasonic therapy as a valuable therapeutic adjunct in the field of medicine.

DR. HUETER: May I ask one question with regard to the numbers you gave in the very first part of the paper stating, for instance, that the ultrasonic therapy unit should have an area about 4.5 or 5 square centimeters. Don't you think these numbers should be taken with a grain of salt since some manufacturers might be happy about it and others rather unhappy?

DR. ALDES: I only say that, in our experience, we feel the best radiating head is between 4.5 and 5 cm. In five years experience with 4,000 cases, where we have not seen any damaging results or any pathological changes indicated in blood or x-ray tests, we found that the best radiating head has an area of 4.5 to 5 cm. In addition, we found that the average intensities used for treatment were 0.5 to 1.5 watts. I do not believe in the series of 4,000 cases, there were 10 percent of the cases which got over 1.5 w/cm.^{2} The only time that higher intensities were used was in the case of Marie-Strempell disease. In this disease there is considerable calcium deposit within the soft tissue of the spine.

DR. HUETER: If you only use 1.5 watts, perhaps you may advocate a machine that has a maximum intensity of about 7 watts.

DR. ALDES: It is my personal belief that the machine does not have to have more than a total output of between 12 to 15 watts.

DR. SCHWAN: A further question about the area of the soundhead. I do not understand the reasons for using the massage technique. There can be only two reasons for employing the moving techniques of the soundhead. One is to prevent too high a dosage in a local area for a prolonged time interval. Obviously, however, this could be taken care of in another way by simply reducing the energy output of the generator. The second reason would be to apply the generated heat to a greater area than is provided by the soundhead. If the second reason is valid, this would indicate that a soundhead of greater area would be beneficial.

DR. ALDES: It is our experience that a massage type is less dangerous.

DR. SCHWAN: Why is it used? It is less dangerous. In other words, you feel in the stationary technique the output is too high? Why don't you reduce the output of the generator with the stationary technique instead of moving the transducer?

DR. ALDES: Because we have to treat such conditions as cervical arthritis. In that condition the entire cervical spine must be treated and we do not want to use the stationary treatment over each little area.

DR. SCHWAN: Could not this be taken care of also by a greater area of the soundhead?

DR. HUETER: Dr. Pohlman advocates using three soundheads and pulsating them.

DR. VON GIERKE: There is some difference between the massage technique and a stationary head technique in which the head has a large radiating area. This rotating motion amounts to a kind of pulsing of the sound.

DR. HUETER: You could take care of that by a stationary head which you pulse.

DR. VON GIERKE: The rotating method is the equivalent of pulsing very slowly.

DR. SCHWAN: In other words, the only explanation would be that a nonthermal component is affected in the treatment.

DR. VON GIERKE: By pulsing you allow the heat to be carried away.

DR. ALDES: We only use the stationary method in calcareous deposits and in comparing stationary methods for calcareous deposits against the massage method. We do feel that the massage method is far superior. As far as the three-headed cushions are concerned, we are in the midst of an investigation at the present time.

DR. LEHMANN: If you use the massaging technique in the dogs, as previously described, a rise in temperature is definitely produced, which is in the area of a biologically effective rise in temperature.

Dr. Bendler put thermocouples in various areas of the thigh of the dog, and as far as I remember, he used the massaging technique and moved the sound head back and forth. It was surprising to me to see how smooth the curve of the temperature rise was. There were ripples up and down, whenever he went over the spot where the thermocouple was, but the temperature never, if the technique was performed in that fashion, dropped down to the initial temperature. The variation in temperature was approximately 10 to 20 percent, so that you got a gradual increase of temperature with some wavy ripples on top. So under those conditions we definitely produce a rise of temperature. It has also been found that if the massage technique is used improperly, in other words, if the strokes become very long and are not circular, or if you move rapidly from one spot to the other, then you get only a little temperature increase and after that the temperature drops back to body temperature and nothing happens for a long period of time. No biological effects were observed in the laboratory, and the clinicians also obtained the impression that no clinical improvements were obtained under such circumstances. So this massage technique definitely produces a rise of temperature and whether or not there are nonthermal effects cannot be decided by this method as it is used. In summary, I would like to answer the question of Dr. Schwan. I believe, for clinical application, the massage technique is used, one, because of the necessity of heating a larger area than that of the sound applicator. This technique is simpler and cheaper than the use of a multiple base head, multiple beam, or other apparatus; two, because of the pain safety factor which Dr. Aldes mentioned. You know that the rise of temperature is critically dependent on the output. This is true especially of the rise of temperature in bony substances and periosteum, where the rise of temperature occurs very fast. With just a slight increase of the dosage, burns can occur very rapidly. Dr. Bendler and Dr. Herrick measured a temperature rise of 40 degrees Centigrade within two minutes in the periosteum of the femur of dogs. That is a tremendous temperature rise as far as biological tissues are concerned and would destroy everything. If the technician were to turn his back to the patient, and were to forget the movement of the sound head, the patient would be burned. I think those are practical reasons why massaging technique is used at the present time in preference to other methods.

Dr. Herrick: I think we are omitting a very important point. I am amazed at the confidence with which a therapist assumes that he hits the desired site at which he intends to apply his therapy. How can you be certain the correct area is being reached? If you visualize your irradiation pattern, all you have to do is just make a small rotation, and the target point is completely missed. In our experimental laboratory we feel that we have to have a probe in order to have any degree of confidence that we are giving the treatment. Therefore, the massage method is used because the probability of hitting the site you wish to hit is greater by this method than by using a stationary technique.

Dr. Aldes: In addition to the stationary method we always use a massage method. Even though I indicated to you that we used stationary methods with calcium deposits, I do not think that is the method of choice. I still think that the method of choice is the massage type for calcium deposits. We try the stationary technique for calcium deposits when the normal type of treatment does not help.

Dr. Busnel: Ultrasonic irradiation has a specific effect on the nervous system as has been demonstrated by the German Physiological School and also in France at my laboratory.

The nervous system can be considered as being composed of the central nervous system and the sympathetic system. If it is desired to irradiate the root of the sciatic nerve it is not necessary to move the ultrasonic head since the specific area can be designated. If, on the other hand, it is desired to irradiate the sympathetic nervous system (the celiac plexus for example) it is necessary to move the ultrasonic head over a very large area. The irradiation procedure is determined by the specific nervous system you wish to affect. It is not necessary to employ ultrasonics for the dispersion of the injected Hydrocortone. You can obtain the same result with 50 cycle per second waves.

I do not agree completely with the report of Dr. Lehmann on the heating action of ultrasonics. Certainly there is a thermal action but we have demonstrated that ultrasonic irradiation of the left sciatic nerve causes an action in the left but also a reflex action on the right sciatic. Giving the same thermal value by means of short wave diathermy results in no reflex action in the other nerve. This certainly demonstrates a difference between the action of ultrasonics and of short wave diathermy which produces the same amount of heat. I believe the ultrasonics have a specific action, especially on the nervous system.

Dr. Aldes: I do not think that the action of ultrasonics is all thermal. We have proved this point before. If it was all thermal, we might as well use diathermy to give the same action.

Dr. Schwan: It seems to me any comparison between sonic diathermy and any one of the electrical forms of diathermy is superficial unless you recognize the vast difference in performance between the different kinds of diathermy, the depth of penetration, the development of heat in various parts of the body, and dosage problems. It is all vastly different with each of those types of diathermy, so you simply cannot argue that, if you get a certain effect with sound and not the same effect with the diathermy, then it therefore must not be a thermal effect. It is simply that the heat in the diathermy case is more likely developed in a completely different location than in the sonic case. Any argument that does not consider the great variability between the different forms of diathermy in this respect is subject to criticism. There is another point I would like to bring up. I am always very much surprised by the rather small intensity levels which are quoted. Dr. Aldes mentioned intensities as low as 0.2 watt/cm.^{2}, which would provide an extremely small amount of energy in the body as compared to other forms of diathermy. A simple calculation indicates we almost have to have one-half square centimeter to get any substantial heating at all. I would like to inquire about this point. It seems to me if the low intensity levels really cause an effect they must be nonthermal.

DR. ALDES: We made a note in the previous discussion that the range is from 1.5 to 2 watts/cm.^{2}, but the average range that we have always used is 0.5 to 1.5 watts/cm.^{2}

DR. HUETER: Dr. Schwan brought up a very interesting point, indeed, that if there are such effects at such low intensities, and there are some others who state that we can obtain results at 0.2 watt/cm.^{2}, this is an indication there are nonthermal components.

DR. HERRICK: I do not know why we are arguing about this thermal effect versus nonthermal. I think all of us agree that there are both thermal and nonthermal effects. I do not think any of us who emphasize the thermal effect are trying to exclude the other effect. All that we are saying is that there are certain conditions in which the thermal effect predominates. That is quite an objective point of view, and I think substantiated theoretically.

DR. BALLANTINE: Following along the thoughts of Dr. Herrick and Dr. Schwan, in Dr. Aldes' talk he mentioned biological effects of ultrasound. He mentioned two. One was heat, and the other was cavitation which would release the vapors and gases. Does Dr. Aldes feel cavitation plays a role in his treatments at all, or in the usual therapeutic use of ultrasound?

DR. ALDES: I think that all those effects play a role.

DR. BALLANTINE: You think then there is cavitation?

DR. HUETER: At levels of 0.5 watt/cm.^{2}?

DR. ALDES: I do not think so. When higher wattages are used, then you probably have cavitation as a destructive mechanism. I do think, however, there is a great deal of dispersing power of ultrasonics in fibrous tissues which takes care of the exudates in that area and the small calcium you have in the soft tissue. I do not think the cavitation is there under small dosage conditions.

DR. BALLANTINE: What dosage do you feel you would have to use to get cavitation in living tissues?

DR. ALDES: I would think in the higher doses.

DR. FRY: In the case of cavitation you certainly can go to 1,000 watts/cm.^{2}

to get dosages suitable to destroy tissues without cavitation. I do not think you have to worry about 0.5 watt/cm.^{2}

DR. NAGLER: The heat question has been discussed quite a bit. I do not think it is solved, but in this connection I would like to ask, did you make any comparative study in your bursitis cases with those treated with x-ray, which is apparently non-heat treatment, and cortisone? The other question I have, is the pain an indicator of toxicity or damage? Pain is a rather subjective indicator. As we go to higher intensities in the lower tissues where pain is considered rather unreliable, do you have other indications guiding you in the possibility of damaging factors in your treatment, other than pain?

DR. ALDES: First of all, on the bursitis, in all our series we always use controls against the conservative type of treatment that exists at the present time, such as diathermy, microthermy, hot-packing, flushing of the shoulder area, x-ray therapy, and so forth. These were blind studies. Whoever evaluated them did not know what the other person had been given. We used cortisone injections, procaine, xylocaine, and so forth, and compared the results against using Hydrocortone alone for injection and against Hydrocortone plus ultrasonics. We felt, at the end, that the best treatment was Hydrocortone injections plus ultrasonics. We did not give the injections all the way through. We only gave three injections and held the fourth one off, but we gave the radiation for a period of six to eight average sonations until the patient had a complete free movement of his arm plus relinquishing of pain. As far as this pain syndrome is concerned, you are absolutely right. You might have a greater pain syndrome than I have. Although I use that term "the patient has pain," as the stopping point for my staff who are applying the ultrasound, yet I wonder whether this is a good point to use, even though the individual may be neurologically normal. But we feel in our clinic since we have a maximum of 1.5 watts/cm.^{2} intensity that we are not going to cause any damaging effects. However, there are some patients—we had a group of about 10—that cannot even take 0.5 watt/cm.^{2} on the side of the pathology, for example, on the side of the bursitis, but can take it on the opposite shoulder. In these cases we must reduce the intensity and consequently it takes a longer time. So you are perfectly right, and I am very happy you brought that point out.

DR. BALDES: Could I ask you a question about the lesions on the pig? Have you had any observation of damage done below the surface?

DR. ALDES: Dr. Freedman who is in charge of a pathological laboratory, had histological sections prepared all the way through the series, and we found areas all the way down to the periosteum using 3 watts for 10 minutes stationary. But in therapeutic doses we did not find any changes at all.

DR. BALDES: 3 watts/cm.^{2}?

DR. ALDES: As a maximum in the modalities we were using. In all this pig work we were trying to find whether in therapeutic doses there were damaging effects to the individual. We used 200-pound pigs to get the closest to the average human as possible. The knee joints of a pig are similar to ours. A 200-pound pig's knee joint anatomically is close to the ones that we have.

DR. HUETER: Is that a burning lesion?

DR. ALDES: Yes.

DR. HUETER: Do you get excessive heat?

DR. ALDES: It is a caustic thing. We produced them also by caustic medicinals, and by removing a plastic adherent to the skin.

DR. HUETER: Is there one particular reason why you make the lesion with ultrasound rather than directly?

DR. ALDES: No, just as an experiment.

DR. HERRICK: I would like to ask a general question among the physicists, and also the therapists: Have we a right to discuss cavitation in terms of the dosage when we consider that there are multiplications due to reflections? I am quite sure that at certain interfaces the internal intensities have been multiplied so that we do not know what levels they reach, but we do know that the intensity may rise to the point where, as Dr. Lehmann has indicated experimentally, he does get cavitation with a dosage that at one time was acceptable. Therefore, let us consider multiplications of intensities at interfaces when we are trying to correlate dosage with effects.

DR. HUETER: We are all still lacking a good definition of cavitation in tissues.

DR. LEHMANN: First of all, I do not find thermal reactions exclusively. I have found reactions in test tubes which are not thermal in origin and which may occur under therapeutic conditions, but we do not know whether or not they are of any therapeutic significance. Second, we have to specify what kind of cavitation we expect in tissues; as long as the tissue is alive there is gas present, so you will have degassing occurring at much lower intensities than true cavitation. This has been pointed out. I think you can expect that the reactions to degassing or cavitation can be prevented by pressure and that they consist of local lesions. The gas bubbles visualized under microscopic observation by O. Hug et al. tend to confirm this opinion and the threshold of intensity which has been found to produce such lesions in our experiments.

DR. HUETER: Call it a non-linear effect.

DR. LEHMANN: The thresholds to produce gas bubbles in tissues are very low if you use the stationary technique; the order is 1 to 2 watts/cm.^{2}—if we divide the total output by the surface of the crystal. That does not take into consideration the peak value of intensity in the center of the beam. One has to multiply the above mentioned value by 1 or 2—in other words the peak value is approximately 4 watts. At the same time the temperature goes up, because the tissues absorb ultrasound, so that the solubility of the gases changes at the same time. If gas bubbles are produced, local lesions are formed. The most severe destruction of tissues is confined to the center, and spaces are found histologically which indicate probably the presence of gas bubbles. In addition the damage to the tissues quickly subsides with increasing distance from the center of the lesions.

I do not know the details of how the lesion is produced. The appearance of these lesions and the occurrence of the gas bubbles have been observed recently under the microscope by O. Hug and his colleagues.

DR. HUETER: That paper ought to be translated so everybody can read it.

DR. WILD: I would like to throw in two quick suggestions to Dr. Aldes. One is that nobody mentioned the possible use and value of pulsing the therapeutic agent. As we know, we are up to 70 watts/cm.^{2} and a peak intensity of one microsecond. The other is, I used to be an orthopedic surgeon, and I used to inject needles into our ladies. In the first series I just injected them with a needle and took it out, and they got remarkably better. Then I used to put a needle in and put a little saline in it, and they would hop around nicely and statistically. Then I would put some buffered material in which was aimed at bringing back the pH of the sinovial membrane and sinovial fluid, and they did remarkably better—about 2 percent better. I was just suggesting that perhaps in evaluating these with the Hydrocortisone subfusion or entering the joint with your therapeutic agent, i.e., the ultrasonic agent, you might be careful about the psychological aspects of it, as well as the effect of the needle.

DR. ALDES: We did a blind study of injecting the patient with a solution that looked like Hydrocortone. We have used controls all the way through.

DR. VON GIERKE: I just wanted to come back to Dr. Herrick's question. I think we all agree that at the interface we have some increase. I would not call it increase of energy, but increased absorption probably due to such sheer wave mechanism as Dr. Oestreicher discussed at the last Symposium here. This investigation shows that absorption changes quite a bit with the angle of incidence on such interfaces. It is possible that one of the reasons for using this non-stationary massage is to avoid low heat in spots. I agree with you, naturally, the total heat cannot be carried away in this time. You get some average heating, but by this non-stationary massage you might avoid local heating spots and equalize this effect.

DR. SCHWAN: I would like to comment on the order of magnitude of time which is necessary in order to carry heat away. It depends on the size of the heating body. If you have a sphere of 1 cm. diameter, you will need a few minutes before you get your heat properly down. For larger spheres you may need a few hours to carry the heat away. To comment on Dr. Von Gierke's remark, the localized spots must be extremely small in order for the massage technique to allow the heat to be carried away. However, if we investigate the stationary temperature which can be achieved in very small spots we find it is very small. In other words, the smaller the area, the more difficult it is to elevate it very significantly in temperature.

DR. HUETER: May I at this point, ask a question of Dr. Schwan, Dr. Carstensen, and others interested in absorption. Are we not a little bit too pre-occupied with this notion of heat? Why do we get the heat? Because these molecules are squeezed in a weird fashion, and we do not even understand how they are squeezed. It is like dislocations in the metal and holes that move around, and it may be bonds that break or switch over. Could not this very mechanism which produces the heat, i.e., the particular way of producing the heat, could not that be something specific to ultrasound as compared to some of the diathermy ways of producing heat, and could not the heat just activate or potentiate this primary ultrasonic effect?

DR. SCHWAN: I very definitely think this is a possibility. I would like to come back to a statement Dr. Herrick made some time ago—that we all know there are thermal effects and nonthermal effects. I would personally like to modify this a little. We certainly all know that there ARE thermal effects and that there MAY BE nonthermal effects.

DR. HUETER: Does it really make sense in the final molecular analysis to distinguish between thermal and mechanical effects?

DR. SCHWAN: I cannot see any basic difference between the ordered molecular movement in the sonic case and the unordered movement.

DR. HUETER: I have a slide that I will show tomorrow. There is some difference. Namely, the one in amplitude, not in energy, but in amplitude, and that may do something.

DR. CARSTENSEN: It seems to me there is a difference between them. You can define a thermal effect, because you can measure the degree rise in temperature or calories or whatever you like, so it is something you can define. Of course, the purpose of our investigation with blood was to determine as much as we could about the mechanism of absorption to see if this would lead to some understanding of possible nonthermal effects.

DR. LEHMANN: I think there is also a difference in the conclusion. If something like Dr. Hueter has suggested exists . . . and molecules are destroyed by such a mechanism, the parameters which influence this mechanism would be different from those which perhaps produce a temperature increase of so many degrees Centigrade. Since we want to produce a therapeutic effect under optimal conditions, we must consider the possibility that these conditions are dependent upon the mechanism by which the therapeutic result is produced.

Dr. Hueter: I do not quite understand your point.

Dr. Lehmann: The effect might go with the square or square root of the intensity, to give an example.

Dr. Hueter: Not necessarily. It would be all the same thing to produce heat, but the fact that you squeeze the molecule to produce the heat could be significant biologically. Even Dr. Fry in lesion-making would produce heat if he did not turn off the sound for a while and cool it down, but this very exposure of tissue to ultrasound will always produce heat, but it may even damage tissue without evidence of heat, of heat-destruction.

Dr. Lehmann: If you increase intensity the temperature will increase so much at the same time. If you increase intensity again to the same level, the amount of destruction or the number of destroyed molecules might not necessarily be the same, if a nonthermal mechanism, as you suggested, produces the effect.

Dr. Hueter: What of Dr. Bushnel's findings that he can use vibrations of 50 cycles to do some of these things?

Dr. Lehmann: I only want to make the point the optimal condition of a therapeutic application might be different in the case a nonthermal mechanism produces the results, rather than a heating mechanism.

Dr. Schwan: I would like to make a historical remark, concerning the introduction of short wave diathermy. At that time about the same struggle went on quite viciously, and actually the majority of the people almost believed in nonthermal effects and all sorts of specific effects. This field is now 30 years old and none of the effects have been proven to exist. In the ultrasonic field, beside speculation which is certainty impressive, I would like to see something concrete.

Dr. Hueter: Maybe it is the wrong question to ask, thermal or nonthermal or mechanical. Maybe it is the same thing.

Dr. Von Gierke: We have to make a difference between thermal and nonthermal effect; otherwise we could not make a difference if we apply the same energy at 50 cycles or at 5 meg.

Dr. Hueter: In some cases apparently we can.

Dr. Von Gierke: Only the absorption coefficients would make the difference. If we apply the same energy at low frequency we do not get this.

Dr. Busnel: But if you produce heat by several different treatments on the excised nerve—with warm water, diathermy, infra-red, and so forth, you always have an action on the nerve, but no reflex action. However, with very low frequency, 50 or 100 cycles, or with ultrasonics of very low power, 0.002 watt/cm.^{2} you always have a reflex action on the other nerve.

Dr. Rioch: I think you have to pay attention to heat and mechanical results in molecules. With very high velocity missiles you get tremendous areas of destruction of cells, so that they stain totally differently. It is practically impossible to fix and stain them. They are just soup—but with no temperature change at all. With mechanical energy you get destruction of cells, and as soon as you get destruction of cells you get many chemical effects you do not get otherwise, and this, of course, is not cavitation in that sense.

I want to ask Dr. Aldes if he had done any work with regrowth of peripheral nerves and applied ultrasonics to this problem, and if you know about the changes, i.e., the histological changes of healing that ultrasound brings about that other methods do not.

Dr. Aldes: Regarding nerves, we haven't done anything. As far as the healing power of ultrasound is concerned, I can only say that we have found in the experimental animals that the healing capacity was faster than with the regular medicinals that we apply on caustic burns of any kind or eradication of tissue. Less time occurs between the original trauma and the healing over the skin.

Neurosonicsurgery

W. J. Fry and F. J. Fry

Bioacoustics Laboratory, University of Illinois, Urbana, Illinois

Editor's note: Dr. W. J. Fry presented a 16 mm. sound, color motion picture entitled "Neurosonicsurgery." The following is an abstract of the film.

RESEARCH conducted during the past six years at the Bioacoustics Laboratory of the University of Illinois in the design of precision ultrasonic focusing instruments and their application in biological investigations has made it possible to employ ultrasonic energy in research in neuroanatomy, neurophysiology and neuropathology and now opens the way for extensive application of this tool to therapeutic procedures in clinical neurologic disorders. By proper monitoring of ultrasonic dosage, relatively reversible as well as enduring lesions of predetermined size, shape, selectivity and loci in the cortical ribbon, sub-cortical and deep-lying structures (e.g., internal capsule and mammillo-thalamic tract) have been produced in cats and monkeys. Over 250 animals have been subjected to such experiments and it has been possible to establish (a) that the procedure is extremely well tolerated by the animals and (b) that, when judged by currently available histologic criteria, structures not intended for alteration by ultrasound energy can be spared.

A serious limitation in the field of bioacoustics is the complete lack of precision ultrasonic instrumentation and auxiliary equipment designed specifically for biological research. To surmount this difficulty, a completely new laboratory designed specifically for ultrasonic irradiation of selective regions of the central nervous system of mammals has been constructed in the Bioacoustics Laboratory at the University of Illinois. The electrically shielded irradiation room (Fig. 1) contains apparatus for supporting the animal, calibration instrumentation for determining the acoustic output of the transducers, and controls for positioning the focused ultrasonic beam, as well as stimulators, amplifiers, oscilloscopes and cameras and other recording devices for observing electrical activity of central nervous systems during irradiation. Projecting through the ceiling of this room is a metal tube (10 feet long and 7 inches in diameter) which supports the focusing transducer. The precise positioning of the sound beam is accomplished by the motor-driven coordinate system supporting the transducer. This system permits translational motion in three mutually perpendicular directions and

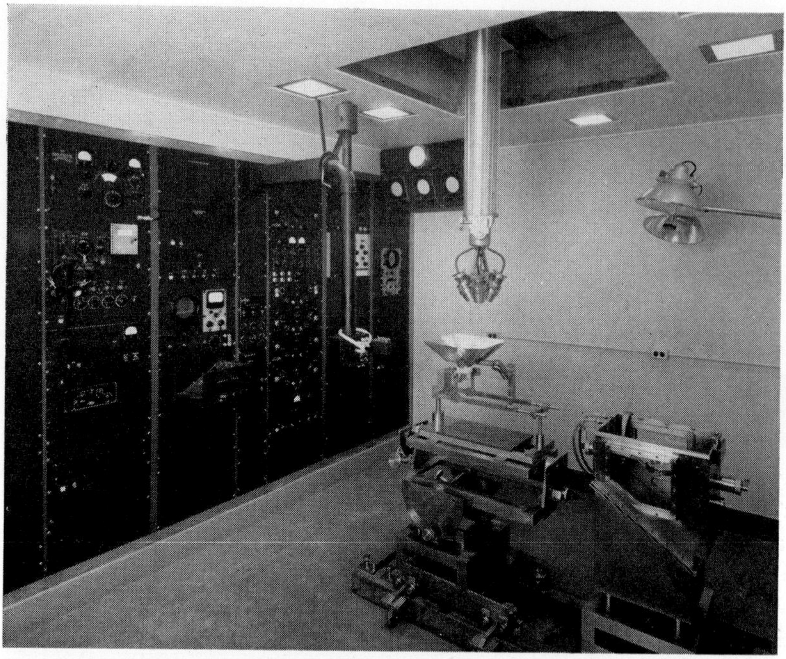

FIG. 1. Instrumentation for focused ultrasonic irradiation of tissue.

two rotational motions. The coordinate system itself, which weighs about 3500 lbs., is mounted on a steel girder framework in the room (Fig. 2) directly over the irradiation room. The controls for the coordinate system are placed in the irradiation room below. The upper room also houses the electronic driver for supplying electrical power to the transducer.

This instrumentation setup makes possible accurate location of the acoustic radiation in any desired region of the central nervous system under precisely controlled dosage conditions.

A four-beam ultrasonic focusing irradiator (Fig. 3) has been designed and is in routine use in this laboratory. In this instrument the focusing beams from each of four transducer heads are adjusted so that the focal regions are brought into coincidence. The most intense region of the ultrasonic field can produce lesions as small as a few cubic millimeters.

To produce a precisely localized lesion by ultrasound, the head of the anaesthetized animal (cat, monkey) is engaged in a stereotaxic substructure in which the usual interaural, Frankfort and midsagittal planes are employed as "zero-references." The skull cap is removed and the dura mater exposed. The bone must be removed because of its high acoustic absorption coefficient, which results in excessive heating, and its disturbance

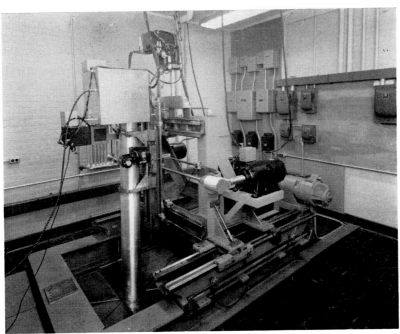

FIG. 2. Coordinate and positioning system for control of the placement of the focus of the ultrasonic beam(s) in the tissue.

of the beam shape. At this point of the procedure no definitive surgical measures, beyond those of achieving hemostasis, are required.

The next step consists of attaching the skin of the animal to a special metallic hopper in such fashion as to provide a "pan," the bottom of which consists of the exposed dura mater. This "pan" holds the degassed physiological saline which acts as the transmitting medium for the sound.

The substructure of the stereotaxic instrument (and the engaged animal) is now moved under the superstructure which supports the four-beam ultrasonic focusing transducer which generates the acoustic waves.

The sterilized four-beam transducer is supported on and moved by a single carriage (Fig. 2). All parameters are suitably checked at this point. The ultrasonic dosage is now delivered. At the highest intensities used the duration of irradiation is usually in the range from one to three seconds. The frequency employed is close to 1 megacycle. For the smallest lesions the tissue is irradiated with the focal spot in a single position but for larger lesions the focal spot is placed successively in a number of positions.

The substructure is now disengaged from the superstructure and the animal returned to the operating room where closure of the cranial muscles and scalp is accomplished.

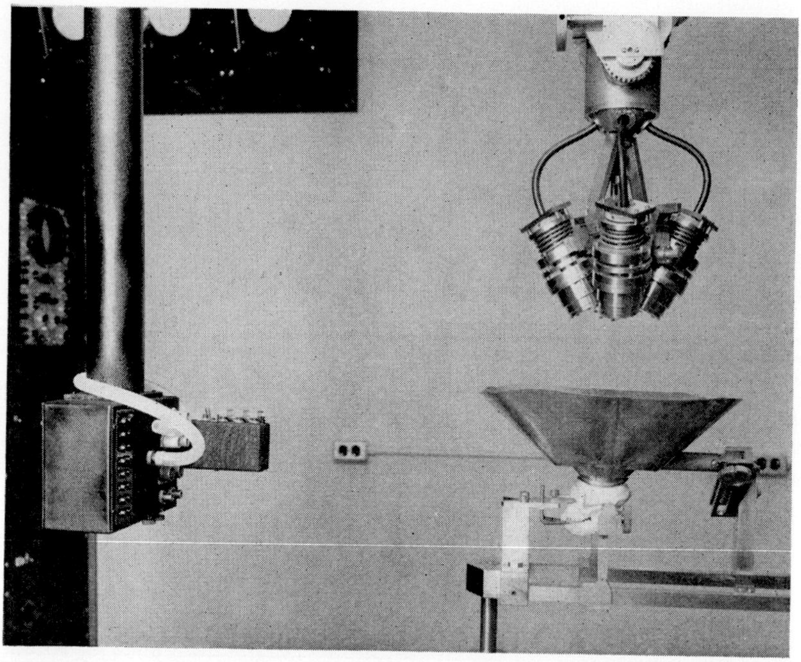

FIG. 3. Four beam focussing irradiator shown above the "pan" which supports the coupling liquid which transmits the sound from the irradiator to the tissue.

The animals are observed for varying periods of minutes to weeks following such experiments, during which time physiologic and/or psychologic aberrations may be noted. The animals are sacrificed minutes to hours, days or weeks after irradiation, the brains removed, fixed and ultimately sectioned, and stained.

A unique advantage of such a procedure is the susceptibility of the fiber tracts of the nervous system to alteration by ultrasound as compared with gray matter and blood vessels at the irradiated locus. This makes it possible to make anatomic, physiologic and pathologic differentia among neural components which, when attacked by the older mechanical, chemical and electrolytic technics inevitably underwent non-differentiated alterations. The advantages of this to research endeavors are self-evident.

It appears that at the parameters employed reversible and irreversible lesions are produced by direct alteration of intercellular structures of the tissues rather than by indiscriminate coagulation by heat. Blood vessels running through a felt-work matrix of ultrasonically damaged tissues are left intact and exhibit no hemorrhaging.

It is envisioned that a variety of neurosurgical procedures can be implemented by ultrasound. These include the hyperkinetic and hypertonic disorders (e.g., Parkinsonism, athetosis, ballism, chorea, dystonia); psychosurgery and intractable pain.

References

Fry, W. J. and R. B. Fry. 1954a. Determination of absolute sound levels and acoustic absorption coefficients by thermocouple probes—Theory. J. Acoust. Soc. Am. *26:* 294–310.

Fry, W. J. and R. B. Fry. 1954b. Determination of absolute sound levels and acoustic absorption coefficients by thermocouple probes—Experiment. J. Acoust. Soc. Am. *26:* 311–317.

DR. W. J. FRY: Before answering questions, I would like to present a few illustrations. Fig. 4 illustrates a lesion in the sub-cortical white matter of a cat brain. The tissue section is stained so that the nerve fibers stain darkly and the gray matter or regions of cell bodies are practically unstained. In this animal, we chose dosage to produce a change in the fiber tracts without affecting the gray matter. The lesion was produced by moving the beam laterally in a number of adjacent overlapping positions spaced ½ millimeter apart. This sharp boundary between the affected white matter and the neighboring unaffected gray matter is realized, as just indicated, by the choice of dosage, but you also observe that a sharp boundary between the affected white matter and the unaffected white matter is also obtained. This is illustrated at the lower border of the lesion. In such a lesion with all the neural components of the white matter destroyed, the blood vessels remain unbroken and functional.

DR. BALDES: Do you sometimes irradiate with the transducer rotating?

DR. W. J. FRY: The apparatus is designed to permit operation in that manner, but we have not used the procedure. Different dosage relations would obtain if the transducer were moved continuously along a path. We have done some work with the common focus of the beams moving, tracing out a path, but we have not emphasized this procedure, because we have been interested in producing both small lesions and lesions of different shapes. We have restricted ourselves primarily to the procedure of irradiating in one spot, and after a fixed time interval irradiating in an adjacent overlapping spot.

DR. BALDES: What do you find is the most advantageous way of degassing water, vacuum or boiling?

DR. W. J. FRY: We use the boiling procedure. We have not compared the two methods.

We dilute the normal physiological saline by the amount of distilled water that is evaporated during the boiling process.

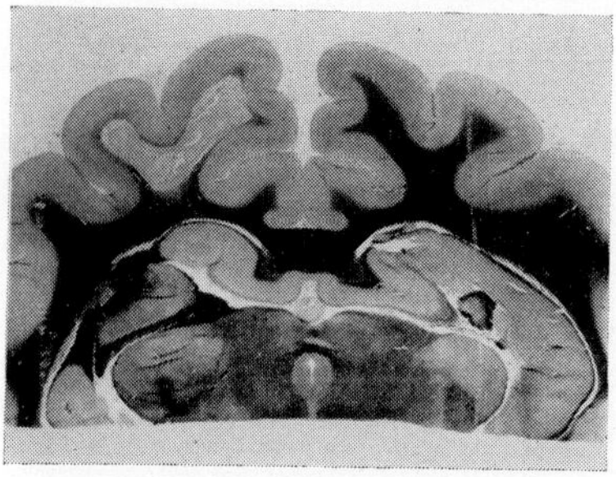

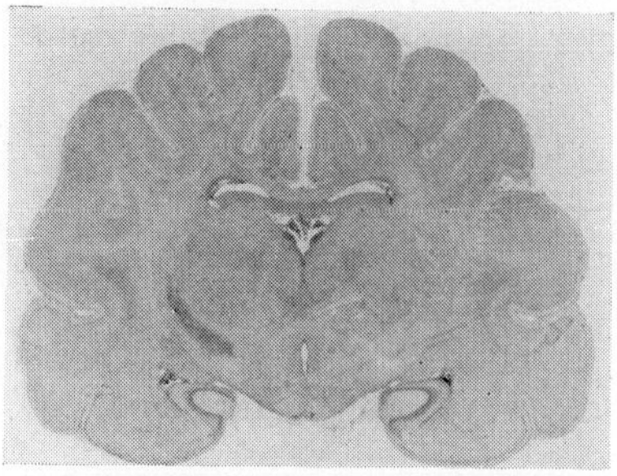

FIG. 4. Large shaped lesion in the subcortical white matter of the brain of a cat. The gray matter bordering the destroyed fiber tracts is not disrupted. This large lesion was produced by placing the focus of the beam successively in a number of adjacent positions.

FIG. 5. A small ultrasonically produced lesion in the cortical gray matter of a cat brain.

DR. HERRICK: Dr. Fry, could you explain from a standpoint of pure physics, the relative selectivity of various parts of the brain structure, particularly the blood vessels to ultrasound i.e., why you do not get damage in the blood vessels, or any degassing effects?

DR. W. J. FRY: We have made dosage studies and have observed the graded selectivity for various dosages. These results will be reviewed in the next paper. At the present time, we do not yet understand the physical mechanism. We have studied temperature and cavitation as possible contributing factors, but we have not yet isolated the physical variable(s) responsible for the primary action.

DR. NYBORG: Can you briefly describe the focussing system?

DR. W. J. FRY: We use two types of focussing systems. The system you saw in the movie is a lens type, four intersecting focussed beams produced by x-cut quartz crystals with polystyrene lenses placed in front of them. We also use a parabolic reflector type of focussing system.

DR. NYBORG: Could you state the beam size?

DR. W. J. FRY: I do not wish to imply that the half-power beam width is a critical value from the viewpoint of dosage. A factor of two change in, for example, intensity, would be quite large. However, in order to indicate the size of beam, it is convenient to state the half power width which in this case is 1.5 millimeters. The animal in Fig. 4 received 70 or 80 shots of radiation with such a beam to produce the lesion illustrated. The next illustration (Fig. 5) shows a lesion in the gray matter produced by irradiating in a single position. The length of the oval-shaped area is about 2 millimeters. This animal was sacrificed four days after irradiation.

DR. HUETER: What is the ratio of the intensities of ultrasound used in these two cases?

Dr. W. J. Fry: The animal of the previous illustration (Fig. 4) was irradiated at a lower level. At 1,000 watts/cm.^{2} the time required to produce a lesion in gray matter is about a factor of 2 greater than that required for a white matter lesion.*

Dr. Bell: Have you any explanation for the differential susceptibility of white matter as opposed to gray matter?

Dr. W. J. Fry: No explanation. It might be noted that gray matter has a lower acoustic absorption coefficient than white matter, but we do not know that this is related to the minimum dose required to produce a lesion.

Dr. Quimby: You do not know for certain that the irradiated gray matter in the tissue of the first illustration (Fig. 4) was unaffected. You only know that it does not appear to be affected on histological examination?

Dr. W. J. Fry: We have in some instances utilized tests other than histological change. We have irradiated animals in which we produce functional changes. The particular animal in the first illustration was not irradiated in a region where you would expect to observe obvious functional changes. However, we have irradiated animals in the motor cortex, for example.

Dr. Hueter: Have you ever used the same duration but varied the intensity in order to get the selectivity between gray and white?

Dr. W. J. Fry: The animal in Fig. 4 was irradiated at 200 watts/cm.^{2} for 4.00 seconds. For the animal in Fig. 5 the dosage was 1,000 watts/cm.^{2} for 2.00 seconds. To produce a change in white matter at 1,000 watts/cm.^{2}, the required duration of exposure would be about one second.

Dr. Bell: What is the " gain " of the multibeam system?

Dr. W. J. Fry: The gain in intensity for this particular multiple beam, compared to a single beam, is about 12 times. The pressure gain is four times, if each irradiator contributes equally. The particle velocity gain is somewhat less than four because of the angle of convergence of the beams, so that the intensity gain is approximately 12.

Dr. Quimby: What is the degree of reproducibility in your lesions, such as a small lesion in the gray matter?

Dr. W. J. Fry: I believe generally we would say they are quantitatively reproducible. If you choose a dosage, you cannot only produce a lesion, but you can grade the lesion in degrees by choice of dosage. This aspect will be discussed in more detail in the next paper by Dr. Barnard. We classify the white matter lesions into three categories, and also the gray matter into three separate categories, depending on the extent of the damage and the selectivity obtained. It is interesting to note that in two cases we have seen

* Specification of the acoustic intensity alone does not completely describe the acoustic field. However, for a particular field configuration the intensity values constitute an indication of relative dosages.

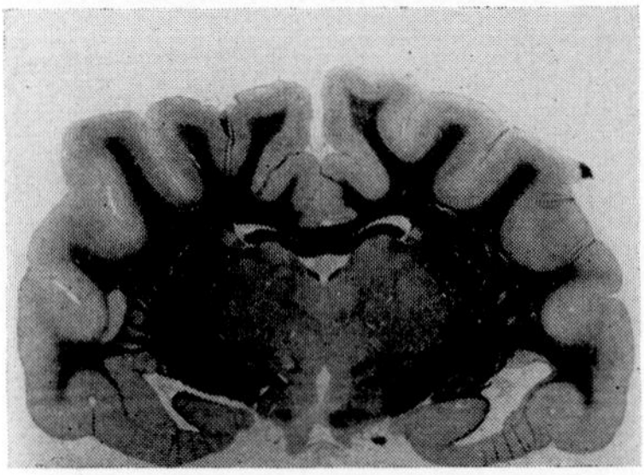
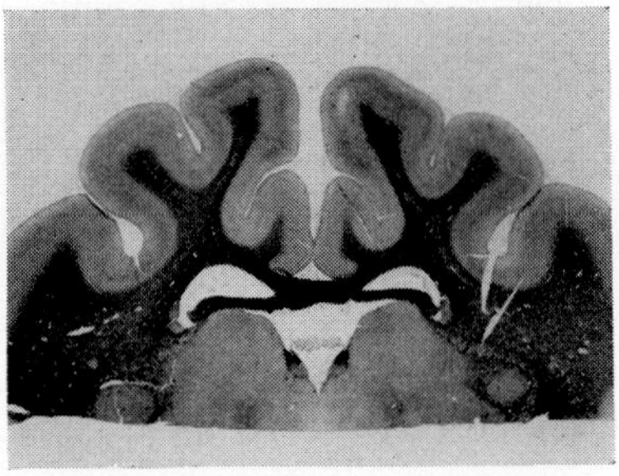

Fig. 6. Large shaped lesion in the white matter of the internal capsule of a cat brain. The dark staining material is a glial scar which has developed in the lesion region 30 days after exposure. None of the tissue intervening between the common focus of the beams and the area of entry of the sound into the brain, was disrupted.

Fig. 7. Interruption of a small (1 mm. diameter) fiber tract deep within the brain without interference to surrounding or intervening tissue.

demyelination of nerve fibers without destruction of the axis cylinders. This has been seen in both gray and white matter.

Dr. Bell: What is the center thickness of the lenses that you use?

Dr. F. J. Fry: 1/32 of an inch and 1 3/8 inches in diameter. The radius of curvature is about 3 inches.

Dr. W. J. Fry: This illustration (Fig. 6) shows a large lesion in depth without effect on intervening tissues. The four beams entered the brain from above. The animal was sacrificed 30 days after irradiation. A glial scar is apparent in the portion of the internal capsule which was irradiated. The irradiation procedure was accomplished by moving the beam laterally and exposing the tissue in a number of adjacent overlapping positions. Fig. 7 illustrates the precision with which you can place a lesion in a deep structure. In this case we were interested in hitting the mammillothalamic tract of a cat. This tract is about a millimeter in diameter and the beam must traverse about 4/5 of the brain thickness before coming to a focus. The four beams entered from above. Coordinates were chosen from standard neuroanatomical maps. The gray matter surrounding the tract was unaffected. This is accomplished by a proper choice of dosage.

Dr. Schwan: If you are interested in experimenting with 10 animals and trying to destroy the same area in each, how often would you succeed?

Dr. W. J. Fry: If one is interested in destroying a small fiber tract such as the mammillothalamic one can irradiate, at a dosage which does not affect gray matter, in a number of adjacent positions and thus interrupt the tract practically every time. Position variation of a specific deep structure with respect to external landmarks is of the order of 1/2 millimeter in cat brain. The focus of the beam can be placed within any desired geometric location within a couple tenths of a millimeter every time.

Dr. Schwan: Do you use bony landmarks only, or do you also look at the surface of the brain?

Dr. W. J. Fry: On cat and monkey, we use the ear bar position and the base of the orbits as references.

Dr. Schwan: I should like to inquire about the margin which exists between the minimum dosage required to cause the lesion and the optimum dosage to spread out the lesion beyond the area which you want to destroy.

Dr. W. J. Fry: You mean, for example, if you are hitting a fiber tract, what would be the ratio between the minimal dosage required and that necessary to cause the lesion to spread out into the neighboring gray? This ratio varies with the sound level. For example, at 200 watts/cm.^{2}, the ratio is quite high, but at 1,000 watts/cm.^{2} the ratio would be something like 1¼, that is a 25% increase in time would be sufficient to pass from a lesion with a sharp border at the gray matter interface to a lesion which starts to invade the gray matter.

Dr. Schwan: You may anticipate at least a certain variation in the absorption coefficient from one cat brain to another. The margin I was asking about is then sufficiently large to permit variations in acoustic properties.

Dr. Nauta: I should like to ask Dr. Fry if, in his experience, the difference in absorption rate between white and gray respectively is such that it would be difficult to produce a selective gray matter lesion close to heavy bundles of myelinated fibers.

Dr. W. J. Fry: The problem is to produce and use a beam which falls off sharply enough to restrict the high level sound entirely to the gray matter. In other words, it is easy to produce a lesion in white and preserve neighboring gray matter, but more difficult to produce a lesion in gray and simultaneously preserve neighboring white matter.

Dr. Nauta: My second question concerns the possible production of inadvertent damage to fiber bundles proximal to the focal point. Is it conceivable that a relatively low concentration of ultrasonic energy, such as would prevail, say, 5 millimeters from the focus of the beam, would suffice to damage fibers passing through the area?

So far, from two limited observations in our own material, I have the impression that we should take account of such possibilities. In these cases, using parameters of exposure too low to produce visible tissue destruction at the focal point, a fairly large number of scattered degenerating axons were present in and around regions proximal to the focus. I want to make one suggestion. It is unlikely you will pick up such diffuse changes with conventional stains. I think your best chance to find them is to employ a stain for degenerating axons, because they can be identified with absolute certainty. Damaged cell bodies will be terribly difficult to detect if there are only a few of them.

DR. HERRICK: Dr. Fry, what is the minimum time between irradiation and the study of histology?

DR. W. J. FRY: We have made histological studies of the irradiated brains of cats sacrificed five minutes after exposure. At this time, no histological changes are evident with the stains employed. The first changes appear at 10 minutes

DR. BELL: When the target is deep in the brain do you have to substantially raise the intensity level or extend the duration of exposure?

DR. W. J. FRY: You raise the intensity level to get the desired value at the lesion site. The intensity absorption coefficient is approximately 20% per cm., and the resultant loss must be offset. We raise the driving voltage to compensate, and maintain constant the duration of exposure. A dosage study in the subcortical white matter thus furnishes the dosage information required for the production of lesions in deep structures.

VOICE: How do you explain the delayed evidence of lesion production?

DR. W. J. FRY: Histologically there is a delay, I don't know why. We are obviously not tearing things apart on a cellular level. We have other observations showing that electrically the lesion can be detected much sooner. We have done some work on rats' spinal cords in which we made measurements of 2 neuron arc response changes. In this case, one finds that the electrical changes occur in seconds or less.

VOICE: Have you done any electron micrography on these various animals?

DR. W. J. FRY: No.

VOICE: Do you hope to do it?

DR. W. J. FRY: Yes. It would be very interesting to see what structural components of the tissue are changed by the ultrasound. It may be that we change structure on the level of organization which is closely associated with function.

VOICE: Why do you use four concentrated beams rather than one?

DR. W. J. FRY: A single beam with the crystal and lens diameter used, has a long focal length. This beam is narrow, but the sound intensity does not vary very rapidly as one moves along the axis of the beam. By employing four of these beams, one can realize a considerable reduction in the length of the high intensity region. I again do not wish to imply that intensity is the important variable. It may be, for example, that particle velocity is much more important than intensity, but I am using the variable intensity to describe the sound levels we are talking about.

DR. FINCH: Do you feel that after four beams have traversed the material that they are still in phase?

DR. W. J. FRY: Yes, if you are speaking about brain tissue. The acoustic velocity does not vary much with position in the brain.

Dr. Baldes: You indicated how you adjusted a knob to change the phase. What does that adjustment do?

Dr. W. J. Fry: There are tilt adjustments which bring the beams into coincidence at a common point. The wheel adjustment or knob moves the beam in the direction of its axis.

Dr. Von Gierke: Did you ever consider the following procedure? After you produce the lesion you irradiate with a low intensity ultrasonic pulse in an attempt to receive an echo from the lesion to see if you really produced a lesion.

Dr. W. J. Fry: We never attempted the possibility you suggest. You would probably have to wait for a period of time ($\geqslant$ 15 minutes) after irradiation because histologically you do not see the changes immediately after exposure. If you were willing to wait for such a period, such a procedure might work.

Dr. Von Gierke: You could observe the echo pattern before you produce the lesion, then produce the lesion and observe the pattern again.

Dr. W. J. Fry: It is a possibility. We have been interested in producing reversible changes to use as a method of locating position functionally. After identification of position by this means, the dosage could then be increased to produce a permanent change.

Dr. Busnel: Have you observed any modification of the animals' behavior after the treatment? You explained you kill the animals after 20 days. Through the 20 days period, have you observed some modification in the behavior in relation to the region where you destroyed the tissue?

Dr. W. J. Fry: In the internal capsule, for example, depending upon the position irradiated we produced motor deficits which are apparent as soon as the animal recovers from the anesthetic.

Dr. Busnel: Is it possible that you can produce some modification in the behavior without complete destruction of the tissue?

Dr. W. J. Fry: This is possible. In fact, we are interested in examining ultrasonically demyelinated systems to see if they are still functional.

Histological Study of Changes Produced by Ultrasound in the Gray and White Matter Of the Central Nervous System

W. J. Fry, J. F. Brennan[1] and J. W. Barnard[2]

Bioacoustics Laboratory, University of Illinois, Urbana, Illinois

THE PURPOSE of the study reported in this paper was the determination of the ultrasonic dosage conditions required to produce very small white and gray matter lesions of different degrees of selectivity with respect to the various tissue components of the brain. Usually more than one position was irradiated in the brain of each animal, but the separate positions were spaced five to ten millimeters apart to permit observation of each site uninfluenced by the other lesions.

This procedure is in contrast to our previously reported work on white matter lesions of a variety of shapes and sizes produced by irradiating the brain in a relatively large number of overlapping positions.

Previous publications from this laboratory have described the design of the ultrasonic transducer employed, the thermocouple probe developed for accurate calibration of the acoustic field, and the experimental procedure used for surgical preparation and irradiation of the animals (Fry et al., 1954; Fry and Fry, 1954; Barnard et al., 1955; Fry et al., 1955a; Fry et al., 1955b).

Methods

The ultrasonic gray matter lesions were produced in the midline gray matter of the lateral gyrus of the cat. The center of the focal spot was positioned two millimeters below the surface of the dura and one-half millimeter from the midline. The white matter lesions were usually placed in the subcortical white matter of the lateral gyrus, three to four millimeters from the midline. The focal spot was positioned three millimeters below the dura at the designated lateral position.

The animals were sacrificed under sodium pentobarbital anesthesia at times after exposure varying from a minimum of five minutes to a maximum time of twelve days. They were exsanguinated and perfused with neutral ten percent formalin in physiological saline under one meter of

[1] Now, Glen L. Martin Company, Baltimore, Maryland.

[2] Deceased.

water pressure. The pertinent parts of the brain were imbedded in paraffin and sectioned at ten microns. A series of every fortieth section was prepared in Weil's myelin stain and studied to locate the position of the lesions. Serial sections from the center of each lesion were then mounted and alternate series prepared with thionin, Romanes' silver, Heidenhain's hematoxylin and Mallory's phosphotungstic acid hematoxylin.

The procedures and instrumentation used in the studies pursued at this laboratory are distinctly different from the ultrasonic diathermy method and apparatus employed by various other investigators in irradiating the brain with ultrasound (Heyck, 1952; Heyck and Hopker, 1952; Lindstrom, 1954). The results reported in this and preceding papers of this series cannot be obtained with diathermy procedures and apparatus.

Results

Tables 1 and 2 summarize the dosage conditions, survival times and a brief description of the histological response of the white matter (Table 1) and gray matter (Table 2). The histological results of white and gray matter irradiations are presented in Tables 3 and 4, organized to indicate the time sequence on the vertical scale and divided into columns representing specific tissue components horizontally. The three weights (thicknesses) of lines denote the three subdivisions of response observed in the white matter (Table 3 *) and gray matter (Table 4 *). Single solid vertical lines indicate that no histological change is observed in the tissue, and dotted lines denote an absence of information. Crosshatching indicates that a particular tissue element, normally present, is absent. The following designations apply to the necessarily brief terms employed: very few—ten percent or less; few—twenty-five percent; some—fifty percent; many—seventy-five percent; most—ninety percent or more.

Effects of Ultrasound on the White Matter of the Cerebrum

The lesions produced in white matter by ultrasound and described in Tables 1 and 3 are classified as *light, medium,* or *heavy,* although a continuous gradation of severity of tissue damage may be obtained by varying the ultrasonic dosage. Lesions in these three categories, as defined below, present an adequate picture of the type of selectivity and graded damage that has been observed.

A lesion possessing a relatively homogeneous field of necrosis is called *light* (Fig. 1a). A lesion which contains a central region (island) staining like normal tissue, surrounded by peripheral necrosis (moat) is called *medium* if the moat does not encroach on neighboring gray matter (Fig. 1b). A lesion is classified as *heavy* if it possesses an island and moat and also infringes on adjacent gray matter (Fig. 1c). In general, increased

* As folder in the back of this book.

TABLE 1
White Matter

Irradiation and Cat No.	Acoustic Pressure Amplitude* (Atms)	Acoustic Particle Velocity Amplitude* ($cm/sec/10^2$)	Irradiation Time (Sec)	Survival Time	Lesion Classification
222-1	46	4.3	1.00	7 min	none
222-2	46	4.3	1.50	6 min	none
222-3	46	4.3	1.75	5 min	none
209-1	48	4.4	1.00	9 min	none
209-2	48	4.4	1.50	8 min	none
209-3	50	4.6	1.75	7 min	none
223-1	44	4.1	1.00	14 min	none
223-2	48	4.4	1.50	13 min	heavy
223-3	48	4.4	1.75	12 min	heavy
207-1	48	4.4	1.00		none
207-2	48	4.4	1.50	1 hr	light
207-3	48	4.4	1.75		heavy
215-1	48	4.4	1.00		medium
215-2	50	4.6	1.50	2 hr	heavy
215-3	49	4.5	1.75		heavy
205-1	50	4.6	1.00		light
205-2	46	4.3	1.50	6 hr	light
205-3	50	4.6	1.75		medium
212-1	46	4.3	1.00		none
212-2	48	4.4	1.50	6 hr	none
212-3	45	4.2	1.75		light
211-1	46	4.3	1.00		light
211-2	48	4.4	1.50	12 hr	medium
211-3	48	4.4	1.75		heavy
218-1	46	4.3	1.00		light
218-2	48	4.4	1.50	1 day	medium
218-3	48	4.4	1.75		heavy
219-1	48	4.4	1.00		light
219-2	49	4.5	1.50	2 day	medium
219-3	48	4.4	1.75		heavy
199-1	48	4.4	1.00		none
199-2	48	4.4	1.50	4 day	medium
199-3	48	4.4	2.00		heavy
221-1	45	4.2	1.00		none
221-2	46	4.3	1.50	12 day	none
221-3	46	4.3	1.75		medium

* The differences in the numerical values are significant on a comparative scale. However, the probable error in the absolute values of pressure and particle velocity does not exceed 10%.

TABLE 2
Gray Matter

Irradiation and Cat No.	Acoustic Pressure Amplitude* (Atms)	Acoustic Particle Velocity Amplitude* (cm/sec/10^2)	Irradiation Time (Sec)	Survival Time	Lesion Classification
225-1	48	4.4	2.00	8 min	none
225-2	48	4.4	2.50	7 min	none
225-3	48	4.4	3.00	6 min	none
226-1	49	4.5	2.00	8 min	none
226-2	46	4.3	2.50	7 min	none
226-3	48	4.4	3.00	6 min	none
210-1	48	4.4	2.00	13 min	none
210-2	48	4.4	2.50	11 min	none
210-3	48	4.4	3.00	10 min	moderate
208-1	48	4.4	2.00	16 min	none
208-2	48	4.4	2.50	15 min	moderate
208-3	48	4.4	3.00	14 min	severe
206-1	49	4.5	2.00		none
206-2	46	4.3	2.50	1 hr	none
206-3	48	4.4	3.00		severe
214-1	48	4.4	2.00		none
214-2	48	4.4	2.50	2 hr	moderate
214-3	48	4.4	3.00		severe
200-1	48	4.4	2.00		none
200-2	48	4.4	2.50	6 hr	none
200-3	48	4.4	3.00		severe
201-1	46	4.3	2.00		mild
201-2	48	4.4	2.25	6 hr	moderate
201-3	48	4.4	2.50		severe
197-1	50	4.7	2.00	12 hr	none
197-2	50	4.6	2.50		severe
216-1	48	4.4	2.00		mild
216-2	48	4.4	2.50	1 day	moderate
216-3	48	4.4	3.00		severe
220-1	46	4.3	2.00		none
220-2	46	4.3	2.50	2 day	none
220-3	46	4.3	3.00		severe
202-1	49	4.5	2.00	4 day	none
202-2	48	4.4	2.50		mild
187-1	45	4.2	1.50	12 day	none
187-2	45	4.2	2.50		moderate
194-1	46	4.3	2.00	12 day	none
194-2	50	4.6	2.50		severe

* The differences in the numerical values are significant on a comparative scale. However, the probable error in the absolute values of pressure and particle velocity does not exceed 10%.

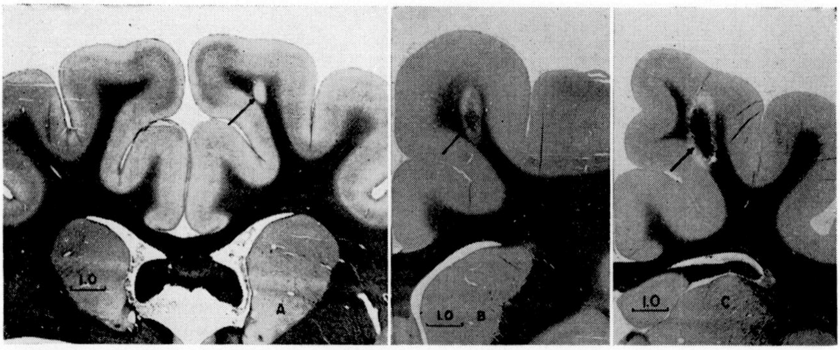

FIG. 1. (a) Frontal section of a cat brain illustrating a *light* ultrasonic lesion in the subcortical white matter. Weil stain. (b) A *medium* ultrasonic lesion in the subcortical white matter. Weil stain. (c) A *heavy* ultrasonic lesion in the subcortical white matter (invading the cortical gray matter). Weil stain.

dosages are manifest by an increase in the size of the lesion area for lesions produced by single isolated shots of ultrasound.

Early Changes

No histological disturbance is observed in the irradiated tissue of animals sacrificed within five to nine minutes after exposure (six irradiated regions in two cats). Twelve to fourteen minutes after treatment the first evidence of lesion formation is visible. A *heavy* lesion twelve minutes after

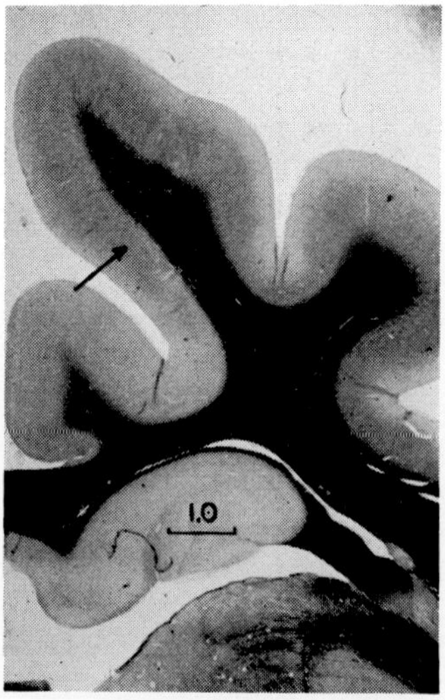

FIG. 2. A *heavy* lesion in the subcortical white matter of a cat brain, twelve minutes after irradiation. Weil stain.

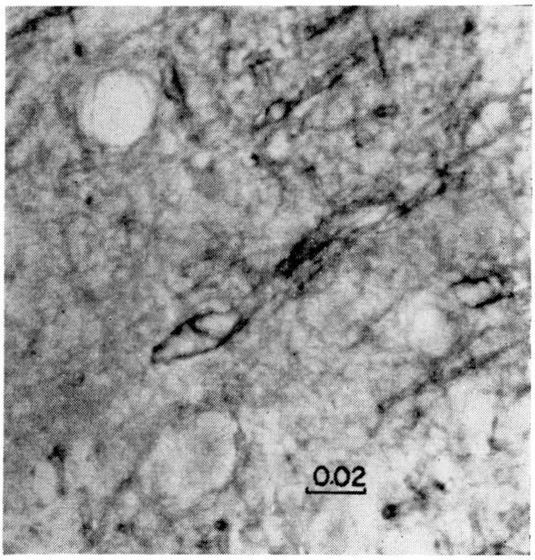

FIG. 3. Swollen myelin sheaths in invaded gray matter. Heavy lesion 13 minutes after irradiation. Weil stain.

irradiation is evident macroscopically as a lightly staining band which delineates, with its oval cross-section, the area enclosing the island (Fig. 2). All tissue components of the white matter in the island appear normal. Structures within the moat are characterized by their poor staining quality. In these perfused preparations, no blood elements are seen in the blood vessels or in the tissue spaces and the blood vessels appear normal.

Although *heavy* lesions in the white matter are clearly evident macroscopically fifteen minutes after irradiation, it is difficult to observe specific

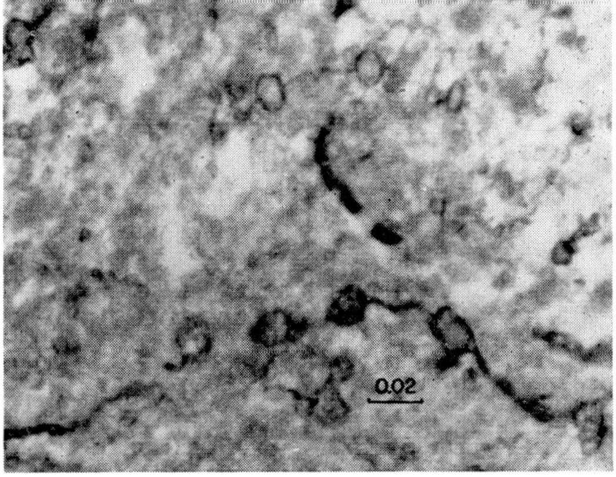

FIG. 4. Bulbous myeline sheaths and isolated spheres in the invaded gray matter one hour after irradiation. Weil stain.

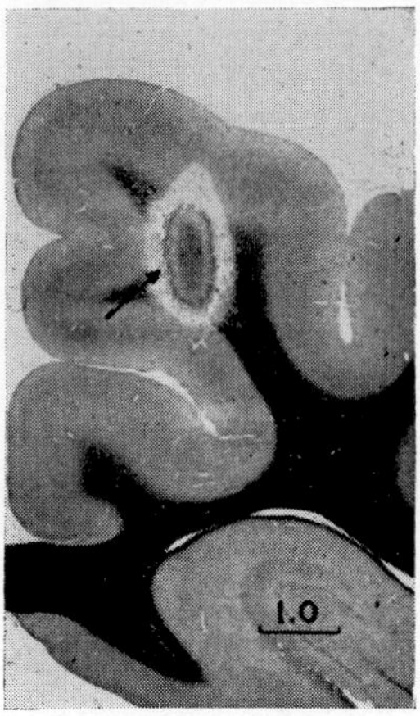

FIG. 5. A *heavy* "laminated" lesion in the subcortical white matter of a cat brain sacrificed four days after the exposure. Weil stain.

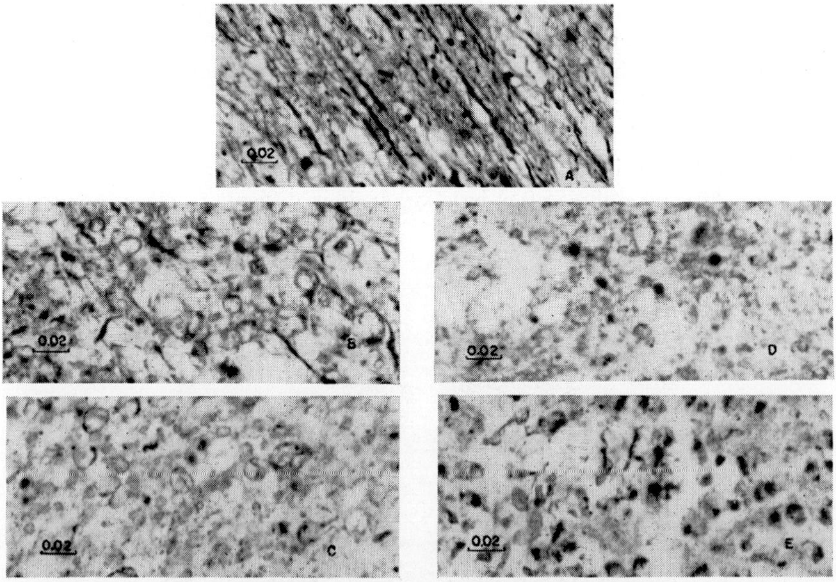

FIG. 6. Stages of axis cylinder degeneration in subcortical white matter of cat brain following ultrasonic irradiation. Romanes silver. (a) Normal axis cylinders. (b) Early stage showing axis cylinder fragments, connected spheres and debris. (c) Intermediate stage showing isolated spheres and detritus. (d) Advanced stage showing detritus and large clear spaces. (e) Terminal stage showing glial scar and clear spaces.

microscopic changes in the tissue structures by examination of the dense fiber tracts. In the neighboring gray matter, where discrete myelin sheaths can be discerned, it is possible to detect changes at this early stage. The sheaths exhibit swellings along their length which give them a nodal appearance (Fig. 3) and at later times develop into connected or isolated thin-walled spheres (Fig. 4).

Some astrocytes and oligodendrocytes in both island and moat stain more palely than normal, and a few show slight swelling and even fragmentation in the moat region.

The discussion of the subsequent changes is organized into descriptions of individual tissue components in the following order: matrix, axis cylinders, myelin sheaths, glia, blood vessels and blood cells.

Matrix

The first change in the irradiated locus is observed ten to fifteen minutes after exposure. The affected area stains weakly and this reaction constitutes the current method of locating early lesions. The oval form of the focal region of the ultrasound beam is reproduced by the shape of this pale

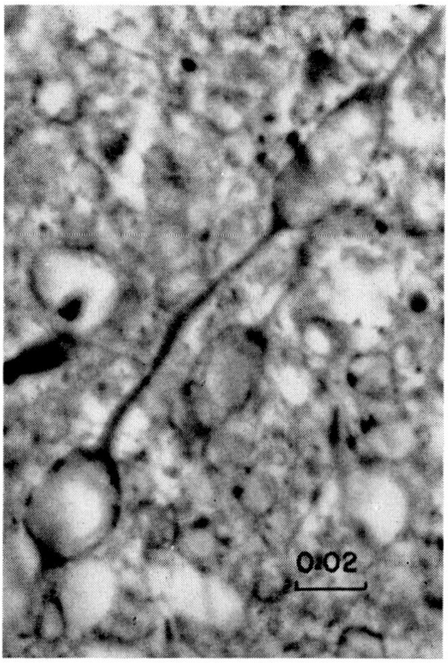

FIG. 7. Bulbous axis cylinder in the moat region of a *medium* lesion in the subcortical white matter twelve hours after irradiation. Romanes silver.

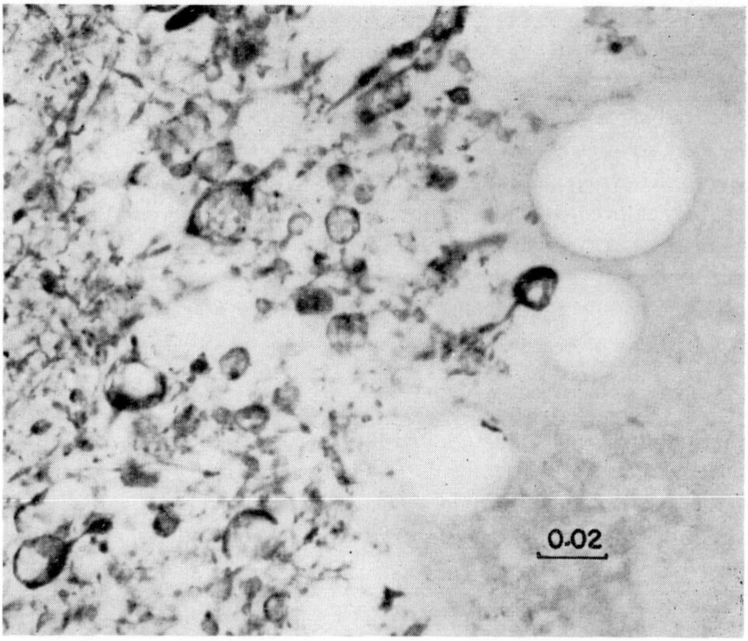

FIG. 8. Retraction bulbs and digestive chambers at the periphery of a *heavy* lesion twelve hours after irradiation. The pale structureless substance containing the clear spaces is the moat region of the lesion. Romanes silver.

area. A *heavy* lesion at this time exhibits a rim of paleness which extends into the gray matter without distortion of the oval shape (Fig. 2). Close examination reveals that the fiber elements are unchanged in the pale rim area which will develop into the moat. The island matrix is normal in all respects.

One hour after exposure the moat area stains more lightly and fluid filled holes may be seen. At two hours the moat has enlarged and clefts or large irregular fluid filled spaces containing debris are found. Some of the fluid filled spaces persist through the twelfth day which was the maximum survival period used in this study. Larger lesions (multiple shot irradiations reported upon previously (Barnard, Fry, Fry and Krumins, 1955)) produced in animals which were sacrificed thirty days after exposure, showed either cyst-like cavities or closed glial scars.

Some *heavy* lesions exhibit the staining characteristics illustrated in Fig. 5. The island is composed of concentric lamina with an innermost core of almost normal staining tissue surrounded by a zone of lighter staining fibers which are, in turn, enclosed by a shell of fibers which stain like the inner core. The whole structure is surrounded by a moat similar to that of lesions containing unlaminated islands. Close examination reveals no morphological differences in the elements of each of these lamina.

Axis Cylinders

With the exception of the preserved fibers in the islands, the sequence of changes which occur in the axis cylinders is similar but with different time rates for all classifications of lesions. This sequence is illustrated in Figs. 6a through 6e. The normal axis cylinders (Fig. 6a) initially became swollen and tortuous, developing ovoid and spherical forms which assume the appearance of a string of beads (Fig. 7). Further reaction causes the fibers to dissociate into free spheres and twisted fragments (Fig. 6b). The spheres alone are visible at later times (Fig. 6c) and are significantly reduced in number in Fig. 6d leaving a necrotic field of cellular detritus and some cleared spaces. After the debris is ingested by phagocytes (gitter cells), a glial scar is formed (Fig. 6e).

At the periphery of the lesions the severed axis cylinders form retraction bulbs which may persist for two weeks after exposure. The clear structureless moat (Fig. 8) is surrounded by these retraction bulbs and digestive

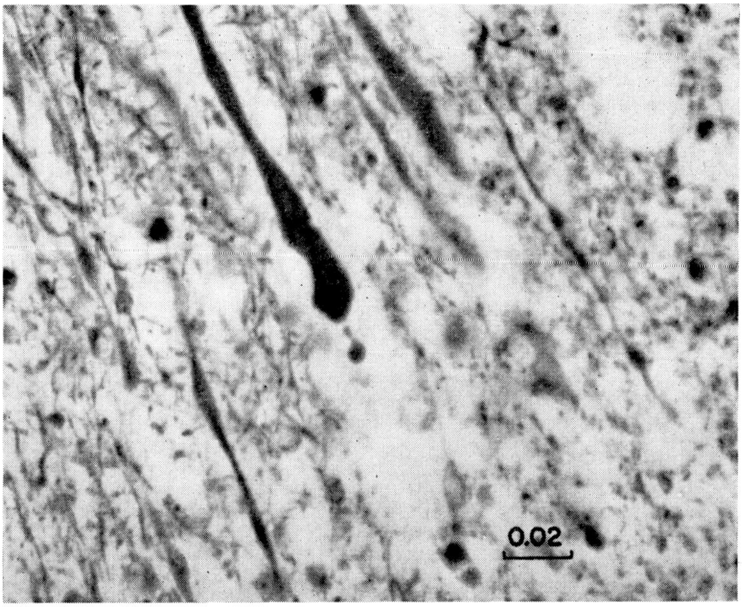

FIG. 9. Retraction bulbs on nerve fibers of various calibers in the border zone of a *heavy* lesion one day after irradiation. Romanes silver.

chambers. The larger caliber fibers retract further into the border zone of the lesion than do fibers of smaller diameter. This can be observed in Fig. 9 in which a small pendulous retraction bulb marks the termination of a large fiber while smaller fibers exhibit only swellings at the same depth.

Myelin Sheaths

The initial response of the myelin sheaths occurs twelve minutes after irradiation in heavy lesions (both island and moat). The sheaths, as seen in Weil's stain, are slightly swollen (Fig. 3). One hour after exposure some of the myelin in the island has a nodal character but the myelin in the moat has already been reduced to hollow spheres. These myelin spheres enclose the spheres resulting from axis cylinder degeneration which may be seen in silver preparations. The myelin sheaths, similar to the axis cylinders, change more slowly in the island than in the moat with the principal difference that the response of the myelin can be recognized earlier than can that of the axis cylinders.

Glia

Changes in the microglia appear earlier in lesions produced by higher dosages but, one day after exposure, all grades of lesions exhibit damaged cells and a reduced population. On the second day, however, they are more numerous than is normal and some are enlarged into phagocytes. Four days after treatment the microglia (macrophages) dominate the field and are enlarged and laden with debris. At twelve days a huge population of microglia is still present but the debris is considerably reduced. From earlier studies it is clear that at thirty days they are greatly reduced in number.

Within ten minutes the astrocytes undergo a slight swelling and paleness of the nuclei and exhibit a few broken membranes. One hour after exposure the changes are similar in nature but more pronounced. At four days the surviving cells have enlarged and are preparing to undergo division. By twelve days there are large astrocytes throughout the interior of the lesion, particularly in close proximity to the blood vessels. They are more concentrated toward the periphery of the lesion and a few are seen in the dividing stage.

The oligodendrocytes undergo degenerative changes which appear ten to fifteen minutes after irradiation: pale staining nuclei in the island and the moat and a few fragmented nuclei in the moat. One hour later these changes have progressed and at one day many cells have disappeared while the remainder are swollen and fragmented. By four days most of the oligodendrocytes have disappeared and only some doubtful fragments remain, while all are gone after twelve days.

Blood Vessels and Blood Cells

The blood vessels in white matter lesions do not appear to be altered morphologically by ultrasound. In all lesions no erythrocytes appear in the matrix of any white matter lesions, even twelve hours after exposure, but by twenty-four hours some erythrocytes have escaped from the vessels in *heavy* lesions. Only in the heaviest lesions are some clusters present which consist of as many as 100 cells in a section, but never more than one or two such clusters have been seen in any one lesion. Occasional erythrocytes are seen in the tissue of *light* and *medium* lesions during the time interval one to four days after exposure.

Perivascular cuffing is first evidenced at twelve hours in the *heavy* lesions. The highest level seen, in the material available, is at four days. By twelve days it has regressed and only residual signs are present. The hematogenous response, of which cuffing is a part, is evidenced by the presence of a few agranulocytes in the tissue beginning at six hours. These reach their numerical peak at two days and then subside, none remaining, at twelve days. Granulocytes are first seen at twelve hours, increase to a maximum at two days, and have disappeared at four days.

Effects of Ultrasound on the Gray Matter of the Cerebrum

The dosage parameters of the ultrasonic field used to produce gray matter lesions were approximately the same as those employed for the formation of white matter lesions but the duration of irradiation required to effect a lesion is one and one half to two times as long.

The lesions produced in gray matter by ultrasound and described in Tables 2 and 4 are classified as *mild, moderate* or *severe*. It has not been possible during the course of this investigation to formulate criteria for the classification of gray matter lesions which can be as readily applied as those formulated for the classification of white matter lesions. The assigning of a gray matter lesion to a particular class is decided primarily on a comparative basis. This method has the disadvantage that, given an arbitrary single lesion, it is difficult to assign it to a class without having available either a graded series of lesions with which to compare it or a detailed description of such a series. However, the comparative method does constitute a consistent one.

It is possible to formulate a few brief criteria which permit a rough assignment of a lesion to a class without using the comparative method. Ten to fifteen minutes after exposure a *mild* lesion is not seen histologically. A *moderate* lesion in this same interval appears macroscopically as a uniform light staining area, and a *severe* lesion exhibits a pale staining band (moat) enclosing a central darker staining area (island).

This island-moat formation is similar to that characteristic of *medium*

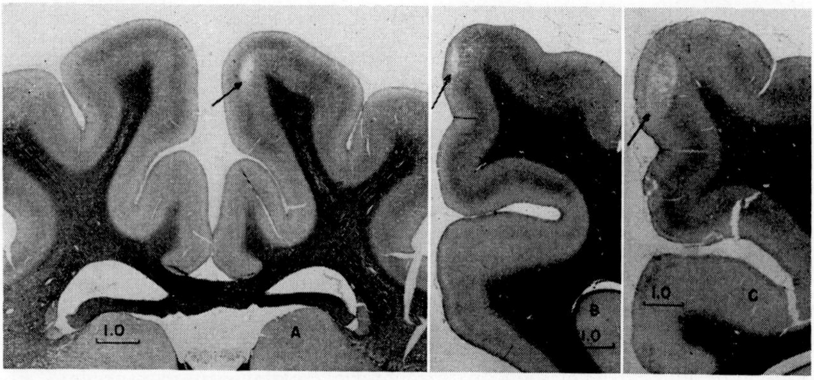

FIG. 10. (a) Lesion produced by ultrasound in the intermediate layers of the cortical gray matter of a cat brain PTAH. (b) Lesion produced by ultrasound in the surface layers of the cortical gray matter of a cat brain. PTAH. (c) A *severe* lesion in the cortical gray matter of a cat brain fourteen minutes after irradiation. PTAH.

and *heavy* white matter lesions. From one hour to several days after irradiation *mild* lesions exhibit some holes which may be as large as 150 microns in diameter. In moderate lesions the density of holes is high and some as large as 500 microns are present. *Severe* lesions are characterized by the presence of large irregular connected clear spaces.

After the glial response is well developed (one to two weeks after irradiation) it is difficult to formulate even rough, non-comparative criteria for classification. A simply applied comparative criterion at these later stages is the relative size of the lesion (for single discrete irradiations). As in the classification of white matter lesions, the categories are arbitrary subdivisions of a continuous series.

Examples of gray matter lesions in the intermediate layers of the cortical gray (Fig. 10a) and in the superficial layers (Fig. 10b) illustrate the precise character of the ultrasonic lesions. Figure 10c shows the similarity of the gray matter island formation with the islands of the fiber tracts.

Early Changes

Two cats irradiated at a total of six positions (single isolated shots) were sacrificed and perfused within six to eight minutes after exposure to ultrasound. None of the irradiated tissues showed any histological change although serial sections were carefully examined for signs of a lesion. Animals sacrificed and perfused from ten to sixteen minutes after irradiation show microscopically visible lesions characterized by a slightly pale staining background in the *moderate* response. Early chromatolysis is observed in some nerve cells. Many of the myelin sheaths are still normal ten minutes after exposure, but some appear bulbous. The axis cylinders stain spottily. In a *moderate* lesion minimal changes appear in the nuclei of astrocytes and oligodendrocytes but all microglial nuclei appear normal.

In the *severe* lesion, ten to sixteen minutes after irradiation, a pale staining region surrounds a normal staining central island. The perivascular spaces are slightly enlarged, but no blood cells are present in the vessels or in the tissue matrix of these perfused cat brains, either in normal or irradiated areas. Some nerve cells are swollen and show diminution of the Nissl granules, and a general lack of staining ability of all parts of the cell. A few normal appearing cells are still present in the lesion area. Many myelin sheaths are swollen and bulbous and some spheres are present. Many axis cylinders are fragmented into dust-like granules, and the remainder stain spottily. The glia in a *severe* response appear normal with the exception of some pale staining nuclei of astrocytes and oligodendrocytes and a few pale staining microglial nuclei.

The discussion of the subsequent changes is organized into descriptions of individual tissue components in the following order: matrix, nerve cells, nerve fibers, glia, blood vessels and blood cells.

Matrix

The pale staining background is obvious as early as ten minutes after irradiation in *moderate* and *severe* lesions. It is accompanied by the ap-

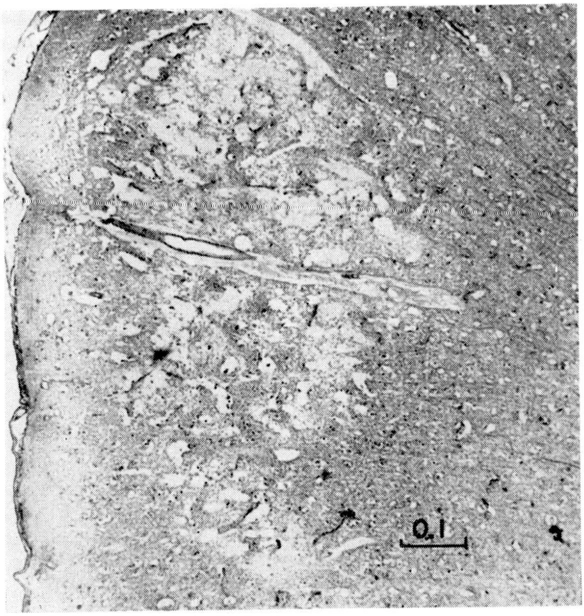

FIG. 11. Clefts in *severe* lesion six hours after irradiation. Romanes silver.

pearance of small perineuronal spaces. One hour after exposure small holes containing clear fluid appear in the tissue. Two hours after treatment in the *severe* lesions this fluid is present in clefts in the matrix (Fig. 11). *Mild* responses are evident histologically six hours after irradiation by the presence of perineuronal spaces and fluid filled holes and clefts which become larger and at one to two days after exposure are quite prominent. At later stages (twelve days after treatment) when the lesion aera becomes densely populated with glia, these spaces are no longer present.

Nerve Cells

The nerve cells show no histological changes within five to eight minutes but definite effects appear ten to fifteen minutes after irradiation in *moderate* and *severe* lesions. Hyperchromatism, paleness and chromatolysis of the affected neurons are apparent (Fig. 12b). The normal appearance of the cortical gray matter is illustrated in Fig. 12a. These cellular changes are succeeded rapidly by advanced chromatolysis, granulation of the cyto-

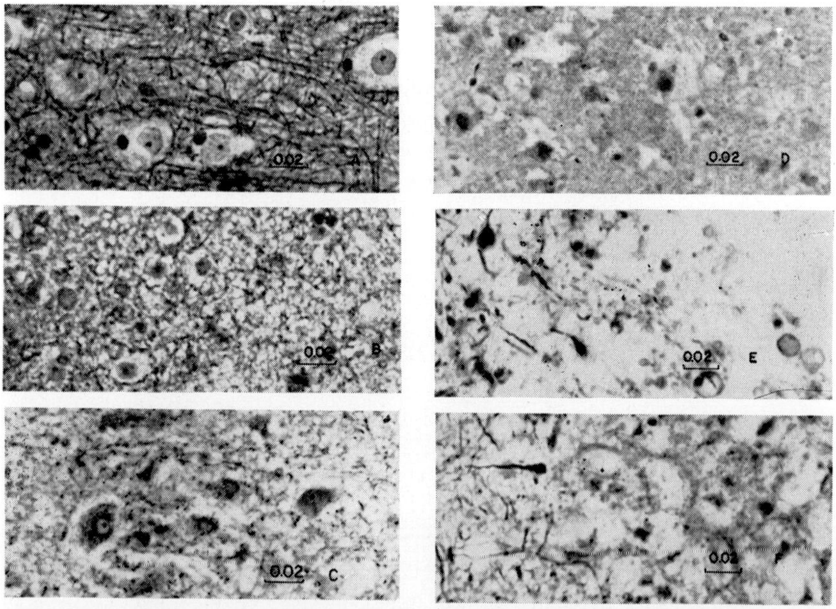

FIG. 12. Stages of neuron degeneration in the cortical gray matter of a cat brain following ultrasonic irradiation. Romanes silver. (a) Normal cortical gray matter. (b) Spottily stained axis cylinders ten minutes after irradiation. (c) Granular cytoplasm in nerve cell bodies, fragments of axis cylinders and small holes in the matrix. (d) Debris of axis cylinders, free nerve cell nuclei with shreds of cytoplasm, holes in the matrix. (e) Border zone of lesion showing retraction bulbs. Adjacent portion distinguishable neural or glial components. (f) Border zone of lesion showing retraction bulbs and adjacent region showing glial scar (twelve days after irradiation).

plasm (Fig. 12c) and liquefaction (Fig. 12d). Six hours after irradiation only a few ghost cells are left in *severe* lesions, and at one day all cells have disappeared (Fig. 12e). Figure 12f illustrates the border zone of the lesion delineated by the presence of retraction bulbs and the glial scar occupying the lesion area twelve days after irradiation.

The nuclei and nucleoli exhibit a series of changes which accompany those of the cytoplasm. The nucleus stains more darkly than normally and persists with intact nuclear membrane after the rupture of the cellular membrane and dissolution of the cytoplasm. The nucleolus becomes indistinct and finally unstainable before complete destruction of the nucleus occurs.

The cellular changes are similar to those described by Nissl, Spielmeyer and Bielschowsky except that in the case of ultrasonic irradiation the rate of dissolution of the cells is somewhat faster.

Nerve Fibers

The axis cylinders and myelin sheaths of the cortical gray matter show morphological changes within ten to sixteen minutes after exposure in *moderate* and *severe* lesions and have completely disappeared from *severe* lesions after two hours. In *mild* lesions, the effects are first seen at six hours and the fibers may be observed as late at one day following irradiation. This rapid dissolution, as compared to the time course of white matter lesions, may be a result of the relatively small amount of fiber debris present in the gray matter or it may be due to the more extensive vascularity of the cortical gray.

Glia

A few of the microglia react by becoming paler-staining one hour after irradiation in the *severe* lesions, by six hours most are absent from the lesion area and at twelve hours all have disappeared. One day after exposure they are present and beginning to metamorphose so that by two days they are fully developed as "gitter" or fat granule cells. The density at this stage is approximately equal to the normal population of microglia. By twelve days their number has increased enormously and they dominate the field of the lesion. In *moderate* lesions the microglia never entirely disappear and at one day many exhibit metamorphic changes. By twelve days the gitter cells are very numerous as in the *severe* lesion. In *mild* lesions only a few microglia disappear, at one day the population (macrophagic stage) has doubled and at four days these cells are present in large numbers.

The astrocytes react ten to fifteen minutes after irradiation by staining less intensely, and twelve hours after exposure all have disappeared from the *severe* lesions. In the *moderate* lesions they are absent after one day. In both grades of lesions they are numerous at twelve days. *Mild* lesions show a reduced number of astrocytes by six hours but at four days the population has increased to normal.

The oligodendrocytes are reduced to approximately one half their normal population two hours after irradiation in the *moderate* and *severe* lesions. Many of the remaining cells are hyperchromatic and shrunken. By two days all are absent in the *severe* lesion. At four days most have disappeared from even the *mild* lesion and at twelve days no oligodendrocytes are present in the centers of any of the lesions.

Blood Vessels and Blood Cells

In animals sacrificed within ten to fifteen minutes after irradiation all blood vessels are cleared of blood elements by perfusion with mammalian saline at a pressure of one meter of water. At one hour, however, many of the vessels in the *severe* lesion contain cells although the perfusion emptied all vessels in the normal tissue. The presence of these blood cells may possibly be explained by hemoconcentration and even sludging of the blood, but the absence of obvious volume changes in the irradiated tissue should be considered in postulating any such mechanism. The occurrence of many filled vessels is only in some *severe* lesions; the *moderate* and *mild* lesions contain only a few such filled vessels. More erythrocytes are found free in the tissue in lesions which have many filled vessels. In general, the free erythrocytes reach their numerical peak between the first and second day in the *severe* lesions. In these instances there are occasional clumps of erythrocytes of fifty to one hundred cells in a section. In the *moderate* and *mild* lesions only scattered red cells are seen and an occasional small cluster of a dozen cells. A few granulocytes and agranulocytes make their appearance at six hours and some are still present at four days.

Perivascular cuffing is barely perceptible at one day but is easily observed two to four days after exposure and consists of a row or two of cells around the vessels. The cuffing is more prominent at the periphery of the lesion. At twelve days only slight residual signs are present. This response is not nearly as marked as was reported in the case of larger multishot white matter lesions (Barnard, Fry, Fry and Krumins, 1955).

As far as a discussion of these results is concerned, we would like to make the following remarks:

Although the island of the white matter lesions represents the center of focus of the converging ultrasonic beams, the rate of morphological alteration of the fibers within the island is much slower than that of the fibers in the immediately surrounding tissue. Accurate measurement of the sound field by thermocouple probes in water and within the brain show that passage through brain tissue does not distort the field. The island-moat formation may occur in the following manner. Ultrasonic dosages only slightly above threshold levels cause damage to the irradiated tissue but do not interfere with the autolytic mechanism. When the dosage is sufficiently intense, the autolytic enzymes are denatured at the center of the lesion and the tissue is preserved since normal dissolution cannot take place. The removal of the preserved tissues is delayed until phagocytic processes can operate. The moat region is less strongly affected and, for this reason, is capable of normal autolytic absorption.

The preserved fibers may be similar to those observed and reported by Cajal (1928) who recognized them as essential concomitants to traumatic lesions. Cajal noted that contusion, tension or compression involved in lesion production resulted in the subsequent presence of a large number of morphologically intact fibers. If the brain tissue was cut with a sharp blade, as contrasted with the use of a dull instrument, and consequently tension and compression stresses minimized, only a few preserved fibers were produced. By means of two transverse cuts in the brain, whole blocks of tissue containing preserved fibers, which extended across the entire block, could be obtained. The histological appearance of fibers within the islands of ultrasonic white matter lesions compares quite closely with the description of Cajal.

The holes and clefts which appear in the matrix as the tissue undergoes dissolution may result almost entirely from autolysis and liquefaction. No obvious swelling of the lesion area occurs, as evidenced by absence of compression in the surrounding tissue, although some small amount of fluid may be transported by the vascular system to the necrotic region. The extravasations of erythrocytes may be the result of vascular embarassment caused by the extensive tissue necrosis.

The physical mechanism of the action of ultrasound to produce tissue damage of the type reported herein is not sufficiently understood. Although it is not felt that heating is the principal factor, it certainly is important, because the primary process is temperature dependent. As described in an earlier paper (Barnard, Fry, Fry and Krumins, 1955), sound is absorbed at almost twice the time rate for equal sonic intensities in white matter as in gray matter, so that this property must be considered in any analysis of the differences in ultrasonic dosages required to produce lesions in gray matter as compared to white matter. It is specifically noted that single myelinated fibers in the gray matter are not aflected at dosages which produce lesions consistently in the white matter, that is, in masses of myelinated fibers.

That heat is not the principal factor acting to produce the changes in the tissue is shown by experiments performed on frogs and new-born mice.

These animals, whose body temperatures are lowered before and during irradiation, have lesions produced in their nervous systems by ultrasound, even though the peak temperatures reached during irradiation are well within the physiological limits for the animals. The work on frogs has been reported previously (Fry, Tucker, Fry and Wulff, 1951) and that on mice is currently in progress.

The phenomenon of cavitation in an intense sound field, that is, the growth of cavities from gas nuclei, with consequent tearing of the tissue fabric, can probably be eliminated as a factor in the production of lesions in the experiments reported here since no animals show any tissue disturbance until at least ten minutes after irradiation. Careful microscopic examination of stained sections of irradiated regions from animals sacrificed less than ten minutes after exposure fails to reveal any changes. Cavitation tears in the tissue would show immediately. Additional evidence that cavitation does not contribute to the mechanism is forthcoming from previous frog experiments, as shown by the fact that irradiation under hydrostatic pressure sufficiently high to completely prevent cavitation does not eliminate the effect of the ultrasound on the tissue.

Two lesions, four days and twelve days after irradiation, exhibit normal appearing axis cylinders in silver stains, yet in Weil's stain these same fibers show no trace of a myelin sheath. The nerve cell bodies are absent as in other lesions at these survival times. These lesions appear to be minimal, that is, close to the ultrasonic dosage threshold necessary to produce a histological change. These axis cylinders do not resemble those of the preserved fibers previously discussed in this paper because they appear normal along their entire length, including the portion in the border zone of the lesion. In addition, these naked axis cylinders occur in the minimal lesion whereas the preserved fibers in white matter lesions are found most abundantly and longest preserved in the heavy response. Apparently a demyelinating process is operative and the axis cylinders may be alive rather than preserved. Further study of these minimal lesions is planned with the intention of comparing them with the demyelination occurring in certain pathological conditions.

When a tissue component is irreversibly affected by ultrasound the consequent degenerative changes are not pathognomonic for the ultrasonic method. Similar changes occur in response to various other physical agents although the rate of the necrotic processes may be different. The ultrasonic method, however, has the distinction of possessing a cetrain amount of selectivity which alters the overall histological pattern of degeneration. This specificity permits lesions to be produced in myelinated fiber tracts passing through gray matter without damage to the surrounding nerve cell bodies. Although some petechial hemorrhages are observed in animals subjected to high doses of ultrasound, it is possible to produce complete destruction of the nervous tissue elements without damage to the circulatory system in that area. For the sound pressure amplitudes and particle velocities used in these studies, the blood vessel damage occurs at roughly twice the duration required for a threshold effect in gray matter. The duration required for the threshold effect in gray matter is, in turn, nearly twice that required for white matter minimal damage.

Additional merits of the ultrasonic method are: the absence of long delayed responses which have been observed following conventional and high energy x-irradiation (Arnold, Bailey and Laughlin, 1954; Clemente and Holst, 1954; Tobias et al., 1954); the complete asepsis of the lesion area, the ability to realize isolated lesions deep within the brain structure without complications resulting from needle tracts; the small size of the affected region; minimal shock; and accuracy of lesion placement, which is as precise as the variation in brain geometry of a given type of animal permits.

Summary

High level (acoustic particle velocities of the order of 5×10^2 cm./sec. and pressure amplitudes of the order of 50 atmospheres) focused ultrasound (frequency 980 kc.) can produce selective lesions in either the gray or white matter of the brain. The following characteristics of such lesions have been determined:

1. The volume of affected tissue can be controlled to restrict the lesion to a few cubic millimeters. Larger lesions can be produced by moving the focal spot of the beam through a prescribed path.
2. A lesion can be produced deep in the brain without affecting any intervening tissue.
3. The dosages of ultrasound necessary to affect irreversible changes in the gray matter are higher than those required for white matter. At 50 atmospheres pressure amplitude and 5×10^2 cm./sec. particle velocity the minimal durations are in the ratio of approximately two to one. Because of this specificity the fiber tracts can be interrupted without damage to adjacent or intervening gray matter.
4. Tissue components of the white matter exhibit the following order of susceptibility to change by sound: myelin sheaths, axis cylinders, glia, blood vessels. The same order is seen in the gray matter with the addition that nerve cell bodies are approximately as sensitive as the axis cylinders. At dosages which induce minimal histological changes an apparent demyelination can be accomplished without morphological alteration of the axis cylinders.
5. Ultrasonic radiation does not produce long delayed effects which have been observed in tissue treated with x-rays.

References

Arnold, A., P. Bailey and J. S. Laughlin. 1954. Effects of betatron radiations on the brains of primates. Neurology *4:* 165–178.

Barnard, J. W., W. J. Fry, F. J. Fry and R. F. Krumins. 1955. Effects of high intensity ultrasound on the central nervous system of the cat. J. Comp. Neurol. *103:* 459–484.

Clemente, C. D. and E. A. Holst. 1954. Pathological changes in neurons, neuroglia and blood-brain barrier induced by X-irradiation of heads of monkeys. A.M.A. Arch. Neurol. and Psychiat. *71:* 66–79.

Fry, W. J., J. W. Barnard, F. J. Fry and J. F. Brennan. 1955. Ultrasonically produced localized selective lesions in the central nervous system. Am. J. Phys. Med. *34:* 413–423.

Fry, W. J., J. W. Barnard, F. J. Fry, R. F. Krumins and J. F. Brennan. 1955. Ultrasonic lesions in the mammalian central nervous system. Science *122:* 517–518.

Fry, W. J. and R. B. Fry. 1954. Determination of absolute sound levels and acoustic absorption coefficients by thermocouple probes—Experiment. J. Acoust. Soc. Am. *26:* 311–317.

Fry, W. J., W. H. Mosberg, Jr., J. W. Barnard and F. J. Fry. 1954. Production of focal destructive lesions in the central nervous system with ultrasound. J. Neurosurg. *11:* 471–478.

Fry, W. J., D. Tucker, F. J. Fry and V. J. Wulff. 1951. Physical factors involved in ultrasonically induced changes in living systems: II. Amplitude duration relations and the effect of hydrostatic pressure for nerve tissue. J. Acoust. Soc. Am. *23:* 364–368.

Heyck, H. 1952. Ultraschall und Zentralnervensystem. Schweiz. med. Wchnschr. *82:* 97–99.

Heyck, H. and W. Höpker. 1952. Hirnveränderungen bei der Ratte durch Ultraschall. Monatsschr. Psychiat. u. Neurol. *123:* 42–64.

Lindstrom, P. A. 1954. Prefrontal ultrasonic irradiation—A substitute for lobotomy. A.M.A. Arch. Neurol. and Psychiat. *72:* 399–425.

Ramón y Cajal, S. 1928. Degeneration and regeneration of the nervous system. Vols. I–II. Oxford Univ. Press. 769 pp. Trans. and ed. by Raoul M. May.

Tobias, C. A., D. C. Van Dyke, M. E. Simpson, H. O. Angler, R. L. Huff and A. A. Koneff. 1954. Irradiation of the pituitary of the rat with high-energy deuterons. Am. J. Roent., Rad. Therapy and Nucl. Med. *72:* 1–21.

On the Problem of Dosage in Ultrasonic Lesion Making

T. F. Hueter,[1] H. T. Ballantine, Jr. and W. C. Cotter

Massachusetts General Hospital, Boston, Massachusetts

ULTRASONIC IRRADIATION of live animal tissues at low intensities (1–3 watts/cm.^{2}) and CW, as used in physical therapy, produces effects which are considered to be mainly thermal in origin (Lehmann, 1953). At high intensities (50–1500 watts/cm.^{2}), using focused ultrasound, there is some indication (Fry, 1953) that cell destruction can be produced by a proper choice of the time sequence of irradiation, even if the temperature of the tissues is kept at safe levels. If a different biological response mechanism is operative in each of the two cases the resulting effects will be governed by different relationships between the physical parameters of the ultrasonic irradiation; i.e., the meaning of the term "dosage" will not be the same at high and at low intensities.

Applications of ultrasonics in neurosurgery involve the production of lesions of a specified size at a specified location and in a reliable, reproducible fashion. To do this, one must be able to correlate the size and the location with the measurable physical quantities such as frequency, intensity, duration and time sequence (for multiple shots). Some amount of reproducibility has been achieved by some investigators for one frequency and for one particular type of equipment (Fry et al., 1954). However, no true and exact dosage relationships have yet been worked out which would enable one to vary the physical quantities such that predictable variations of the degree of destruction can be produced in all types of nervous tissues, and in all parts of the anatomy of the brain.

Dosage control in ultrasonic lesion making depends on the following factors:

a. Geometry of the focal region.
b. Determination of focal intensity.
c. Relationship between the physical irradiation conditions and the biological effect.
d. Mechanisms involved in tissue destruction by ultrasound.

[1] Now, Ratheon Corporation, Waltham, Massachusetts.

The value of neurosurgery of the ultrasonic method depends largely on the precision with which tissue destruction can be produced at a predetermined site by focused ultrasonic irradiation of that particular site. It is often difficult to ascertain whether this goal has been achieved by a given irradiation: depending on the kind of nerve tissue irradiated the damage induced by the ultrasound may or may not spread out to areas outside the region of focal irradiation. From our present knowledge it appears that there are two different approaches to the problem of controlling lesion size and shape: (1) One approach would utilize any existing selectivity (Wall et al., 1951) among the various kinds of nerve tissue, and thus produce damage to structures containing only tissue elements that are readily affected by ultrasound. In this case the outline of the lesion is more or less controlled by the anatomical structure of the brain itself (see Fig. 1 a), provided that the dosage is adjusted to lie within the margins of tissue selectivity. (2) In the other approach one would attempt to control lesion size and shape primarily by the physical properties of the ultrasonic focal spot, irrespective of tissue selectivity (see Fig. 1 b). In this case one would be interested in the smallest possible lesion to be placed, if necessary, even in a tissue structure more resistant to ultrasound than its surroundings (see Fig. 1 c). This approach is obviously the more difficult one, but it may lead to results of more general validity. Let us then adopt the latter view in discussing the above mentioned four groups of problems that arise in connection with dosage.

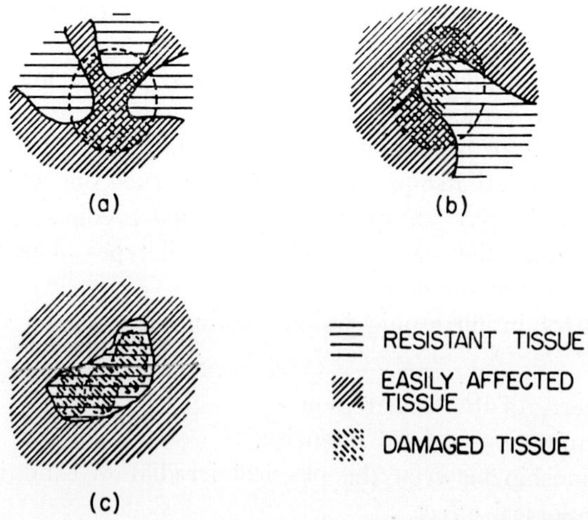

FIG. 1. Influence of tissue selectivity on focusing requirements. (a) lesion size controlled mainly by tissue selectivity; (b) lesion shape determined mainly by focal geometry but modified by tissue selectivity; (c) lesion controlled entirely by focal geometry (triple exposure) against prevailing tissue selectivity.

A. Geometry of the Focal Region

For a given intensity and duration of the ultrasonic irradiation both the diameter and the shape of an ultrasonically produced focal spot depend on the beam aperture a/F and the wavelength λ. The lateral diameter of the main lobe of the diffraction pattern which constitutes the focus is

$$d \simeq 1.2\, F\lambda/a \tag{1}$$

where F is the focal length and a the transducer radius. The shape of the focal spot is an ellipsoid whose axis ratio $r = l/d$ depends on the solid angle of irradiation. In brain work the maximum angle of convergence β is limited because of surgical considerations * as shown in Fig. 2. In a cat brain, for example, the maximum diameter of the skull opening that can be obtained safely is about 3 to 4 cm. For deep site of irradiation, such as in the thalamus (1.5 to 2.0 cm. below the dura), the maximum angle of convergence would then be about $\beta = 90°$ and the focal diameter is then limited to $d = 1.2\lambda$.

As an illustration, Fig. 3 presents some preliminary data obtained by our group using a lens aperture $a/F = 0.33$, and angle $\beta = 37°$ and a frequency of 2.5 mcps. In all cases the region of the ventral anterior nucleus (sterotactic coordinates A 12, L 4, $H+2$) was irradiated, using different exposure times. The quantities l and d used in this graph express the measured dimensions of the region of total destruction, as evidenced by cystic lesions found seven to nine days after the irradiation. From the upper graph we find for the ratio l/d a value $r \approx 5$, and we note that the lesion becomes more globular with increasing exposure. The lower graph indi-

* Because of the high absorption of bone at ultrasonic frequencies portions of the skull have to be removed to provide access to the brain.

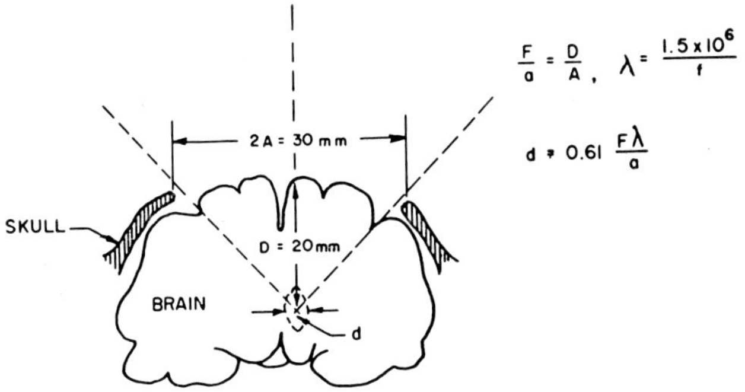

FIG. 2. Dependence of beam aperture on the size of opening in the skull which can be obtained safely, demonstrated for the case of a cat brain.

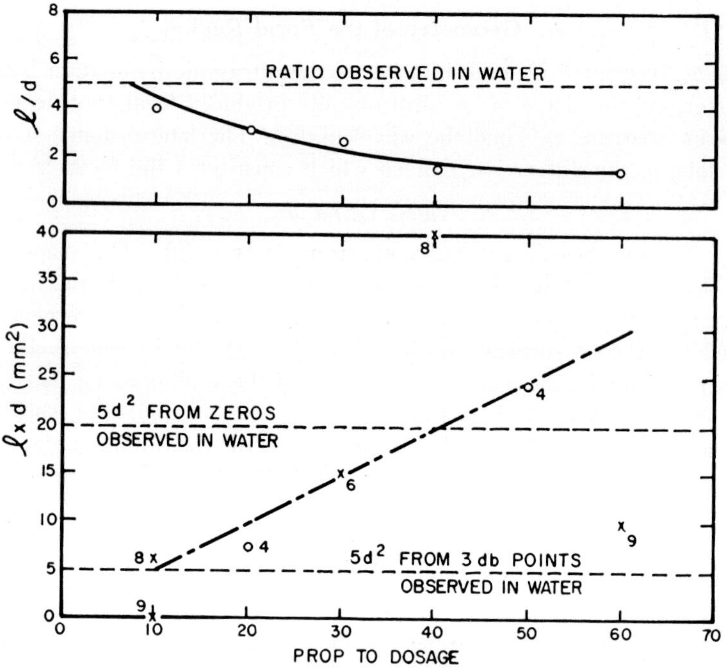

FIG. 3. Some results demonstrating the dependence of lesion size on the time exposure to ultrasound.

cates that there is a minimum dosage, necessary to produce the smallest demonstrable lesion of this kind.

The deeper the location of the lesion, the larger the minimum size of the lesion becomes for a given size of the skull opening and a given focal peak intensity. If several crossed beams (Fry and Barnard, 1954) are used instead of a single converging beam of the same overall aperture, both r and d will be somewhat larger.

According to diffraction theory about 84% of the energy irradiated from a single focusing transducer flows through the ellipsoidal focal region. To know the actual sound intensity to which the tissues are exposed at the focus, at least the wattage W actually delivered by the transducer and the focal diameter d must be determined by appropriate measurements. Such measurements are rather difficult to perform for non-planewave fields and require the use of calibrated probes which are small enough to resolve the focal field distribution.

Further, the absorption within the medium between the transducer and the focus effects both the amount and geometrical distribution of the ultrasound at the focus. The reduction of focal intensity by the absorption of the

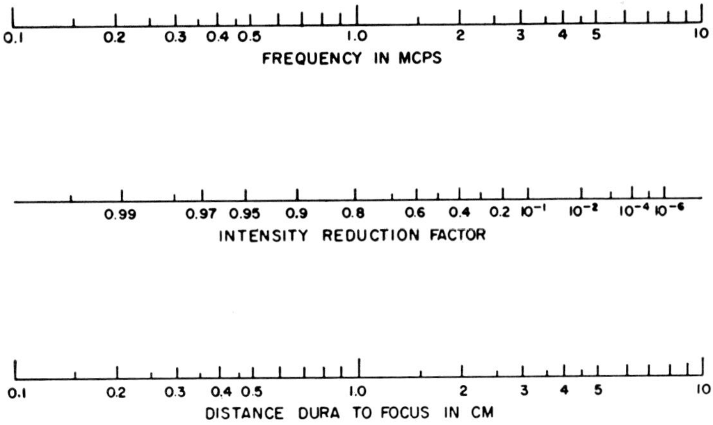

FIG. 4. Nomogram for the determination of the intensity reduction factor from the location of the focus below the brain surface and the frequency.

intervening tissue can be determined by the nomograph of Fig. 4. For example, for a depth of 2 cm. below the surface of the brain the focal intensity is reduced to 62 percent at 1 mcps and to 30 percent at 2.5 mcps from the value which would prevail in the absence of absorption (e.g. in water).

Actually, as the frequency is increased for a given focusing system both the gain of the lens and the absorption of the intervening tissue are increased. The gain Γ may be defined as the ratio $(I_F/I_0)_{av} = 0.84\ S_0/S_F$ in which I_F and I_0 are the average intensities at the focus and at the transducer face, respectively, and S_0, S_F are the associated beam cross section. Using Eq. (1) this becomes

$$\Gamma_\alpha = 0 \simeq 2.4 \frac{a^4}{F^2 \lambda^2} \qquad (2)$$

The effective gain Γ_a will be smaller by a factor e^{-2ax} due to tissue absorption, where a in brain tissue is about 0.12 nepers/cm. per megacycle, and x is the mean distance between the focus and the brain surface. The quantity Γ_a is plotted versus x for a number of frequencies in Fig. 5, assuming a lens system of convergence $\beta = 45°$ and a radius $a = 3.3$ cm. We recognize that an optimal frequency is associated with a given depth x and that the maximum attainable gain decreases rapidly with depth.

Since the effective gain determines the degree to which tissues outside of the focal region are spared the destructive effects at the focus, the geometrical selectivity of the ultrasonic method (as required, for example, for a lesion of the type depicted in Fig. 1c) becomes poor for large depths. This fact results from the geometrical properties of focusing systems, as can be seen from the following argument. Neglecting interference effects

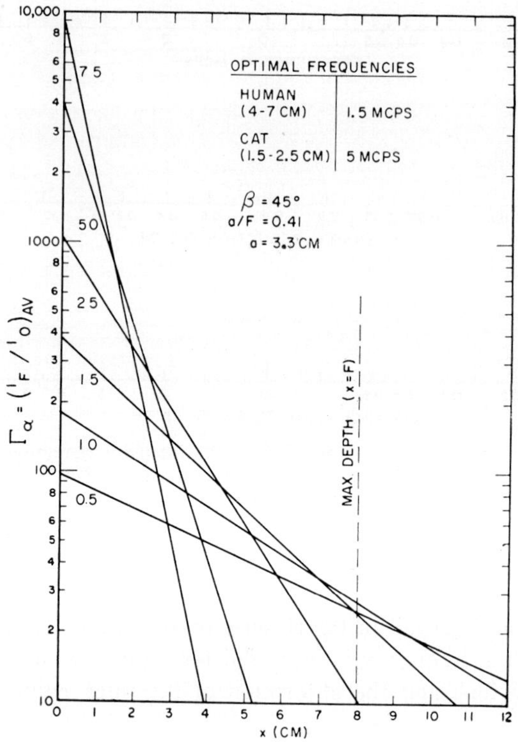

FIG. 5. Focusing gain vs. tissue depth of focus for various frequencies. Envelope of straight line sections determines optimal frequencies.

in the near field of the transducer and at the focus, we may assume that the average intensity decreases proportionally to the square of the distance from the focus. It is then possible to define the gain in intensity from the brain surface to the focus $\Gamma_t \simeq \Gamma_a\, x^2/F^2$, provided that $x \gg d$ (see Eq. (1)). From the optimal gain envelope of Fig. 5 we find that the ratio of the focal depth x to the wavelength λ_{opt} of the optimal frequency is about constant. From Eq. (2) and x/λ_{opt} = const. then follows

$$\Gamma_t \simeq 2.4\, \frac{a^4}{F^2\lambda_{\text{opt}}^2}\, \frac{x^2}{F^2} = \text{const}\left(\frac{a}{F}\right)^4 \tag{3}$$

We note that the tissue gain Γ_t is independent of x; for the system analyzed in Fig. 5 we find $\Gamma_t \simeq 28$. Hence, as x becomes larger the slope of the axial intensity distribution toward the focus becomes smaller. The quantity Γ_t/x is thus a measure of the geometrical selectivity, i.e., the sharpenss with which a focal lesion can be created.

This finding does not mean that it is impossible to create small lesions at large depths by proper grading of the amount of irradiation, but it indicates that the need for accurate dosage control increases with depth because the intensity then drops off more gradually in the directions away from the focus. This must be kept in mind if one is to extend procedures that are found adequate at the smaller depths encountered in cat and monkey brains to the larger depths prevailing in the human brain.

B. Determination of Focal Intensity

The sound intensity at the focus has a distribution of the form $2\,J_1(x)/x$. Hence we must distinguish between the average focal intensity

$$I_{av} = 0.84\,W/(d/2)^2\pi \qquad (4)$$

and the peak focal intensity

$$I_p = (2.2)^2\,I_{av}$$

An indirect determination of I_{av} would involve a measurement of the power W which for a given driving RF voltage across the crystal, is delivered by the transducer. Equation (4) implies that the coupling medium between the source and the focus is non-absorbent and linear, whereas there may be losses, and cavitation-type breakdown may occur at high amplitudes. The latter phenomenon, while well known in liquids, is also ob-

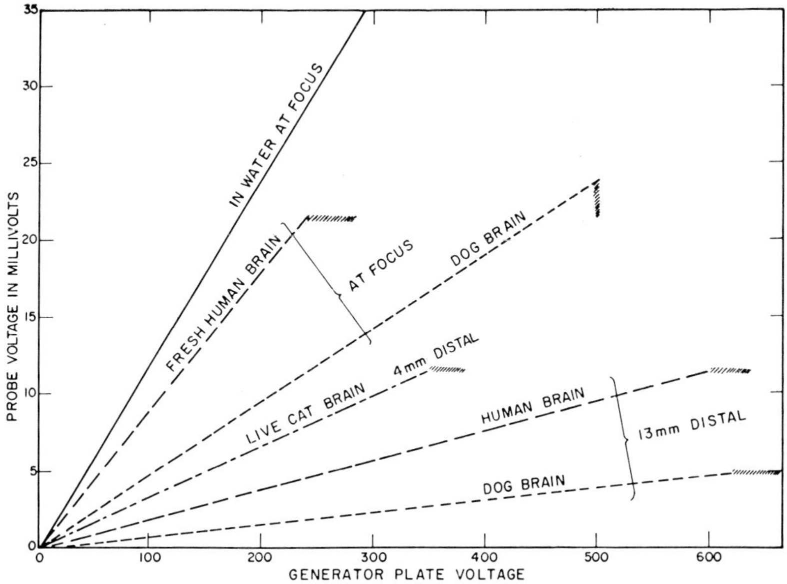

FIG. 6. Probe output voltage detected in tissue at or near focus as a function of generator plate voltage. Shaded regions indicate nonlinear behavior similar to cavitation.

served in tissues (Hug and Pape, 1954). Fig. 6 shows some results obtained by us at 2.5 mcps that are indicative of cavitation. A small probe was inserted into the brain at or beyond the focal point and the relationship between the pressure amplitudes generated by the transducer (proportional to plate voltage) and the pressure amplitudes received by the probe was studied. It was found that in each case there was a limiting amplitude beyond which the probe readings became noisy and erratic. Behavior of this kind suggests that the tensile strength of the medium is exceeded beyond a given threshold amplitude.

These findings lead to the need for direct measurements at the focus by suitable probes. Two types of conversion mechanisms may be utilized if an electrical signal proportional to that of the acoustic field pattern is desired:

i. Piezoelectric pickups sensitive to pressure (p) (Koppelman, 1952; Ackermann, 1953)
ii. Thermocouples sensitive to absorbed energy (aI) (Fry and Fry, 1954)

Some characteristics and relative merits of both kinds of probes are demontrated in Table I. It appears that thermoelectric probes are superior as to resolving power whereas piezoelectric probes give more direct information

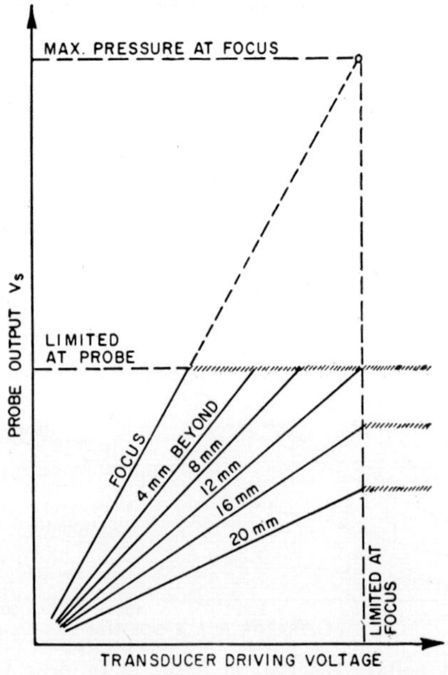

FIG. 7. Extrapolation of focal intensity, required if probe output is limited by cavitation at the probe surface.

TABLE I
Comparison Between Piezoelectric and Thermoelectric Probes

	Type of Probe	
	Piezoelectric	Sensitized Thermoelectric
Smallest possible size for reasonable sensitivity.	$BaTiO_3$ cylinder: 1 mm Crystals with pickup wire: 0.2 mm	Junction diameter 0.013 mm
Scattering artifact at 1 to 3 mcps.	Disturbs focal distribution wire probes useful below 2 mc.	Negligible disturbance by junction.
Field disturbance at high amplitudes.	Cavitation at probe interface.	Cavitation at surface of the enclosure containing absorber.
Calibration	*Direct:* reciprocity *Indirect:* Comparison with other devices, e.g., radiation pressure.	Indirect: Comparison with radiation pressure or using oil of known absorption.
Reading	Instantaneous by VTVM or scope (CW or pulses).	Initial slope of signal vs. time.
Dependence on base temperature.	None with wire probe slight with cylinder.	Strongly dependent (temp. control necessary).
Analysis of waveform.	Possible, e.g., cavitation noise may be detected.	Not possible.
Measurements at site of lesion.	Possible with wire probes mounted in hypodermic needle.	Possible, but calibration depends on knowledge of α at the site of the measurement.

on the signals received. With both types of probes difficulties are encountered at high intensities because of imperfect wetting between the probe surface and the surrounding medium, which may lower the cavitation threshold considerably. This threshold in turn, is frequency dependent; it may increase by a factor of 10 as the frequency is varied from 1 to 2.5 mcps. Thus, even with probes sufficiently small to produce negligible field disturbance it is often impossible to measure focal peak intensities exceeding 100 watts/cm.^{2} directly. Usually the focal intensity must be extrapolated by the procedure shown in Fig. 7.

Again such extrapolations assume linearity over the whole transmission path from crystal to focus. It appears, of course, quite possible to reproduce the irradiation conditions fairly accurately with one given transducer at a given frequency and applied to one type of animal involving a certain range of focal depths. It is rather difficult, however, to correlate the results obtained in one set of such conditions with those of another set, e.g., data obtained on rat cords with those in cat brains, or data obtained at one frequency with those at another.

C. Relationship Between the Physical Irradiation Conditions and the Biological Effect

Let us assume that the magnitude and distribution of ultrasonic intensity at the focal point have been determined as accurately as possible, say with an error not exceeding $\pm 10\%$. There are still many different ways of exposing the tissue to this intensity, and the biological response to a given intensity is found to depend largely on the manner in which the radiation is distributed in time. In this respect the biological response to ultrasound is similar to the response to other physical agents such as ionizing radiation or to some chemicals.

With pulsed ultrasound the temperature rise at the focus can be kept within certain limits (Barth et al., 1949) by a suitable reduction of the duty factor, i.e., by providing sufficient time between the pulses for the dissipation of heat. Pulsing or similar forms of intermittent irradiation are then a means of exposing the tissue to high mechanical stains without reaching destructive temperatures. To demonstrate this possibility a number of controlled experiments have been devised, of which those of Fry and associates (Fry et al., 1954) seem to be the most elaborate ones. Whereas heating would destroy all types of tissues indiscriminately, simply by coagulation, mechanical wear and tear is hoped to affect tissues selectively.

It appears that heating would produce a biological response proportional to $I\ \alpha(\omega) \left[\frac{\text{watts}}{\text{cm.}^3}\right]$, the energy absorbed by the tissue per unit volume and unit time, whereas the effects of mechanical fatigue would be proportional to the strain amplitude $s = 2\pi\ A/\lambda$ and some function of the time of exposure to the cyclic strains. At a given frequency, dosage could thus be expressed in terms of $I \times t$ in the first case, and as $A \times t$ in the second case. There are, of course, complicating factors such as heat transfer, threshold amplitudes and recovery phenomena. In any case, some knowledge of how the observed destructive effects are related to these two basic dosage laws is required if lesions are to be produced with a sufficient degree of control.

Such knowledge may be gained with small animals, such as frogs or mice, that are readily available in the large numbers required to obtain statistically meaningful results. We have irradiated the spinal cords of mice with paralysis of the hind legs as a physiological end point. A dual exposure, locating the beam ¾ mm. to the right and to the left of the mid-

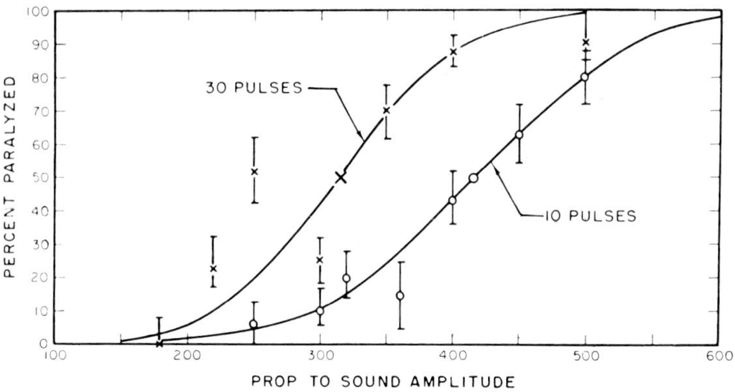

FIG. 8. Probability of paralysis of the hind legs of white mice after irradiation of the spinal cord versus sound amplitude.

line, was used to ensure that both sides of the cord were equally exposed, the lateral distance between half power points at the focal region being only 0.9 mm. at 2.5 mcps. For three different lengths of exposure (10, 30, and 60 pulses, each of 0.4 sec. duration, administered at the rate of 1 per sec.) the probability of paralysis due to an irradiation defect of the cord was determined as function of strain amplitude (which is proportional to the generator voltage).

Some typical data are shown in Fig. 8, in which each point represents a sample of about 30 mice. The slope of the resulting sigmoid curves as well as the probable error of each sample illustrate a rather large biological variation of susceptability to the ultrasound. It appears that it would be difficult to derive values for "a maximum amplitude at which no paralysis occurs," or a "minimum amplitude at which all animals are paralyzed," from such data. The best defined point is the median of the distribution curve, as obtained from a reduction of all the data to a best fitting line on probability paper, assuming a normal distribution. Comparing different lengths of exposure we find the relationship between reciprocal exposure time and sound amplitude shown in Fig. 9. The graph reveals that the paralytic effect produced by ultrasound depends more strongly upon amplitude than upon exposure time, suggesting a relationship of the form

$$(A - A_0)^2 t = \text{const.} \tag{6}$$

This empircial equation obtained with mice at 2.5 mcps, does not agree with the relationship $(A - A_0)t = \text{const.}$ postulated by Fry (1953) who used cooled frogs at 1 mc. but it would agree with the results obtained by Woeber (1949) who irradiated rats with CW ultrasound at 1 mcps and who found $I \times t$ to be approximately constant.

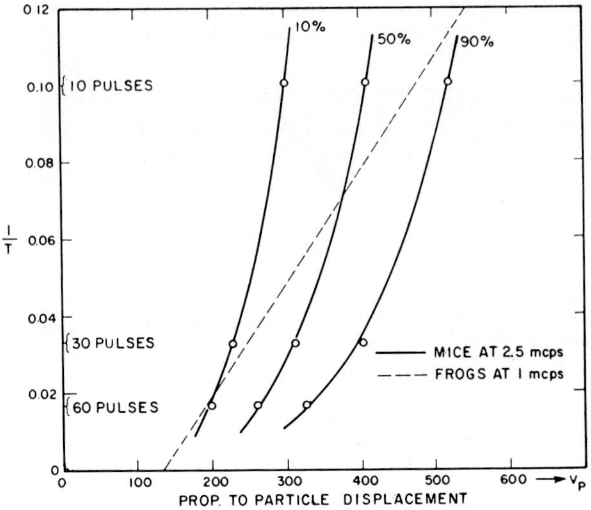

FIG. 9. Plot reciprocal exposure time versus sound amplitude, derived from reduction on probability paper of data presented in Fig. 8.

Comparing these contradictory results, one may at best conclude that the functional connection of the dosage parameters depends on the temperature level prevailing in the irradiated tissue. For example, Fry states that a single 4.3 sec. exposure at an intensity of 35 watts/cm.[2] will not paralyze frogs cooled to 2° C., but will paralyze frogs at 25° C., and Lehmann (1949) has reported similar results. On the other hand, Fry was able to demonstrate nerve damage at high intensities even if the temperature of the spinal cord was kept well below the levels at which denaturation of protein occurs.

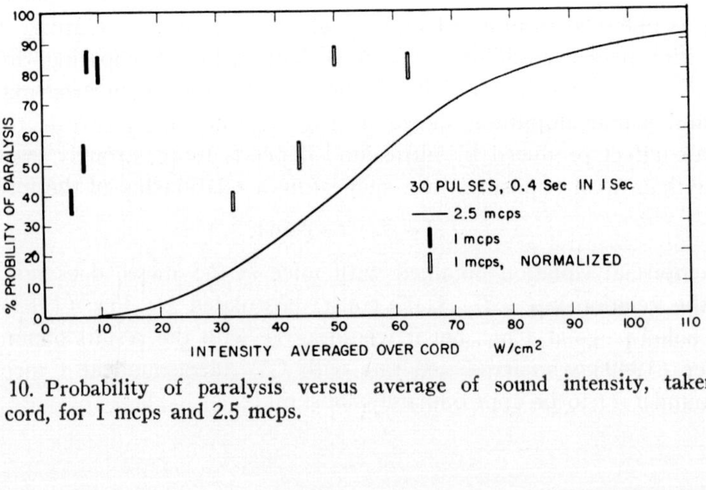

FIG. 10. Probability of paralysis versus average of sound intensity, taken over spinal cord, for I mcps and 2.5 mcps.

To gain further insight into the question of whether the primary cause of tissue damage is mechanical strain rather than energy dissipated as heat we have undertaken a comparison of the intensities required for a given percentage of paralysis at two different frequencies, 1 mcps and 2.5 mcps, for constant exposure time. The result is presented in Fig. 10 from which we note that at 2.5 mcps the median point is located at about 55 watts/cm.^{2} (average over cord), whereas at 1 mcps the median point of the sigmoid is located at about 7 watts/cm.^{2} (cord average). The finding that the intensity necessary to produce the paralytic effect becomes higher with increasing frequency seems to rule out heating as the primary cause of cell-destruction. The increase of the absorption coefficient α with frequency would call for a decrease in sound intensity to produce the same amount of heat $I\alpha$. Neither can the data be explained simply by associating the cell destruction with a given strain s, or sound pressure p, since

$$s = p/\rho c^2 = (2\,I/\rho c^3)^{1/2} \tag{7}$$

which would lead to the requirement that the sound intensity be the same at both frequencies. On the other hand, Fig. 10 shows that normalization of the data with respect to displacement amplitude (by multiplying the abscissa for the 1 mc. data by $(2.5)^2$) leads to agreement (within 10 percent of amplitude) of the results for both frequencies.

It is difficult, however, to visualize a mechanical effect that would depend on displacement amplitude, irrespective of wavelength or frequency. One possible explanation for the observed dependence of the biologically effective intensity on frequency would be in terms of a cavitation type rupture mechanism (Lehmann and Herrick, 1953). As mentioned above, the sound pressure necessary for rupture in liquids increases rapidly in the ultrasonic megacycle region (Esche, 1952). This behavior would account for the observed increase in threshold intensity as the frequency is increased at constant displacement amplitude.

The dependence of the biological response on the acoustical field variables, suggested by this experiment, need not be in contradiction with the finding that no simple $A \times t$ law seems to hold at all temperature levels. One possible explanation would be that the amount and progression of the mechanical cell damage depends greatly on the local tissue temperature, which in turn is a function of the quantity $I\,\alpha\,t$ and the manner of pulsing. The finally observed degree of tissue damage and the selectivity of the various tissue components with regard to a given amount of ultrasonic energy will then depend on the combined action of mechanical tissue fatigue and tissue heating, and this combination effect need not be governed by the simple types of dosage laws which we have examined so far.

It is then of importance to obtain some knowledge on the magnitude of

TABLE II

Mouse Cords: Correlation Between Paralysis and Irradiation Parameters

Run	Peak Intensity I	Pulse Width W	Duty Factor D	Number of Pulses N	ΔT	$I^{1/2}\Delta TD$	Percentage Paralyzed
1	350 w/cm²	0.1 sec	0.2	40	9°C	36	15%
2	300 w/cm²	0.2 sec	0.5	10	5°C	44	36%
3	350 w/cm²	0.1 sec	0.25	40	10°C	50	45%
4	220 w/cm²	0.4 sec	0.4	30	9.6°C	74	70%
5	870 w/cm²	0.1 sec	0.25	10	12°C	89	88%
6	350 w/cm²	1 sec	0.4	4	17.8°C	110	100%

the temperature rise in the focal region at a given set of irradiation conditions. This may be accomplished by inserting small thermocouples into the irradiated region of the spinal cord of mice. Whereas Fry's experiments on cooled frogs at 1 mcps indicate that paralysis does not depend on achieving a critical temperature *level,* our own results with 2.5 mcps on mice at normal body temperature suggest that the probability of paralysis is related to the temperature rise produced by the ultrasound. Some of our results with pulsed irradiation of varying intensity, pulse-width and duty factor are shown in Table II. The temperature rises ΔT that are observed under the irradiation conditions of run 2, 4, and 5 are plotted versus the number of pulses N in Fig. 11.

Comparing runs 4, 5, and 6 we note that a high percentage of paralysis is associated with a large temperature rise although the intensities, pulse widths and pulse numbers were completely different in the three cases.

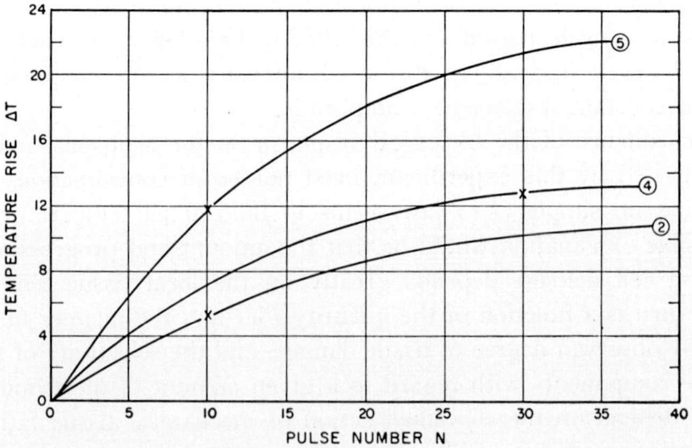

FIG. 11. Measured mean temperature rises ΔT versus pulse number in mouse cord, corresponding to irradiation conditions of runs 2, 4, and 5 in Table II. Crosses indicate pulse numbers used in Table II.

However, a comparison between runs 1 and 2 reveals a greater effect at the lower value of ΔT and makes the pulse width appear as the controlling quantity. Finally, between runs 3 and 5 the intensity seems to be the determining factor. From these and other tests we have been led to define as a tentative measure of biologically effective dosage the following combination of parameters:

$$I^{1/2}\,\Delta T D \sim A\,\Delta T\, w/p \tag{8}$$

in which w is the pulsewidth and p the pulse period. The temperature rise ΔT may be computed from a solution of the heat equation for the focal region (Rosenberg). Calculations based on this theory have been found to agree very well with the measured rises of cord temperature reported by W. J. Fry at 1 mcps as well as those recorded by us at 2.5 mc. Obviously, ΔT depends itself on the intensity absorbed, the duration and the sequencing (if pulsed) of the irradiation; also, the focal diameter enters critically into the equations.

We do not claim that the simple empirical dosage relation of Eq. (8) would hold for biologically abnormal situations such as when the body temperature of the animals is drastically lowered. Under the normal conditions, however, which prevail in most of the anticipated applications of focused ultrasound in neurosurgery Eq. (8) appears to be a workable approximation. This is further born out by our studies in cat brains, some of which are listed in Table III. An illustration of the macroscopic appearance of the kind of lesions that can be produced by focused ultrasound deep within the brain is given in Fig. 12.

D. Mechanisms Involved in Tissue Destruction by Ultrasound

Ultrasonic dosimetry would be much easier if we would have a clearer picture, preferably at a molecular level, of the way in which the tissue and its constituents respond to the applied alternating strains. From the foregoing discussion it seems unrealistic to attempt a clear-cut identification of "Non-Temperature Effects" because most biological reactions are temperature dependent. The complex molecular structure of living tissue may react in a similar way to the disrupting effect of mechanical strain as to the disordering effect of heat. Histological studies of cells affected by either ultrasound or heat do not give many clues on the specific cause of cell death: they reveal the same sequence of progressive decay in both cases (Hoepker, 1952).

The main argument for the existence of an interference of the ultrasound with the cell structure that is primarily mechanical rests with the finding (Fry et al., 1954) that a subliminal dose of ultrasound, which by itself produces neither a substantial temperature rise, nor any histological or physiological effect, has a "priming" effect on the tissue; i.e., the tissue displays a "memory" for such a subliminal dose. It appears that this memory of a subliminal exposure to ultrasound is stored in the form of subtle and reversible structural changes at a submicroscopic level. If the exposure

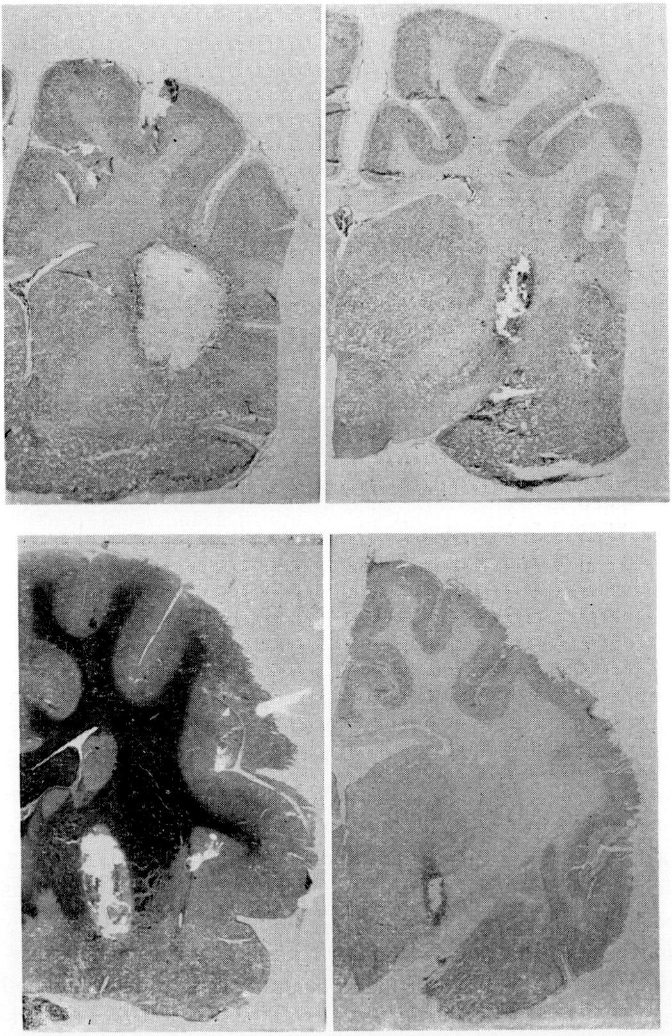

FIG. 12. Stained sections through brains of cats No. 6 and 8. Cell irradiated with pulses of 0.4 sec duration and 1 sec repetition rate. Upper row: Cat No. 8, intensity 225 watts/cm.², left 40 pulses, right 10 pulses. Lower row: Cat No. 6, 30 pulses, left 225 watts/cm.², right 164 watts/cm.²

is repeated at suitable intervals the amount of these changes reaches a level where a decay process is initiated. It is reasonable to assume that the changes and their progression are critically dependent on the temperature prevailing at the site of irradiation.

The mechanical hypothesis is corroborated by evidence shown by Peters (1949) that the morphology of brain damage by ultrasound is similar to that following mechanical concussion. Also, the type of destruction in the central nervous system observed by Catchpole and Gersh (1947) as a result of decompression sickness is quite similar to the destruction caused by ultrasound. These findings, as well as those by Hug and Pape (1954) and by Lindstrom (1954) would even suggest that the tissue is affected primarily at weak points within the tissue structure in a similar way as cavitation occurs at weak spots within a liquid. Fry's finding (1953) that the application of high hydrostatic pressure reduces the biological effect to a given dose would be consistent with this view.

To obtain a suitable model for a process of this kind we recall our finding that both the frequency dependence and the temperature dependence of the biologically effective sound pressure are similar to that observed in the cavitation breakdown in liquids, and we further note that focal lesions in their earliest stages originate at the periphery of the ellipsoidal focal region where strong shearing strains exist (Barnard, 1955).

A model based on viscosity, i.e., on the change in configuration of neighboring molecules due to applied stress, thus seems to be promising. We propose that the processes under consideration are governed by Eyring's theory of viscosity, plasticity and diffusion (Eyring, 1936). Our approach would be analogous to that of Briggs, Johnson and Mason (1947) inasmuch as the basic mechanism would consist in the production of holes (or breaking of intermolecular bonds) in the medium. The number of holes N_H, assumed to be a small fraction of the total number of N of molecules present is given by

$$N_H = N e^{-U/kT} \tag{9}$$

where k is the Boltzmann constant and T the absolute temperature. The activation energy U is defined by

$$U = U_0 + \beta(t)\, p \Delta v, \tag{10}$$

where U_0 represents the energy associated with intermolecular attraction, p is the external pressure, Δv is the average hole size and $\beta(t)$ is a time dependent coefficient. If p varies with time, as in a soundwave, we assume with Mason that $\beta(t)$ be unity for positive pressure and be much larger than unity, depending on the sound frequency and pulse width, for high negative pressures. An intense soundwave will then increase the number of holes N_H until a critical fraction $(N_H/N)_c$ is reached at which the molecular structure of the cellular contents becomes disorganized (Altenberg, 1953). To test this hypothesis we may write

$$\ln (N_H/N)_c = -(U_0 + \beta(t)p\Delta v)/kT, \tag{11}$$

or

$$-AT = B(t)I^{1/2} - C \tag{12}$$

in which A and C are constants, $B(t)$ is a time dependent coefficient and I is the sound intensity. Solving for $I^{1/2}$ we finally obtain

$$B(t)I^{1/2} = C - AT = A(T_l - T) \tag{13}$$

where $T_l = C/A$ is that temperature at which cell life ceases without mechanical interference. Equation (13) may be tested by experiments on paralysis of mice by ultrasonic irradiation of the spinal cord.

Our data on 700 mice, presented in Figs. 8 and 9, may be used for a check on Eq. (13). The temperature T reached at the end of each irradiation was calculated as described above, and confirmed in a number of test runs of the type illustrated in Fig. 11. The result is shown in Fig. 13 for the three probabilities of paralysis of Fig. 9. In the absence of any clues with regard to the time function $\beta(t)$ we have tentatively set $B(t) = t^{1/2}$, where t is the total irradiation time. We do not, however, expect this approximation to hold for runs in which the duty cycle D or the pulse width W differ from the values ($D = 0.4$, $\omega = 0.4$ sec) in which the plots of Figs. 8, 9, and 13 are based. Unless the general form of $B(t)$ is known, no fruitful comparison between Eq. (13) and the similar empirical relation of Eq. (8) can be made.

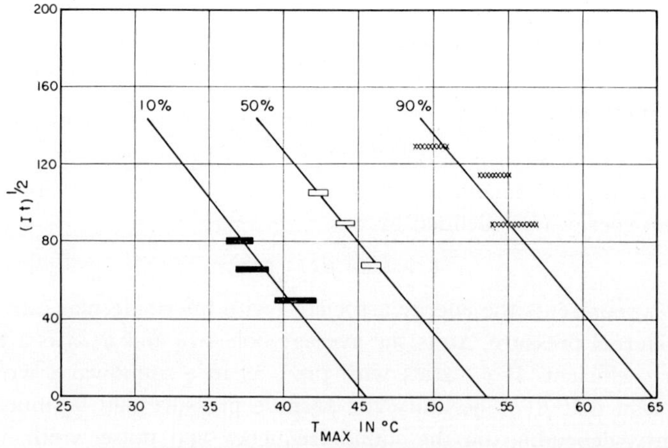

FIG. 13. Plot, according to Eq. (13) of data from Fig. 9 on probability of paralysis in mice.

The fact that our data on paralysis can be presented in the form of Eq. (13) lends some support to the applicability of Eyring's theory to this problem. Moreover, it is gratifying to note that the intersections of the straight lines in Fig. 13 with the abscissa lie in the range of temperatures at which heat alone is found to damage nerve tissues.

Conclusion

From all these considerations emerges the picture of a temperature dependent mechanical effect originating at weak points of the tissue structure and capable of regression or progression depending on the reaction kinetics of the rupture and restitution of molecular bonds. Because of the strong dependence of biological reaction equilibria on temperature, it would be difficult to differentiate between effects that are primarily mechanical and effects that are primarily thermal.

Tissue selectivity, as demonstrated by Fry, might only be expected in a narrow range above dosages that lead to only reversible damage and below dosages at which thermal effects prevail. This range is expected to be a function of such factors as the (frequency dependent) absorption coefficient, the focal geometry, and the location of the site of irradiation. Considering the limited accuracy with which these factors can be evaluated in planning a dosage, it appears that lesions based entirely on tissue selectivity cannot be produced with a reasonable degree of control and safety. In applying ultrasonic lesion making to humans, at the present state of our knowledge, such types of lesions are preferable that do not require an extreme amount of control of localization and size.

Acknowledgments

The authors are grateful to Professor W. J. H. Nauta of the Walter Reed Army Medical Center for histological examination of the irradiated brain material. The help of Mr. M. S. Cohen in design of ultrasonic equipment and of Miss Ann Conant in extensive animal work was invaluable for the success of our investigations. We also wish to acknowledge the use of calibration facilities of the M.I.T. Acoustics Laboratory.

References

Ackerman, E. and W. Holak. 1953. Ceramic Probe Microphones. WADC Tech. Report 52–77. 21 pp.

Barth, G., J. Paetzold and F. Wachsmann. 1949. Über den Wirkungsmechanismus biologischer Ultraschallreaktionen; Möglichkeiten zur Klärung des Wirkungsmechanismus. Strahlentherapie *80:* 305–311.

Catchpole, H. R. and I. Gersh. 1947. Pathogenetic factors and pathological consequences of decompression sickness. Physiol. Rev. *27:* 360–397.

Esche, R. 1952. Investigations on ultrasonic absorption in animal tissues and plastics. (In German) Acustica *2:* Akust. Beihefte No. 2: AB 71–AB 74.

Esche, R. 1952. Investigation of cavitation by sound in liquids. (In German) Acustica *2:* Akust. Beihefte No. 4: AB 208–AB 218.
Fry, W. J. 1953. Action of ultrasound on nerve tissue—A review. J. Acoust. Soc. Amer. *25:* 1–5.
Fry, W. J. and J. W. Barnard. 1954. IRE Convention Record. Part. 6: 102.
Fry, W. J. and R. B. Fry. 1954. Determination of absolute sound levels and acoustic absorption coefficients by thermocouple probes—Experiment. J. Acoust. Soc. Amer. *26:* 311–317.
Fry, W. J., W. H. Mosberg, Jr., J. W. Barnard and F. J. Fry. 1954. Production of focal destructive lesions in the central nervous system with ultrasound. J. Neurosurg. *11:* 471–478.
Hoepker, W. 1952. Die biologischen Wirkungen des Ultraschalls auf das Gehirn. Der Ultraschall in der Medizin *5:* 178–185.
Hug. O. and R. Pape. 1954. Ultraschall in Medizin und Grenzgebieten *7:* 42.
Koppelman, J. 1952. Contributions to ultrasonic measurement technique in liquids. (In German) Acustica *2:* 92-95.
Lehmann, J. 1949. Über die Temperaturabhängigkeit therapeutischer Ultraschallreaktionen unter besonderer Berücksichtigung der Wirkung auf Nerven. Strahlentherapie *79:* 543–552.
Lehmann, J. F. 1953. The biophysical mode of action of biologic and therapeutic ultrasonic reactions. J. Acoust. Soc. Amer. *25:* 17–26.
Lehmann, J. F. and J. F. Herrick. 1953. Biologic reactions to cavitation, a consideration for ultrasonic therapy. Arch. Phys. Med. *34:* 86–98.
Lindstrom, P. A. 1954. Prefrontal ultrasonic irradiation—A substitute for lobotomy. A.M.A. Arch. Neurol. and Psychiat. *72:* 399–425.
Peters, G. 1949. Die Wirkung der Ultraschallwellen auf das Zentralnervensystem. Strahlentherapie *79:* 653–658.
Rosenberg, M. D. Private communication.
Wall, P. D., W. J. Fry, R. Stephens, D. Tucker and J. Y. Lettvin. 1951. Changes produced in the central nervous system by ultrasound. Science *114:* 686–687.
Woeber, K. 1949. Über das Auftreten von Schädigungen am Zentralnervensystem der Ratte durch Ultraschallwellen. Strahlentherapie *79:* 643–652.

Dr. Ballantine: I would like to say at the outset that it is a great pleasure to be here and to open this discussion as a member of the group which Dr. Hueter has represented in a previous paper.

First of all I want to congratulate Dr. Fry on the magnificent presentation that began last evening and is going on through this morning. Dr. Fry's and Dr. Barnard's work, I think, speaks for itself.

To avoid any misunderstanding because we are in a sort of boundary layer between physics and medicine, and at such boundary layers all sorts of refractions and heat can be generated and reflections can be cast, or seem to be cast, I would like to make it clear that we have the highest respect for the work that Dr. Fry has done, and that any questions we may ask, or problems that we may raise, are generally for our help and for no other reason.

I want to make a few summarizing statements, based on the discussions here at the symposium and on our work in Boston. First of all, I believe we know that focused ultrasound can produce lesions in the central nervous system at a distance from the cerebral cortex, if you choose the focal depths correctly. Evidently, the intervening tissue is not damaged, although I do not believe we know for certain the exact limits of the damage to the tissues by the focused ultrasonic beam. I am open to correction on this point if someone wants to do so. I believe we have been shown today that the lesions are, to a degree, selective. How selective, again, is a point for discussion. Selectivity is based on the dosage, and I do not think any of us have a clear idea of what dosage is. I think that the one problem that bothers the neurosurgeon as he considers this method, aside from those that I have raised so far, is that of reproducibility. Now, we have had situations in our own experimental work in which a dosage parameter was chosen consisting of a certain number of pulses at a certain amplitude, which would produce a large lesion. We have gone back and repeated that in another cat and have found no lesion at all. I am wondering if this is a problem which we have to solve uniquely, or whether this has occurred with the work that has gone on at the University of Illinois. I would like to know if we could have a statistical analysis of a given dosage parameter and the percent of reproducibility of a lesion at a given site within the brain of an experimental animal at that parameter. Thank you.

Dr. Schwan: I wish to stress the importance of a knowledge of the variability of the absorption coefficient of the tissues in brain. Dr. Hueter showed one curve which indicates an absorption of about 20 percent in a distance of 15 millimeters for the 1 megacycle frequency. Now, if you assume, just to give an example of the importance of variability in the absorption coefficient, that the coefficient is uncertain by a factor of 2 then we could conclude that for this depth of about 15 millimeters, the dosage specification is uncertain by 25 percent. In other words, for lesions very near to the surface of the brain an uncertainty in absorption coefficients obviously does not affect the totally applied dosage very much. But for deeper brain lesions the absorption coefficient must be known much more exactly. Therefore, there must be a critical relationship between the acceptable uncertainty in the value of the absorption coefficient and the depth at which we can produce lesions within the 25 percent margin stated by Dr. Fry.

Dr. Fry: As far as variability in absorption coefficient is concerned, the only comment I can make at the moment is that in some experiments which we performed on rats' spinal cords, we had a variation (from one animal to another) in the absorption coefficient, of about 10 percent as indicated by the time rate of temperature rise in response to a sound pulse of constant intensity and duration. This was recorded by placing a thermocouple in the spinal cord of the rat. Up to the present time, this is the only data that we have, which indicates the variation in the absorption coefficient from one animal to another. We do not presently have any information on the variation of the absorption coefficient from one position to another within a single cat brain.

Regarding the question of dosage and its meaning, I might say that dosage is defined with respect to some particular end-point. For example, we may describe dosage with respect to histological changes produced by the sound as described by Dr. Barnard this morning. This is one end-point, namely histological change. Another end-point which we have used is electrical response. For example, we have employed an experimental situation wherein we observe a two neuron arc response which is suppressed by an acoustic exposure. We can then describe and determine the dosage in relation to this particular criterion of suppression. Another dosage relation can be described in terms of paralysis of the hind legs of a mouse. There are these three different approaches that we are using at the present time, and I believe the group at M.I.T. is using a couple of different approaches.

It is readily possible to make clear what is meant by a dosage relation and a dosage determination, but in order to do so definite criteria must be formulated which are capable of precise tests. The choice of criteria may be somewhat arbitrary, and there is no assurance whatsoever that each different choice will yield the same type of relation. You must make judgments regarding the criteria to be used, and if your judgment is fruitful, you derive results which have some interesting relation to the biological system and the response you are studying. I do not think that at the present time it is possible to describe a dosage relation, a single, unique dosage relation into which everything of interest can be incorporated.

I want to make a comment on the scattering of the paralysis results that Dr. Hueter discussed. We have done some work with mice and find that under precisely controlled conditions of irradiation, for example precise control of temperature, and accurate localization of the sound beam with respect to the particular section of the spinal cord irradiated, it is possible to reduce the scattering from one animal to another to a rather small percentage. We have been using paralysis of the hind legs of the young mouse as an end-point in a dosage study using a deficit in function as a criterion. An analysis of the data yields the result that at a constant intensity the time of exposure for 10 percent of the animals paralyzed differs by only 15 percent from the exposure time for 90 percent of the animals paralyzed.

There is one other point. I believe Dr. Hueter concluded that it is not, at the present time, too feasible to carry out localized irradiations to produce localized lesions in the depth of the brain. Is that what you indicated?

DR. HUETER: No—lesions where you would want to use selectivity.

DR. FRY: Blood vessels, or what kind of selectivity?

DR. HUETER: Let us assume the case of a small structure of white matter imbedded in grey matter deep down in the brain. We want to irradiate that and use the margin of selectivity between the two types of tissues. We base our dosage on that. In a large mass of white matter you want to hit a specific spot rather accurately. Can you do that?

DR. FRY: Yes. We can remove a fiber tract area out of surrounding grey matter without difficulty at the present time. On the basis of the experience we have, there is no great difficulty in selectively destroying a fiber tract surrounded by a mass of grey matter.

DR. HUETER: May I just go to the blackboard for a moment? There was one very interesting observation last night which I think should be discussed. Some of these irradiations have been made with multiple shots, where you move the irradiator over a small amount in between the shots. There apparently was one slide where you made Shot No. 1 and you got a lesion of a certain size, and you then moved over and made Shot No. 2 with the same intensity and the same duration, and you got a slightly larger lesion. Then you moved over again and made Shot No. 3 after the same interval, and you got an even larger lesion, and Shot No. 4 was perhaps still larger. It was explained that Shot No. 1 had set up a temperature distribution in the tissue which modified the response of the tissue so that Shot No. 2, although given with the same intensity and duration, produced a larger lesion, and this condition again modified Shot No. 3. Is this not a very difficult situation? I believe the conclusion was that it is necessary to wait a long time between shots in order to permit the tissue to cool off, but one would really have to know what the thermal situation, conduction, and so forth is, in whatever region you work in order to plan the duration between the shots. For instance, did you not agree that in one shot at 220 watts/cm.^{2} at 4-second duration you would produce a maximum temperature rise of the order of 10 degrees? Murray Rosenberg has a theory applicable to focal regions within which you can calculate this, and in calculating it for your focal area, Murray has found a 12° temperature rise. A 10° temperature rise would change the biological response of the system appreciably and this would increase the dosage quite a bit.

DR. FRY: Every dosage must be described with respect to the time between shots. For example, in producing a small lesion if you want to accomplish it with one shot or a couple of shots, it is desirable to wait a considerable time between shots, because the overlapping of this residual effect is important. The slides of the cats with the large lesions had a fixed time interval between adjacent shots. In that particular case, I think it was 30 seconds, so we have a whole dosage study in which a 30-second interval was used between shoots for the production of large-sized lesions. At the present time, it appears that the best procedure, for small lesions, when you have to use more than one shot, is to wait a considerable time, say five minutes between shots. However, if you are going to produce a large lesion, then you can decrease this considerably because the following situation obtains. The number of shots interior to the border of the lesion is large compared to the number of shots on the border of the lesion. The dosage, intensity and duration of exposure per shot, is chosen so that the desired tissue change is produced at the interior points. The shots at the peripheral points act to set up an environmental condition for the interior points which is relatively constant from one interior point to another if the time between shots is kept fixed.

DR. HUETER: You have this variable of time between shots and a possible variability in heat conduction that enters the picture—which would influence your selectivity. Is it not necessary to know how this works in all regions of the brain and at all intensities?

DR. FRY: Yes, if the heat conductivity coefficient also varies considerably from one part of the brain to the other. There aren't to my knowledge, any values available of the heat conductivity coefficient as a function of position in the brain. Large lesions can be produced in the subcortical white matter and internal capsule equally well.

DR. HUETER: What is your beam, 2 millimeters in diameter?

DR. FRY: The beam is 1.5 millimeters in diameter.

DR. HUETER: If you apply a hydrostatic pressure how does this effect the dosage for a given change?

DR. FRY: If you plot sound pressure amplitude as a function of the reciprocal of the time for production of paralysis of the hind legs of frogs, then for a hydrostatic pressure of 1 atmosphere we get a straight line and for 13 atmospheres we get a second straight line. The same threshold (minimum sound intensity at which paralysis can be obtained) is obtained in both cases but at values of the sound intensity above threshold the duration of exposure to produce the paralysis in the 13 atmosphere case is greater than the duration required at one atmosphere.

DR. NYBORG: I would like to say something in regard to the physical aspects of the matter. In connection with cavitation, I think it might be worth while to distinguish between the destructive effects which are more commonly regarded as an aspect of cavitation and the milder effects which might nevertheless be important, and which might be associated with the presence of cavities or bubbles or nuclei. I do not believe that there is adequate information as to just how many such nuclei or small gas bubbles may exist in the normal living organism. Since at a megacycle a resonant bubble would be of the order of a micron, it would be hard to carry out such a study to determine how many effective gas bubbles might be present. I mention this not because I have a feeling it is an important one, but it is one that should be ruled out, namely that one might have acoustic stirring, that is some sort of convection, which has an effect on the biological processes. In this case the temperature would have an effect, not only in itself but also in effecting the stirring. The viscosity would tend to be decreased as the temperature is increased, which would, in turn, decrease the boundary layers. One would expect, therefore, an increase effect in convection if it were present and important.

Some Examples of Ultrasonic Frequency Sensitive and Frequency Insensitive Biological Reactions

René-Guy Busnel

L'Institut National de la Recherche Agronomique à Jouy-en-Josas (S.-&-O.), France

I WOULD LIKE TO DISCUSS some experiments in which the effective role of the frequency of the ultrasonic radiation was being specifically studied. Most investigators and especially biologists utilize commercial ultrasonic generators which have only one, two, or three frequencies, as determined by the manufacturer. In addition, the types of apparatus used in the scientific studies are quite different. Therefore, a comparison of results obtained by various investigators employing such diverse generators and procedures is a difficult project. Despite these shortcomings I would like to report on some work which we have accomplished in our laboratory. As indicated, we are particularly interested in a systematic study of the role of frequency in ultrasonic action. Frequencies from 19 kilocycles to 1 megacycle in liquids and from 1 to 100 kilocycles in air have been used to determine in what kind of reactions the frequency was a determining factor and in what kind it was of no importance. I would like to discuss a few cases in which these two types of reaction are demonstrated.

Experiments with Preferential Action of the Frequency

In those cases in which the frequency shows a preferential action, it has been found that cavitation is generally involved. We studied the oxidation of potassium iodide under conditions of known power output determined by calorimetric measurements. The following frequencies were studied under exactly identical conditions: 192, 240, 320, 412, 612, 640, 720, and 960 kilocycles. The results of these experiments, expressed in amount of iodine released as a function of frequency, showed a definite influence of wave length. As indicated in Fig. 1, the reaction increased with increase of frequency, reached a plateau between 240 and 412 kilocycles—the reaction is maximum at approximately 300 kilocycles—then there is a flat region or plateau from around 400 kilocycles out to 1 megacycle. Additional experiments performed at low frequencies of 19 and 150 kilocycles gave very low

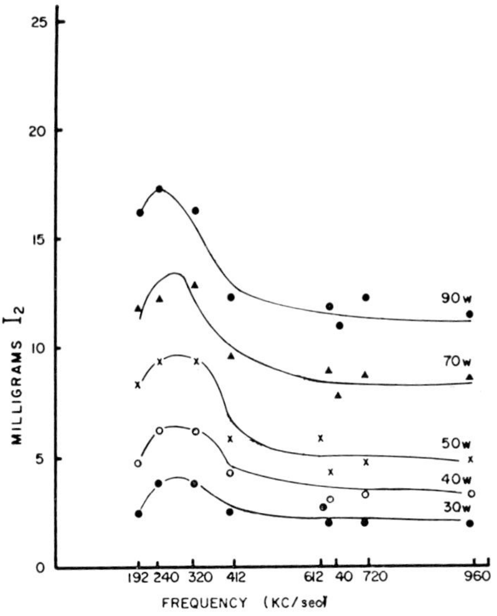

FIG. 1. Released iodine, resulting from the oxidation of KI by ultrasound, as a function of the ultrasonic frequency.

results and at 1, 2, and 3 megacycles evidenced a decrease after the plateau. The long plateau leads us to suppose that the reaction is frequency independent between the limits 400 kilocycles through 1 megacycle. Cavitation may be considered the principal reactive agent in these cases because the mechanism of cavitation, which is a function of the frequency, directly enters into the reaction.

Experiments Where the Frequency Is Not an Essential Factor

As an example of experimentation in which the frequency is apparently unimportant, we may consider the germinative acceleration of ultrasonated barley seeds. This work was done in cooperation with the Canadian scientist, G. Obolensky. The metabolic processes of germination (hydration, absorption, water content, respiration) are all accelerated by treatment with ultrasonic waves (with parameters similar to those used in the oxidative study) but are not influenced by the different frequencies employed (23, 30, 80, 412, 570, 720, 960 kilocycles). The different methods used for these studies in plant physiology (water content, isotopic phosphorus 32, ash content, microcalorimetry) showed that the growth acceleration was due primarily to greater membrane action of ultrasound.

The results of our experiments on young plants (four days after germination) irradiated at 3 watts/cm.[2] for various durations and for three par-

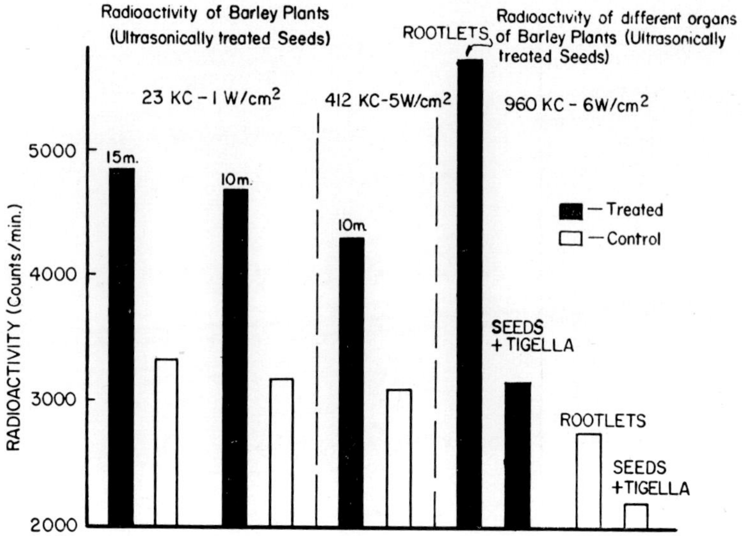

FIG. 2. Radioactivity of barley plants—comparison of plants treated by ultrasound at different frequencies with untreated plants.

ticular frequencies show that the fresh weight versus frequency relation shows no frequency effect. Using the same procedure, but with P^{32} in the nutritive solution, the ashes of the plants were measured for radioactivity to determine the uptake of the isotope and these values were plotted. As indicated in Fig. 2, there was no correspondence between the frequency and the isotopic uptake. Again using the 3 watts/cm.^{2} intensity and the same three frequencies, the respiration of the seeds was studied by means of an automatic recording microcalorimeter developed in France. We obtained no statistical difference between the results at the different frequencies. At the low frequencies, with an intensity level of 3 watts/cm.^{2}, we are quite certain that we do not have chemical cavitation in the seeds. Therefore, this is certainly an example of a purely mechanical action of ultrasonic waves.

Another type of problem that we have investigated is concerned with animal phonotropisms, i.e., reactions of animals to acoustic stimuli. The phonotropisms can be subdivided into: phonotaxis, the attraction or repulsion of the animal; phonokinesis, the reaction of the animal but with no movement toward or away from the source; and phonoresponse, the excitation which induces the animal to reply to the acoustic signal. Phonotropisms have been reported by our laboratory using Orthoptera, Batrachia, and birds, and in the literature by Timm and Schaller (1950) with Lepidoptera. The reactions were provoked by acoustic signals produced by gen-

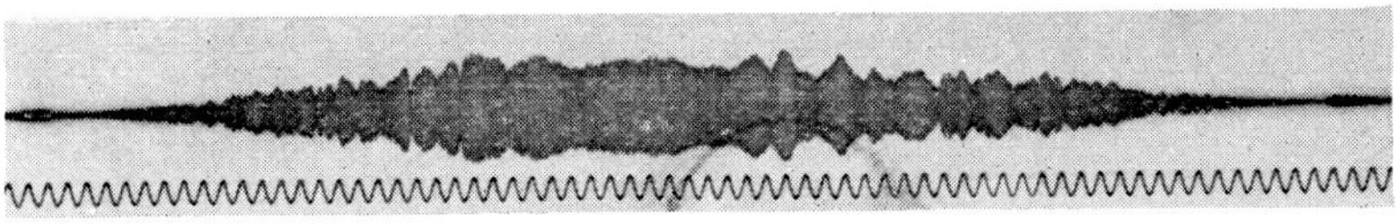

FIG. 3. Waveform of acoustic output from Galton Whistle—no response from grasshopper.

erators and transmitted either in gas or water. These signals provoked a similar reaction for frequencies so widely dispersed that it seems that frequency does not have an essential character. As an example of the method employed in this experimentation, I will briefly discuss the work with the female grasshopper (*Ephippigera*). We used either a Galton whistle or a special loudspeaker giving a very large range of ultrasonic waves (ionophone). The same reaction is observed in either case, namely each sonic emission causes the animal to jump while a steady progression is made in the direction of the sound source. Over the range of frequencies from 2 to 20 kilocycles the same response is always obtained. If you use the form of the signal as indicated in Fig. 3 at the different frequencies between 50 cycles and 50,000 cycles you never get a response from the animal. However, if you cut the magnetic tape so that you get a signal of the form indicated in Fig. 4, you always get a reaction from the animal between the range of 50 to 50,000 cycles. For example, Fig. 5 indicates a particular form of the signal which will always give a reaction when applied at a frequency of 9700 cycles. Fig. 6 shows another form of the signal that will give a reaction in the indicated frequency range. You can get the same reaction from the same signal for many species of insects and many species of moths. Timm and Schaller in Germany have published results on twenty-five or thirty species of moths showing a response of negative phonotaxis, i.e., the moths stop their flight in midair and drop to the floor in response to the signal. During a personal discussion, Schaller indicated the reaction is dependent on the form of the signal and seems to have no relation to the

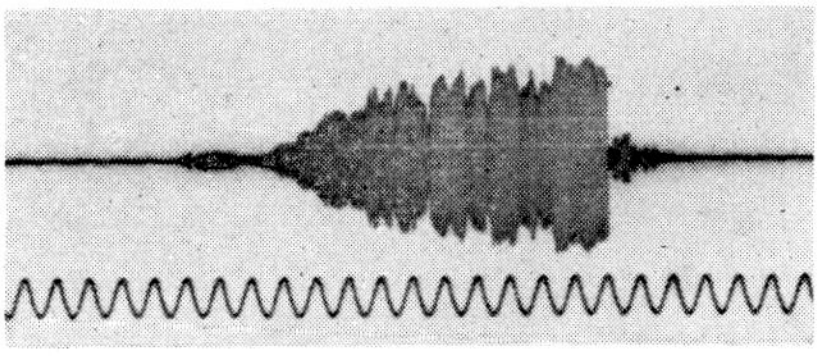

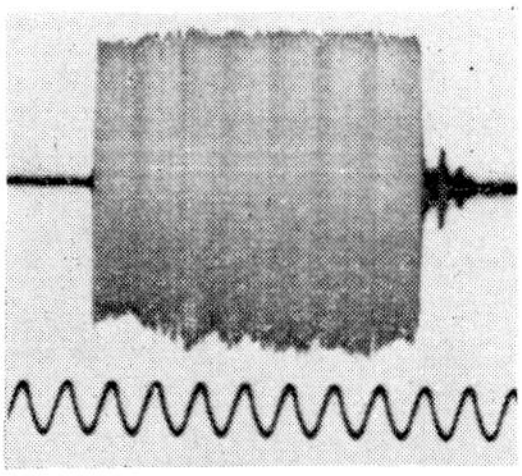

FIG. 4. Acoustic output from Galton Whistle terminated abruptly—always a response from grasshopper.

FIG. 5. Second example of an acoustic signal which always elicits a response from the grasshopper.

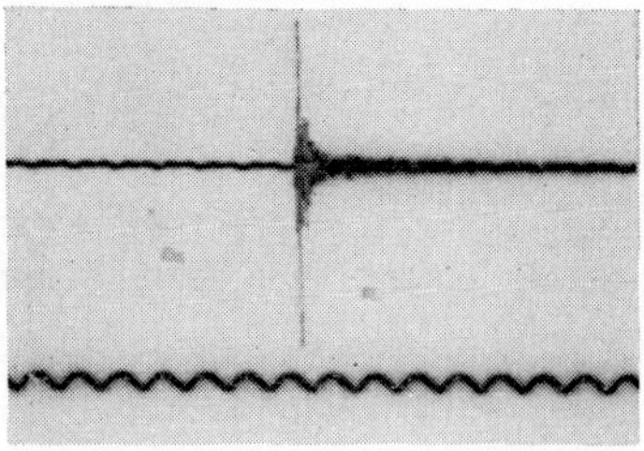

FIG. 6. Third example of an acoustic signal which always elicits a response from the grasshopper.

frequency in the range studied. We obtained the same reaction in other species, especially the frog (*Hyla arborea*) and some other animal forms.

There is one other example where the frequency is not the most important factor, namely in audiogenic seizures in mice. This experiment was first performed by Frings of Pennsylvania State University. It is possible to obtain a seizure between 10 and 25 kilocycles. We repeated this work in our laboratory and obtained the seizures between 100 cycles and 25 kilocycles. The reaction of the animals is not related to the frequency in this range. As a matter of fact, these reactions can be obtained only with a certain intensity level and with a particular form of the signal. It should be of interest to physiologists that the general reaction of animals (phonotaxis and phonokineses) shows points in common with the reaction of neuromuscular preparations to electrical current—namely that it is the break in the excitation process which provokes the reaction and not the current itself—as outlined in the laws of Pflüger and DuBois-Reymond.

The animal reactions to acoustic signals are apparently due to organs which are pressure receptive or at least receptive to variations in sonic pressure. Their sensibility is of the type called "differential" as defined by Loeb, with frequency independence through large limits.

Experiments Where the Importance of Frequency Is Controversial

Studies of emulsions, either of water and organic compounds of the vinyl chloride type or vegetal oil for intravenous injections, obtained by ultrasonic irradiation from magnetostrictive or quartz generators or even an ultrasonic whistle at 23, 240, 640, 960 kilocycles, were performed in conjunction with Degrois, Jobard, and Quaintel. In all cases, independent of the frequency, the proportion of tensio-active agents was reduced in similar proportions. However, other experimenters (Audoin and Levasseur, 1948) have found preferential frequencies or even frequencies at which no emulsification occurred, specifically with 576 and 720 kilocycles. The criterion in these examples of mechanical actions seems to be a factor bound to the nature of the products and probably to their viscosity.

Conclusions

The numerous measurements for each experiment cited here were made under strictly identical conditions of method of treatment, temperature, system of waves, type of generator and intensity. The results obtained indicate that it is necessary to know considerably more about ultrasonic actions before it will be possible to establish particular laws such as the relation between the reaction studied and the wave length. The diversity of the conditions of treatment employed by different experimenters has not assisted in the determination of these laws. It is hoped that systematic measurements will be made in specialized laboratories, in order to aid biologists in the development of better application of ultrasonic techniques.*

References

Audouin, A. and G. Levasseur. 1948. Note No. 158 du C. R. S. I. M. de Marseille. (18 mai 1948)

Busnel, R. G. 1955. Mise en évidence d'un caractère physique réactogène essentiel de signaux acoustiques synthétiques déclenchant les phonotropismes dans le règne animal. Comp. Rend. Acad. Sci. *240:* 1477–1479.

Busnel, R. G. 1955. Probabilité du rôle prédominant d'un des caractères physiques des signaux acoustiques artificiels dans le règne animal. Jour. Physiol. *47:* 123–128.

Busnel, R. G. and B. Dumortier. 1954. Comp. Rend. Soc. Biol. *148:* 1751.

Busnel, R. G. and B. Dumortier. 1955. Comp. Rend. Soc. Zool. *80:* 23–27.

Busnel, R. G., W. Loher, and F. Pasquinelly. 1954. Recherches sur les signaux acoustiques réactogènes pour divers acrididae ♂. Comp. Rend. Soc. Biol. *148:* 1987–1991.

Busnel, R. G. and G. Obolensky. 1954. Action des ultrasons sur la vitesse de germination et la croissance de l'orge. Comp. Rend. Acad. Sci. *239:* 777–778.

Busnel, R. G. and G. Obolensky. 1955. Étude microcalorimétrique de l'accélération de la germination des graines traitées aux ultrasons. Comp. Rend. Acad. Sci. *240:* 1358–1360.

Busnel, R. G. and G. Obolensky. 1955. Recherches préliminaires sur l'action des ultrasons de haute et basse fréquence sur la germination de l'orge. Ultraschall in Medizin und Grenzgebieten *8:* 8–18.

Busnel, R. G. and D. Picard. 1952. Relation between the wave length and the oxidation of potassium iodide by ultrasonics. Comp. Rend. Acad. Sci. *235:* 1217–1220.

Busnel, R. G., D. Picard, and H. Bouzigues. 1953. Relations between the wave length and the oxidation of potassium iodide by ultrasonics. Jour. de Chimie Physique *50:* 97–101.

Degrois, M., M. Jobard, and R. Michallet. 1955. Cong. Internat. sur les traitements par les U. S. a Marseille.

* The experiments summarized in this paper have been previously published in various French scientific journals; readers should check the bibliography for the experimental details and values of results.

Frings, H. and M. Frings. 1952. Acoustical determinants of audiogenic seizures in laboratory mice. J. Acoust. Soc. Amer. *24:* 163–169.
Quaintel, A. 1953. Diplome de radiologie de la Faculte de Medecine de Paris.
Schaller, F. and C. Timm. 1950. Zeits. f. vergl. Physiol. *32:* 468–481.
Schevill, W. E. and B. Lawrence. 1953. Auditory response of a bottle-nosed porpoise, *Tursiops truncatus,* to frequencies above 100 kc. J. Exper. Zool. *124:* 147–165.

DR. BALDES: How did you apply three watts/cm.^{2} to the barley seeds?

DR. BUSNEL: Fig. 1 indicates the set-up used to irradiate the barley seeds in the water. Please note that the liquid under study is placed in the bottle and the power measurements are made right in the bottle by calorimetric techniques.

DR. HUETER: This is fine at a megacycle or at 200 kilocycles, but you quoted frequencies as low as 20 kilocycles. Wouldn't you have a completely different field distribution?

DR. BUSNEL: Yes sir, but we made the measurements only in the bottle, and, therefore, that is not important.

DR. HUETER: Let us say at one megacycle you have a rather good beam which irradiates into your bottle, while at 20 kilocycles, where you have a magnetostrictive crystal, you probably have very large wave lengths. There is probably only one wave length, or two, across the bottle.

DR. BUSNEL: That is true, but if you make the measurement of the power in the bottle with the calorimetric methods which expresses the total degradation of the ultrasonic energy (independently of the frequency) in a determined volume, you always obtain the same value. These measurements are quite reliable.

DR. HUETER: It is a little difficult to define the quantity, let us say, 3 watts/cm.^{2} at 1 megacycle and at 20 kilocycles if the field is so different.

DR. BUSNEL: That is true, but there are not many possibilities for measurements. We measure the frequency, we measure the system of waves and we also control the power. It is impossible to control another parameter. If you can suggest another technique, I would be very grateful. I must add that each author, when he indicates ultrasonic power, refers to watts per square centimeter (w./cm.^{2}), which indicates mostly a mean statistical power and supposes a uniform radiation field of the projectors.

DR. HUETER: You could measure the pressure amplitude in your vessel.

DR. BUSNEL: It is possible, but it is very difficult to obtain a relation between the several frequencies.

DR. SCHWAN: May I interrupt a moment? If I understand correctly, this is a set-up which you used in the studies which you referred to in the beginning of your lecture. In those slides you showed curves which had a rather pronounced peak, around 300 kilocycles, a relatively flat plateau. It seems to me the criticism Dr. Hueter formulates could not substantially alter this response.

DR. HUETER: Unless your phenomenon rests at 300 kilocycles.

DR. SCHWAN: The curves indicate two mechanisms which are involved. There was a sort of resonant peak at about 300 kilocycles and a response which was comparatively frequency independent.

DR. BUSNEL: That is right. However, at very low frequencies (19–20 kc./s.) there is no oxidation as at very high frequencies (2–3 mc./s.).

DR. SCHWAN: My question in regard to the curve was, would it indicate two different mechanisms; one mechanism associated with this sort of resonance peak, and another mechanism associated with this more flat part at high frequencies. I wonder if you have any idea if there are two different mechanisms, and what they are.

DR. BUSNEL: I don't understand why we have this peak in the curve. For the very high and very low frequencies one may think that the absence or decrease of the oxidation values is connected to the absence or decrease of true cavitation; in the frequency range we studied, true cavitation is always present. It is possible that there might be a preferential threshold around 300 kilocycles/s., perhaps associated with a resonance phenomenon which I cannot, as yet, explain. However, this phenomenon would be considered to be within the general physico-chemical actions of ultrasonic cavitation.

DR. HERRICK: The question was the measurement of the energy and not the biologic reaction. Dr. Hueter wanted to know how you could apply a measurement more applicable to a higher frequency, to your power at the low frequency.

DR. BUSNEL: The difference of the frequency between 190 and 290 kilocycles is really the same. Also between 350 and 412 kilocycles. The difference between the frequency is not very high, and the value is very different. It is impossible to make a mistake in the measurements.

DR. NYBORG: I think you said cavitation was present.

DR. BUSNEL: Yes, oxidation of the potassium iodide is possible only when you get true cavitation. It is a mechanism with a luminescence phenomenon.

DR. SCHWAN: Is there a substantial variation between different types of insects, or would you say that all insects respond to the very high frequency?

DR. BUSNEL: In some species, especially in Orthoptera, we use high frequency. In this species all answer to 50,000 c.p.s. Lepidoptera (moths) respond to 15 kilocycles and 175 kilocycles. For the mosquito it is between 10 and 10,000 cycles.

DR. SCHWAN: In other words, there is very substantial variation from one type to the other. We cannot simply say all insects are higher than, let us say, human beings.

DR. HUETER: If you take one of these grasshoppers, they make a particular music of their own. If you put that on a tape and use that to attract them, do they respond more to their own noise?

DR. BUSNEL: To answer your question, I can say that it is a matter of intensity. If the recorded noise is much louder than their own song, they will respond to it. However, the reaction to the synthetic signal is very different than the reaction to the normal signal. The normal signal is attractive between male and female only in the same species. Our signal is not specific. You attract many different species with the same signal. It is a physiological reaction given by the level of the pressure and the transients; that is the term we use for the definition.

A Forum on an Ultrasonic Method for Measuring the Velocity of Blood

E. J. Baldes, W. R. Farrall, M. C. Haugen[1] and J. F. Herrick

Section of Biophysics, Mayo Clinic and Mayo Foundation, Rochester, Minnesota

Presented by Dr. Baldes.

I AM GOING TO INTRODUCE the subject of blood flow, and let my three colleagues give you the details of the possible application of the ultrasonic technique. As the title of this paper indicates, we are interested in the development of a flowmeter for the measurement of blood velocity. What, then, are the criteria that must be sought? First, if the measurement of blood flow is to be achieved in the most nearly physiologic manner possible, then it is apparent that an unopened blood vessel usually supplying an organ of the animal or an extremity must be used. In addition, after application of the unit to the blood vessel, it is most desirable to obtain the value of the flow on the animal after complete recovery from the surgical procedure involved in application of the unit. Only in this manner can we meet the complete physiologic conditions of a normal state.

Various methods, too numerous to mention, for measuring flow have been developed throughout the years of study of the circulation of blood. Many of these methods are adaptations of those employed by physicists and engineers for measuring the flow of Newtonian liquids. To measure the flow of blood without any interference whatsoever with the closed vascular system is a particularly difficult problem. The fact that such a method does not exist today which is generally acceptable to all physiologists is sufficient evidence for the difficulties associated with the accurate measurement of blood flow.

Our experience in the past has involved chiefly the use of the Rein (1928) thermostromuhr unit and its modifications (Herrick and Baldes, 1931; Baldes and Herrick, 1937). The active elements of this unit—a differential thermocouple with a heater unit midway between the thermojunctions—are housed in transparent bakelite. After careful calibration with excised blood vessels, a unit of proper size is carefully sterilized and applied to the blood vessel, and the four leads are brought out through a stab

[1] Milton, Wisconsin.

wound in the skin. Measurements of blood flow can then be made at any time, even weeks after the application of the unit to the blood vessel.

The Rein method is subject to several limitations. Calibration of a unit is effected with excised blood vessels before and after application in an animal. The over-all accuracy usually is ± 10 percent. Rapid variations in blood flow cannot be followed because 20 to 30 seconds are necessary to obtain thermal equilibrium for a steady state. The condition of zero blood flow is indeterminate (Herrick et al., 1938). In the hands of some physiologists, the method has proved to be a hazard.

However, the thermostromuhr approached the ideal method fairly closely because measurements could be made without opening the vascular system. Painstaking care was essential at all times in order to work within the limits which this method imposed. The thermostromuhr is not a method which can be used without considerable experience and without an understanding of the conditions required for reliability. These latter comments are not peculiar to the thermostromuhr. The intelligent use of any instrument requires a rigorous analysis of its "personality." We are interested in a method of blood flow measurement which is definitely more reliable than the Rein thermostromuhr, and we are now looking in the direction of the ultrasonic technique. Dr. Herrick will discuss this further.

Presented by Dr. Herrick.

While attending a course entitled "Acoustics in Testing and Processing" at the Massachusetts Institute of Technology during the summer of 1951, I learned that rates of flow could be measured by acoustic methods. The sound in this case is used as a measuring stick, and the amounts of acoustic power needed for this application are small and incidental. Hence, the biologic effects of ultrasound caused by larger amounts of acoustic power may be considered as negligible. A survey of the application of acoustic flowmeters at this time indicated that reliable measurements could be made provided the order of magnitude of flow was large. Adaptation of acoustic methods to such small flows as those even in the arteries of experimental animals appeared to be questionable.

When the literature was reviewed, a paper published in 1950 by Hess, Swengel and Waldorf, entitled "An Ultrasonic Method for Measuring Water Velocity," was found. Publications by these same authors (Swengel, Hess and Waldorf, 1954; Ibid., 1955) have appeared subsequently. The most recent publication by Swengel (1955) is particularly interesting. Kalmus and his associates (Kalmus, 1954; Kalmus, Hedrich and Pardue, 1954) have described an acoustic flowmeter which is adaptable to liquids having flows within the range of the flow of blood. In fact, these authors suggested the application of their instruments to the measurement of blood flow.

It was the work of Swengel and his associates and also the work of Kalmus and his associates that encouraged us to develop the ultrasonic flowmeter which we wish to describe at this time. The years of experience which we have amassed in measurements of blood flow made us realize that the ultrasonic method has the following outstanding advantages: (1) it is indirect, meaning that measurements can be made without opening the blood vessel; (2) it is fast, meaning that measurements can be made within the interval of the cardiac cycle; and (3) the source of the index observed is foreign to any biologic entity (ultrasonic waves of the order of magnitude of 300 kilocycles and higher do not occur naturally in the usual laboratory animal, so far as we know at present).

The fundamental principle underlying the measurement of the velocity of a flowing liquid by means of ultrasound is relatively simple: measurement of the difference in transit times for the transmission of sound upstream and downstream between two similar transducers (cylindric in our instrument) spaced on the outside of the liquid-carrying tube.

Although the principle is simple, the application of it is difficult to achieve. The requirements for accurate performance of the electronic equipment are so severe that the circuitry is working almost beyond its physically realizable limits. These severe requirements would tend to discourage electronic engineers who are inexperienced in medical electronics. The two members of our team who will describe presently the performance of the flowmeter are largely responsible for its successful performance. Much additional developmental work needs to be done. However, we wished to hold a forum on the flowmeter at this symposium at which constructive and valuable criticism would be forthcoming. Mr. Haugen will now discuss the circuitry and some of the electronic problems.

Presented by Mr. Haugen.

The ultrasonic flowmeter measures that component of sound velocity, caused by flow of the liquid, between two stationary points in a liquid. It employs an ultrasonic-transducer assembly in the path of flow, as shown at the top of the block diagram (Fig. 1), consisting of two cylindric ceramic transducers mounted on the outside of a liquid-carrying tube. The tube may be a blood vessel or some inert plastic material; the liquid may be blood or, for convenience in experimental development, simply water. For this demonstration we have water flowing in a plastic tube.

What we are trying to measure is the difference in time required for sound waves to travel through the liquid between the two transducers when

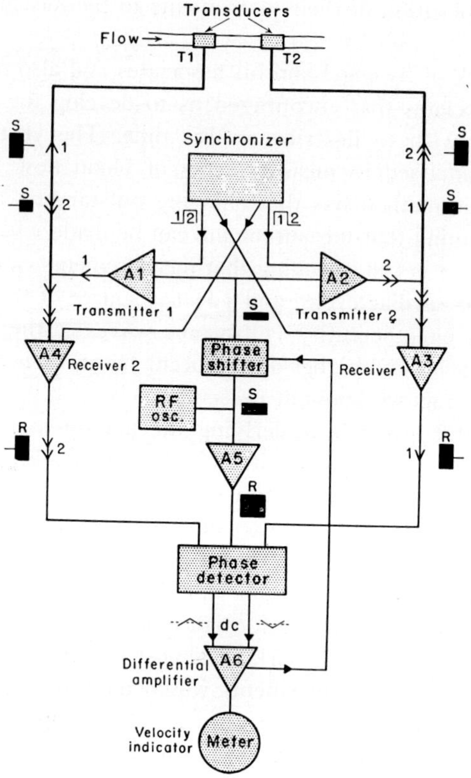

FIG. 1. Block diagram of the ultrasonic flowmeter. Wave forms are shown for one synchronizer cycle. Single and double arrowheads indicate direction of signal flow during intervals 1 and 2 of the cycle. Sinusoidal or rectangular radio-frequency wave forms are indicated by *S* or *R*. *A5* is the reference amplifier.

the liquid is stationary or moving. The difference in velocity of the sound is simply the velocity of flow of the liquid. Because this difference is a very small fraction of the total velocity, a balanced system is employed which is sensitive to the small difference in transit time of signals traveling up and down stream.

In order to measure only ultrasonic signals that travel through the liquid, it is essential that no appreciable sound be transmitted along the walls of the tubing. Experimentally it was found that a very small fraction of the signal is transmitted along the wall of a blood vessel at a frequency in the neighborhood of 300 to 400 kilocycles.

The problem, then, is to send ultrasonic waves of suitable frequency alternately up and down stream, to measure the difference in transit time or phase shift for signals going in the two directions, to process that datum, and to feed it into a meter calibrated in velocity of flow.

Referring again to the block diagram (Fig. 1), an oscillator of about 370 kilocycles feeds a signal through a phase shifter into two amplifiers labeled A1 and A2, which serve as transmitters to drive the transducers. Also connected to the transducers are amplifiers A3 and A4, which serve as receivers for signals generated in the transducers by ultrasonic waves in the liquid. The circuitry must be switched so that the signal goes first in one direction through the liquid and then in the other. This is accomplished by means of the synchronizer, which gates the transmitters and receivers and permits the radio-frequency signal to go through only one transmitter-receiver pair at a time. A phase detector compares the phase of each receiver output with that of the reference amplifier A5 and interprets phase difference of the two receivers in terms of velocity of flow. Phase-detector output is amplified by the differential amplifier A6, and is fed into a meter which indicates velocity of flow, both in magnitude and in direction, on a linear scale.

A unit cycle of flowmeter operation is one cycle of the synchronizer switching cycle, consisting of the two intervals designated 1 and 2. During interval 1 of the rectangular switching signal, which occurs at a frequency of about 100 times a second, the signal path is through transmitter A1, downstream between transducers, through receiver A3, and into the phase detector. During interval 2, the signal path is through transmitter A2, upstream between transducers, through receiver A4, and into a second section of the phase detector.

Each phase-detector tube has two control grids driven, respectively, by radio-frequency signals from the reference amplifier and one of the receivers. The phase shifter is adjusted so that these two signals are approximately in phase quadrature. The tube is biased to cut-off except when both signals are positive. The grid signals are of rectangular-wave form, and act as switches to turn the plate current on for one quarter of each radio-frequency cycle, during one half of a synchronizer cycle. The plate voltage decreases during conduction and increases during cut-off periods. Deviation in average d-c level is proportional to phase deviation from quadrature. When liquid is flowing between transducers, the output of one receiver becomes more nearly in phase with the reference amplifier, while the output of the other receiver becomes more nearly out of phase. Corresponding differences in average plate voltages are amplified by the differential amplifier, and are fed into a meter. Meter deflection is positive for one direction of flow and negative for the other.

Functionally, the circuit is rather simple. A radio-frequency signal alternates in direction between two transducers and the difference in phase shift is converted into a meter deflection proportional to velocity of flow. However, because the phase differences to be measured as as low as a few hundredths of a degree, sensitivity and stability requirements are difficult to meet. The main problems in design are to keep each half of the circuit balanced with respect to the other, and to obtain suitable wave forms.

Rectangular radio-frequency wave forms are required to operate the phase detector. Because there has been some uncertainty as to the best operating frequency, broad-band amplifiers are used throughout the radio-frequency path. This system provides reasonably rectangular wave forms with a fundamental frequency from 90 to 400 kilocycles. There are no tuned circuits except in the oscillator.

The most serious limitation of the equipment is zero drift resulting from unbalance between the two signal paths. Sensitivity to small unbalance conditions is aggravated by imperfect wave forms. This drift amounts to about plus or minus 5 percent of full scale for short periods. The error may be much greater for long-time measurements, unless some provision is made for checking and resetting zero balance during a run. Several methods are being considered to reduce zero drift, such as making the circuits less sensitive to errors in wave form and improving wave forms. Other conditions of unbalance causing drift are unequal phase shifts in the two paths and, especially in the phase-meter circuit, variations in tube characteristics.

An automatic phase control circuit compensates for balanced phase shifts common to both paths, in order to maintain the quadrature phase relations in the phase detector and to keep the phase detector operating at proper d-c potentials.

At present, the sensitivity of the ultrasonic flowmeter seems adequate for the measurement of normal blood flows through the larger blood vessels. Stability should be improved. Noise level is not a serious limitation.

Presented by Mr. Farrall.

At the start of this project several problems came to mind. They all revolved around the acoustic path over which flow was to be measured. First, was it possible to transmit enough energy over the path to give a reasonable signal to noise ratio? Results of early experiments with disk-type transducers were not promising, but they encouraged us to proceed. The later use of tubular transducers gave us much better coupling to the vessel, and resulted in an excellent signal-to-noise ratio.

Another problem seemed to be the amount of signal transmitted through the wall of the blood vessel. Results of experiments with blood vessels, rubber tubing, and plastic tubing convinced us that we would not encounter

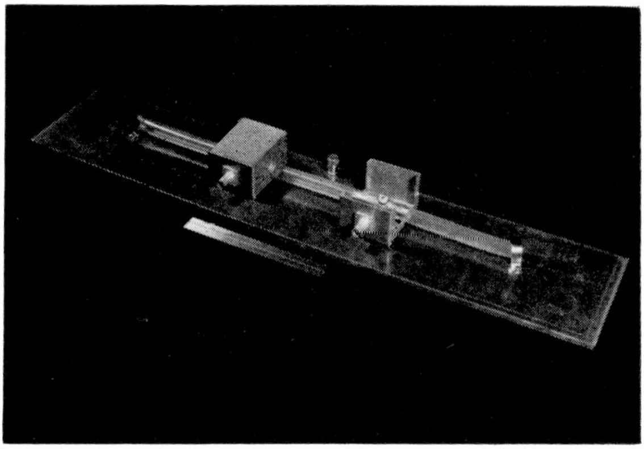

FIG. 2. Transducer assembly, in which disk-type transducers are used on a ½-inch tube.

difficulty with the signal propagated through the wall of the tube. The signal transmitted through the liquid in the tube or vessel was at least 100 times as great as the signal sent through the wall.

Since little is known about the acoustic properties of blood, experiments were conducted on blood and other liquids to ascertain if they exhibited similar properties in this type of acoustic system. Human blood, blood of dogs, isotonic solution of sodium chloride, and water all gave similar results. This encouraged us to use water as a test subject up to the final stages of development.

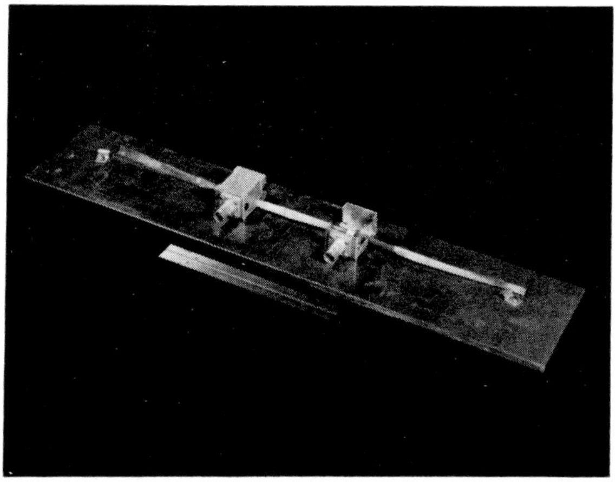

FIG. 3. Transducer assembly used in measurement of flow. Tubular transducers with diameters of $\frac{5}{32}$ inch are applied to a Penrose rubber tube.

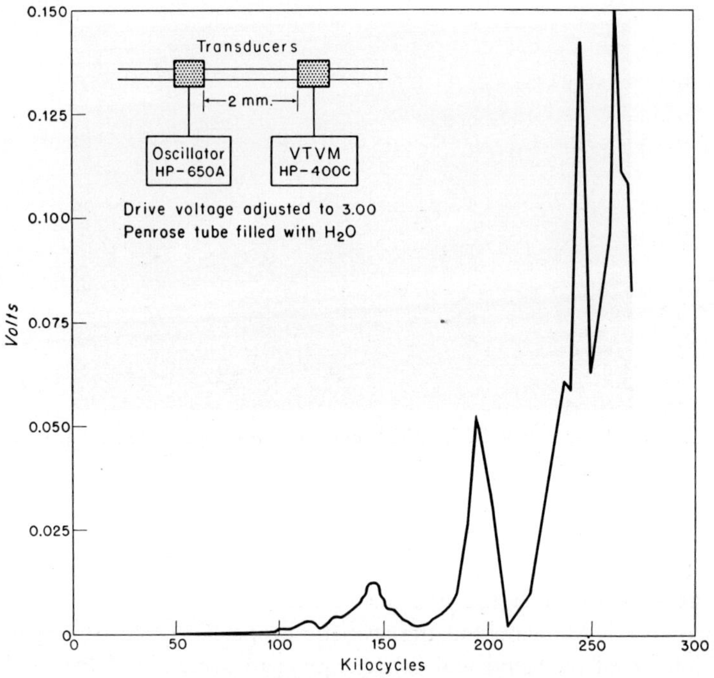

FIG. 4. The transducer system response.

Early transducer experiments were made with 3/16-inch barium titanate disks similar to the ones used by Kalmus. A test set-up in which this type of transducer is used is shown in Fig. 2. Poor acoustic coupling in this set-up gave us a very small received signal.

By the use of cylindric transducers which exactly fit the vessel, it was possible to obtain a good signal level. When this method was used a 200-millivolt signal was received an inch away from the driven transducer. The drive signal was 10 volts. The received signal was more than that required to operate our flowmeter. A transducer assembly which was used in our flow measurement is shown in Fig. 3. Cylindric transducers were used.

Frequency-response curves were obtained from all transducer systems to determine their optimal operating frequency. Fig. 4 shows a typical curve. Note that there are two resonance peaks near 250 kilocycles. These transducers do not have the same resonance frequency. A curve from identical transducers would show only one resonance peak. Of course, there may be other resonance peaks corresponding to different modes of vibration. Operation of the flowmeter was found possible over a wide range of frequency, but most satisfactory operation was obtained near the resonance of the transducer.

A development which has not yet proved satisfactory is the use of a slit-cylinder transducer. When this type of transducer is used, the blood vessel can be collapsed and pushed through the slit. The vessel then expands and holds the transducer on.

Fig. 5 shows the present flowmeter. The flowmeter is constructed in

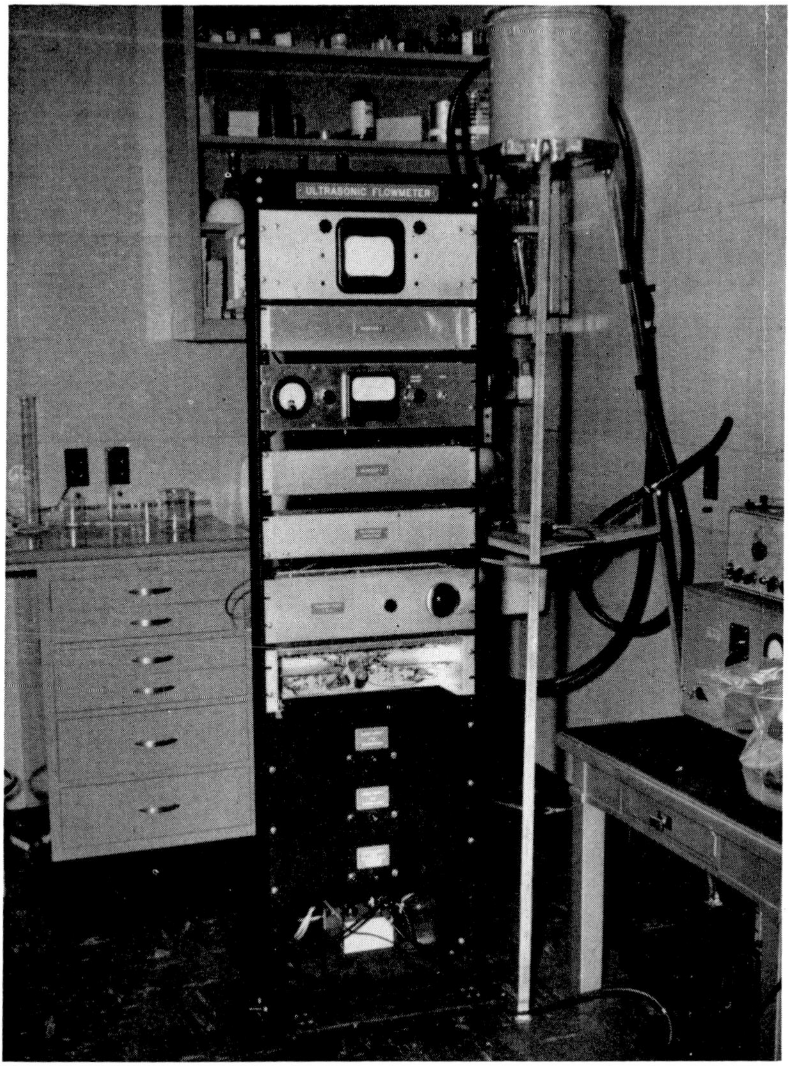

FIG. 5. Present flowmeter. The units from the top down are: oscilloscope, receiver 1, phasemeter, receiver 2, reference amplifier, transmitter, synchronizer, and three regulated power supplies.

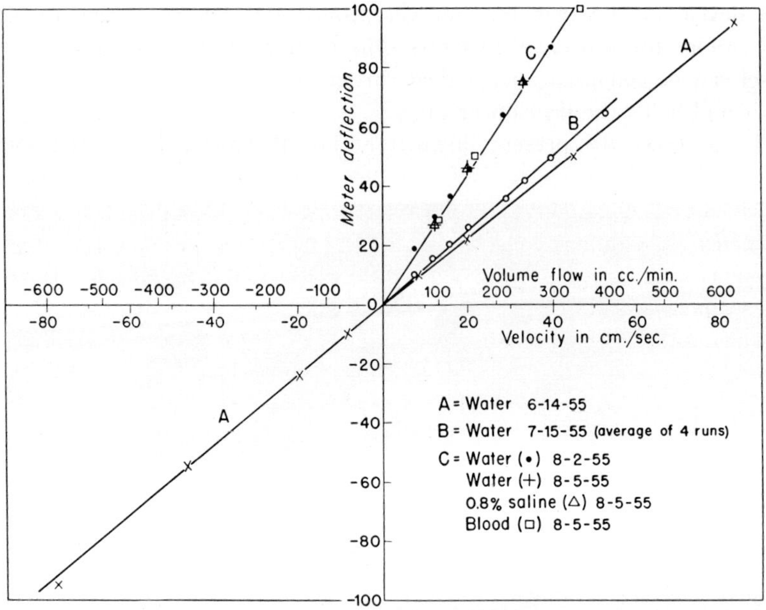

FIG. 6. Velocity calibration. Data corrected for zero drift.

units which are easily removed for modification. These units are mounted in a 6-foot relay rack.

For some time we have been able to detect flow with our flowmeter, but only recently have we been able to measure flow. Zero drift and erratic fluctuations have affected the flowmeter. Fluctuations arose from two different phenomena. As changes in flow occur, transient conditions are set up. The indication of flow follows the transients, but there is a small movement of the transducers along the vessel. This changes the length of the path and thus gives an incorrect reading of flow.

These changes in length of path are compensated for by the automatic phase-control circuit, a recent addition. When a shift in phase occurs in both signal paths, an error signal shifts the phase relationship in the transmitter and thus adjusts for the error. This control has effect over a limited range of transducer movement, and thus will not correct for gross movement.

Another source of erratic indication was traced to bubbles in the fluid. In operation, the flowmeter would give a steady indication until a bubble would come through; then the meter would become erratic until the bubble had passed through the transducers. The meter would then return to its stable state unless the bubble was very large. In that event, it sometimes was necessary to readjust the zero. By the use of boiled water these difficulties were eliminated.

A slow zero drift of unknown origin causes difficulty and makes it necessary to readjust the meter zero every few minutes. The total error amounts to about 5 percent. It appears that it will be possible to reduce the error to 1 percent. The maximal sensitivity is mainly dependent on the amount of drift, and could be increased greatly if the zero drift could be improved.

The present flowmeter has three ranges of sensitivity, 50 cc. per minute, 400 cc. per minute, and 800 cc. per minute full scale for a flow of a diameter of 5/32 inch. The ouput of the phasemeter circuit is linear with flow. Downstream flow is indicated with a positive meter deflection, while upstream flow is indicated with a negative meter deflection. Flow is indicated on a zero center meter with zero deflection corresponding to zero flow. A curve showing this relationship is shown in Fig. 6.

While a completely stable ultrasonic flowmeter for the measurement of blood in vivo has not yet been developed, the prospect is promising.

References

Baldes, E. J. and J. F. Herrick. 1937. A thermostromuhr with direct current heater. Proc. Soc. Exper. Biol. and Med. *37:* 432–435.

Herrick, J. F. and E. J. Baldes. 1931. The thermostromuhr method of measuring blood flow. Physics *1:* 407–417.

Herrick, J. F., E. J. Baldes and F. P. Sedgwick. 1938. Experimental analysis of Rein's thermostromuhr for small flows. (With appendix by Burton, A. C.: Appendix: Theory and Design of the Thermostromuhr.) J. Appl. Physics *9:* 124–131.

Hess, W. B., R. C. Swengel and S. K. Waldorf. 1950. An ultrasonic method for measuring water velocity. American Institute of Electrical Engineers, Miscellaneous Paper 50-214, October, 1950. Digest: Measuring Water Velocity by an Ultrasonic Method. Elec. Eng. *69:* 983.

Kalmus, H. P. 1954. Electronic flowmeter system. Rev. Sc. Instr. *25:* 201–206.

Kalmus, H. P., A. L. Hedrich and D. R. Pardue. 1954. The acoustic flowmeter using electronic switching. Trans. I.R.E. Professional Group on Ultrasonics Engineering, vol. 1, pp. 49–62.

Swengel, R. C. 1955. Antenna-type transducers for ultrasonic flowmetering. I.R.E. Convention Record, vol. 3, part 9, pp. 33–37.

Swengel, R. C., W. B. Hess and S. K. Waldorf. 1954. Demonstration of the principles of the ultrasonic flowmeter. American Institute of Electrical Engineers, Conference Paper C54–470, October, 1954. Digest: Elec. Eng. *73:* 1082–1084.

Swengel, R. C., W. B. Hess and S. K. Waldorf. 1955. Principles and application of the ultrasonic flowmeter. Trans. A.I.E.E., Part 3, April, 1955, pp. 112–118. Winter General Meeting of the American Institute of Electrical Engineers, February, 1955.

DR. SCHWAN: What was your minimum flow level that you registered?

MR. HAUGEN: Roughly in the order of 1 cc. per second.

DR. SCHWAN: You mentioned before you feel this is not your limit.

MR. HAUGEN: Right now our limit lies in the zero drift, and that is something we really have not yet investigated very thoroughly.

DR. REID: Is there any reason why this device could not be made to follow the velocity variations during systole and diastole? It would have to operate at frequencies of the order of 100 per second if the circuits could be worked out.

MR. HAUGEN: There is no reason why we should limit our switching rate to 100 per second. It is possible to operate at a much higher frequency.

DR. REID: Do you think it might be possible to follow the instantaneous velocity?

MR. HAUGEN: We could easily go to 1,000-cycle switching rate with no problem at all.

DR. VON GIERKE: In my opinion the main question here is, are you able with this kind of transducer arrangement to set up compressional waves in the blood? I wonder if you have any information with respect to this.

You have these two transducers reacting on the blood vessel, and this possibly sets up compressional waves, or some bouncing back and forth on the walls. Are you sure that the diameter and the walls of your tube do not enter the whole measurement technique?

DR. HERRICK: We used a small generator and a vacuum tube voltmeter to check that when the tube was empty. No signals went through.

DR. VON GIERKE: The only valid proof on this point, it appears to me, would be to determine, on an absolute scale, the sound velocity, i.e., measure the time that the pulse takes in transit from one transducer to the other. It could then be determined if the resultant sound velocity is approximately that of compressional waves in blood. You cannot consider the walls as rigid in this frequency range. The velocity of propagation you obtain is not the free field sound velocity, and it will always depend on the elastic properties of the wall.

DR. BALDES: It is the transit time difference between upstream and downstream only that we are considering.

DR. VON GIERKE: But this time difference would be different for different vessels. A vessel with a thicker wall would be different from a vessel with a thinner wall. You can have very slow signal velocities when the wall is very thin so that the transit time difference would be very large in this case. For a heart wall, however, you would get very little difference because your velocities are very fast.

DR. OESTREICHER: Did you ever try your method on different tubes?

DR. HERRICK: We are going to have a series of units which are calibrated for use on different size blood vessels. We won't expect to use the same unit over a wide range of vessel sizes.

Destructive Effects of High-intensity Ultrasound on Plant Tissues

J. F. Lehmann,[1] E. J. Baldes[2] and F. H. Krusen[3]

Ohio State University Hospital, Columbus, Ohio, and Mayo Clinic and Mayo Foundation, Rochester, Minnesota

The diagnostic and therapeutic use of high-intensity ultrasound has made rapid progress during recent years (Fry, 1952; Wild and Reid, 1952, Ibid., 1953; Fry, 1953; Wall, Tucker, Fry and Mosberg, 1953; Wakim, 1953; Fischer, 1954; Hueter, 1951; Lehmann, 1953a; Lehmann, 1953b; Lehmann and Krusen, in press). It is now possible to produce pin-point lesions in the brains of experimental animals with great accuracy (Fry et al., 1954). Also, an attempt has been made to substitute lesions produced by ultrasonic energy for lesions previously produced by surgical methods (Lindstrom, 1954).

Information on the detailed effects of high-intensity ultrasound on the various cellular structures is still incomplete, and the biophysical mode of action of high-intensity ultrasound is as yet unknown. Fry and associates (Fry, 1952; Ibid., 1953; Wall et al., 1953) concluded from extensive experimental work that they dealt with a non-thermal reaction of unknown origin which was not caused by cavitation.

Under these circumstances it seemed worthwhile to investigate the effects of high-intensity ultrasound on cellular structures. This investigation also was undertaken in the hope of obtaining perhaps more information on the biophysical mode of action of high-intensity ultrasound.

The tissues of growing onion roots were chosen as objects of this investigation because they exhibit very distinctly the various cellular structures. They are also more uniform in structure than most of the tissues of warm-blooded animals. Finally, previous experimental work provided information on the mechanism by which lesions were produced at low ultrasonic intensities in this type of tissue (Lehmann, Herrick and Krusen, 1954).

[1] Department of Physical Medicine and Rehabilitation, Ohio State University Hospital, Columbus, Ohio; now, University of Washington, Seattle, Washington.

[2] Section of Biophysics and Biophysical Research, Mayo Clinic and Mayo Foundation, Rochester, Minnesota.

[3] Section of Physical Medicine and Rehabilitation, Mayo Clinic and Mayo Foundation, Rochester, Minnesota.

Methods

An ultrasonic frequency of 1 megacycle was used. The sound beam was focused by means of a polystyrene lens (Fig. 1) (Sette, 1949; Bronzo and Anderson, 1952). The focal intensity was measured with a calibrated thermocouple probe (Bergmann, 1949; Fry and Fry, 1954) and was found to be of the order of 110 watts/cm.^{2} The diameter of the focal area was approximately 0.5 to 1 mm. Water carefully degassed by boiling was used as the coupling medium, and the water temperature was kept constant between 0° and 3° C.

The onion roots were exposed in the focus of the ultrasonic beam for 5 minutes. This was done under a pressure of 450 pounds per square inch (Fig. 2). This pressure exceeded the pressure amplitude of the ultrasonic waves and thus prevented the occurrence of cavitation (Bergmann, 1949). The pressure was built up prior to the exposure to ultrasound over a period of 15 minutes and was slowly reduced following the exposure during a period of 30 minutes; then, the onion roots were fixed in formalin immediately. Later on, histologic slides were made and stained as previously described (Lehmann, Herrick and Krusen, 1954).

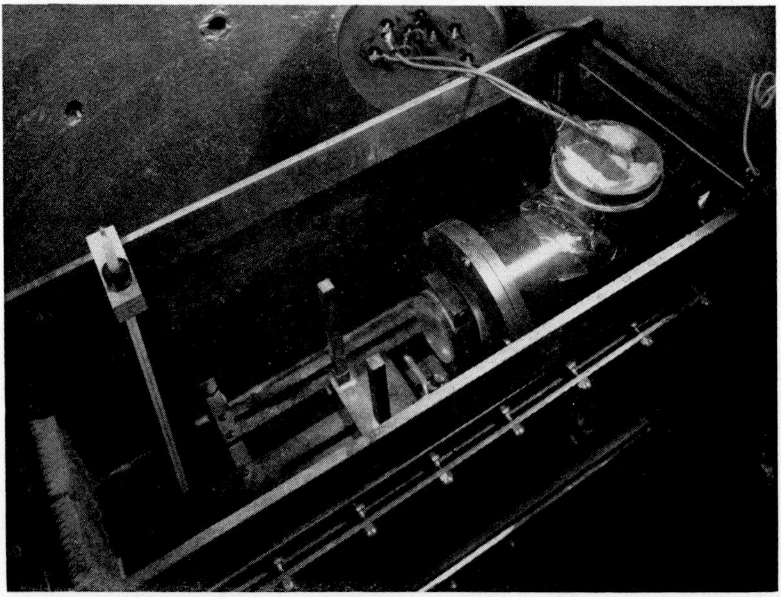

FIG. 1. Water tank for irradiation of the onion roots with sound applicator on the right, polystyrene lens in front of the applicator. Tip of pointer at focal area. On the left, brush absorber. Holder for onion bulb with root has been removed. The entire tank was accommodated within the pressure chamber.

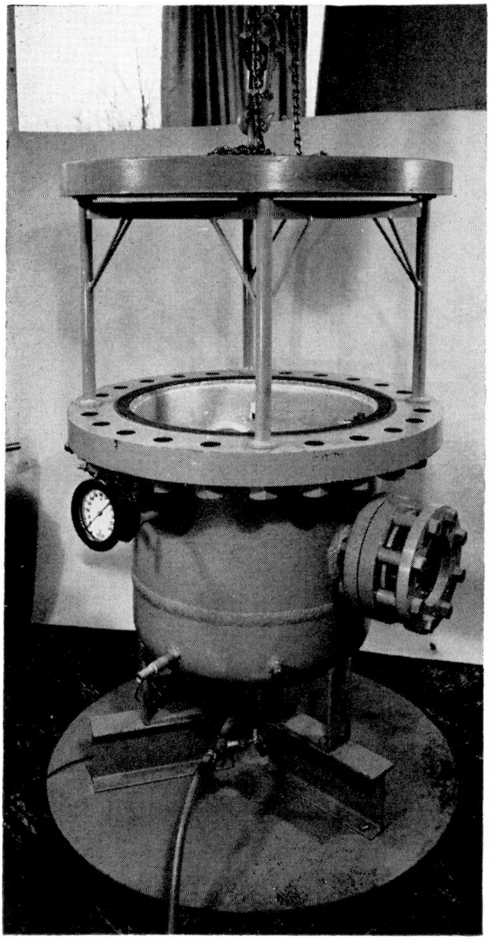

FIG. 2. Pressure chamber with window for direct observation on right.

The temperatures which were developed within the onion roots during exposure to the focused beam were estimated by extrapolation from actual measurements at lower intensities after it had been found that the rise of temperature was proportional to the intensity applied. Direct measurements at 110 watts/cm.^{2} could be obtained only sporadically because the thermocouple wires, as a result of the sound pressure, pierced the onion-root tissue and protruded into the surrounding water. In addition, the rate of the rise of temperature was estimated by kymographic studies. The thermocouples consisted of 5/1,000 inch steel and 3/1,000 inch constantan wires.

In another series of experiments the rise of temperature within the onion roots was produced, not by ultrasound, but by immersing them in water

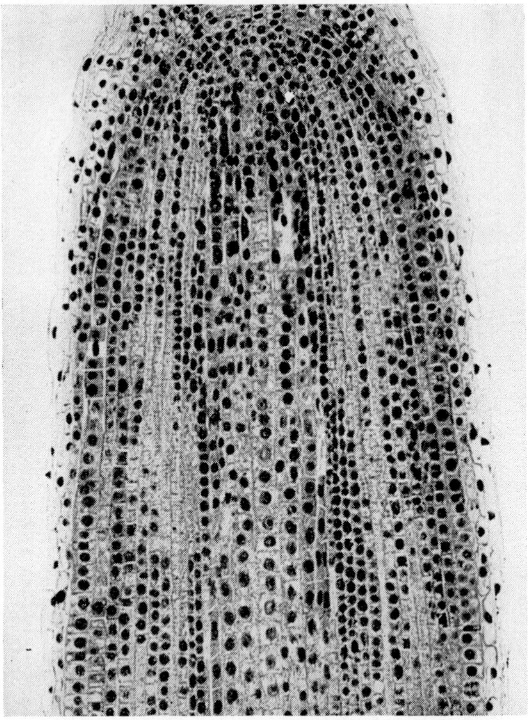

FIG. 3. Control. Intact cellular structures and mitotic figures within the tip of the onion root (iron hematoxylin, Heidenhain; ×120). (Reproduced with permission from Lehmann, J. F., Herrick, J. F. and Krusen, F. H. Arch. Phys. Med. and Rehab. *35:* 141–148. Mar. 1954.)

and mineral oil of various temperatures. These experiments were performed under atmospheric pressure, which was the only variation from the conditions of the experiments performed with high-intensity ultrasound.

Each of the above outlined experiments was repeated nine times.

In all experiments with ultrasound or application of heat, an equal number of controls was kept under the same experimental conditions (pressure, water bath, and so forth) but these controls were not exposed to ultrasound or heat. The histologic appearance of the tissues of all controls was normal (Fig. 3).

Experiments

When onion roots were exposed to the ultrasonic intensity of 110 watts/cm.^{2} the following result was obtained. All structures were destroyed within the center of the onion root. The cells were converted into a homogeneous mass of fine granular debris with some interspersed nuclear fragments. This reaction was uniform throughout the center of the root. The outer cell layers of the onion root were well preserved with regard to the gross cellular structures (Fig. 4). On close examination, marked changes consisting of shrinkage and vacuolization of the protoplasm and of an increase in density of the chromatin structures of the nuclei were observed (Fig. 5).

The rise of temperature within the onion root during exposure to ultrasound was estimated as described and found to be of the order of 154° C. ($\sigma \pm$ 34.4° C.). This estimation is based on a series of 14 experiments. Also, the rate of rise of temperature was estimated and found to be of the order of 30° C. per second.

Next, the question arose whether or not this rise of temperature might explain the occurrence of the destructive lesions observed after exposure to high-intensity ultrasound. A number of onion roots were inserted into water baths of 60° to 80° C. and others into mineral oid of 208° C. In previous experiments (Lehmann, Herrick and Krusen, 1954) onion roots had been

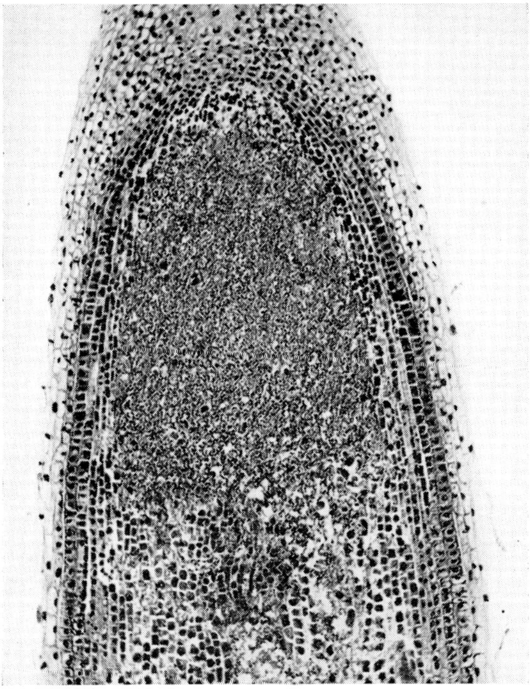

FIG. 4. Destruction of the onion root after exposure to ultrasonic energy of 110 watts./cm.^{2} Uniform and homogeneous fine granular debris is found in the center of the root with interspersed nuclear fragments. Shrinkage and vacuolization of nuclei and plasma at the edges of the root (iron hematoxylin, Heidenhain; ×85).

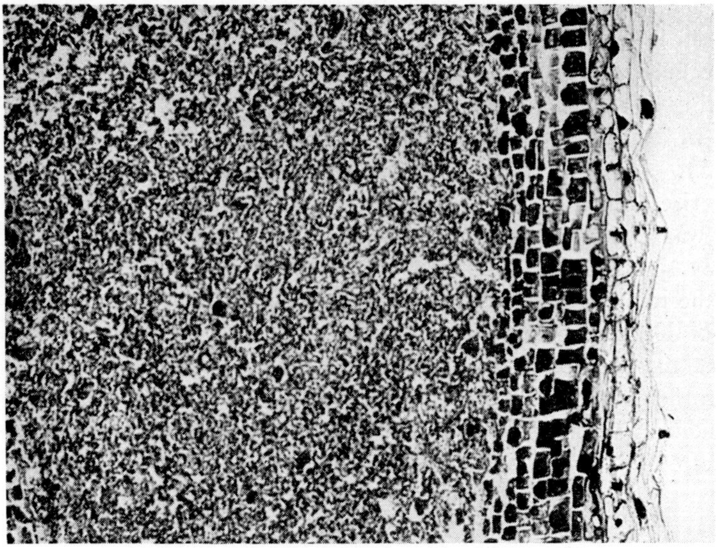

FIG. 5. As Fig. 4 (iron hematoxylin, Heidenhain; ×200). (Reproduced with permission from Lehmann, J. F., Baldes, E. J. and Krusen, F. H. Unpublished data.)

exposed to temperatures of 39°, 41° and 48° C. A surprisingly uniform result was obtained by exposing the roots to such temperatures. The gross structures of tissues and cells were well preserved. In addition there were definite shrinkage and vacuolization of the protoplasm and an increase in the density of the nuclei. This reaction was uniformly distributed all over the root and was indistinguishable from the reaction observed at the edges of the root after exposure to ultrasound (Figs. 6 and 7). However, it was completely different from the destruction occurring in the center of the root during exposure to ultrasound, which resulted in a conversion of all cellular structures into a fine granular debris.

When the roots were exposed to a temperature of 208° C., almost instantaneous vaporization of the fluids in the tissues occurred. The histologic appearance, however, was essentially not altered except for the occurrence of holes in the tissues (Figs. 8 and 9). The surrounding cellular structures were partially pushed aside and compressed, but exhibited preserved gross structures. Again the histologic appearance of these onion roots was entirely different from that observed after exposure to ultrasound.

The reactions observed after exposure to high-intensity ultrasound also differed in appearance from lesions which had been previously found at low ultrasonic intensities occurring as a result of degassing (Lehmann et al., 1954; Lehmann and Herrick, 1953; Hug and Pape, 1954) (Figs. 10 and 11). The lesions occurring at low intensities, as a result of degassing, had

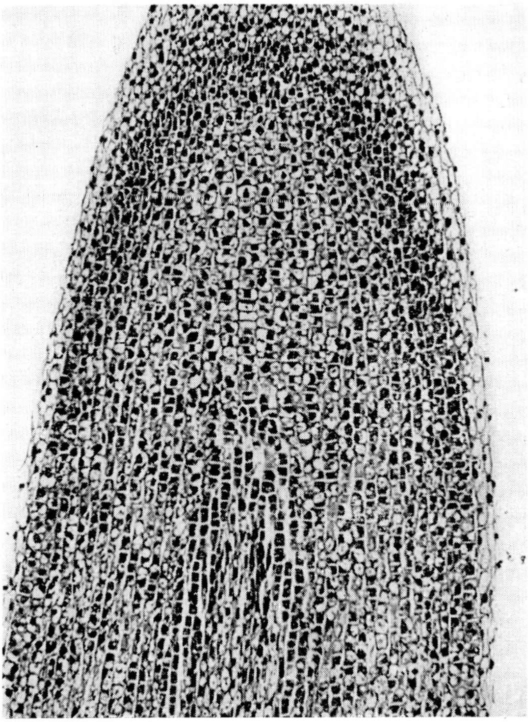

FIG. 6. Reaction with shrinkage and vacuolization of nuclei and plasma after exposure to temperature of 80° C. (iron hematoxylin, Heidenhain; ×90). (Reproduced with permission from Lehmann, J. F., Baldes, E. J. and Krusen, F. H. Unpublished data.)

the following characteristics: they were spotty; the most severe destruction of the cellular structures was found in the center of the lesion; the degree of destruction rapidly decreased with increasing distance from the center of the lesion. Even if those areas were confluent, no uniform destruction was observed. This was in contrast to the lesions observed in the centers of the roots after exposure to high-intensity ultrasound. In this case an entirely uniform, homogeneous mass was found throughout the area.

Summary

The recent use of high-intensity ultrasound for diagnostic and therapeutic purposes has pointed to a need for a better knowledge of the biologic effects and mode of action of high-intensity ultrasound. Experimental investigations of these phenomena could be expected to lead to improvement of therapeutic and diagnostic results.

Onion roots were exposed to ultrasonic intensities of 110 watts/cm.^{2} In

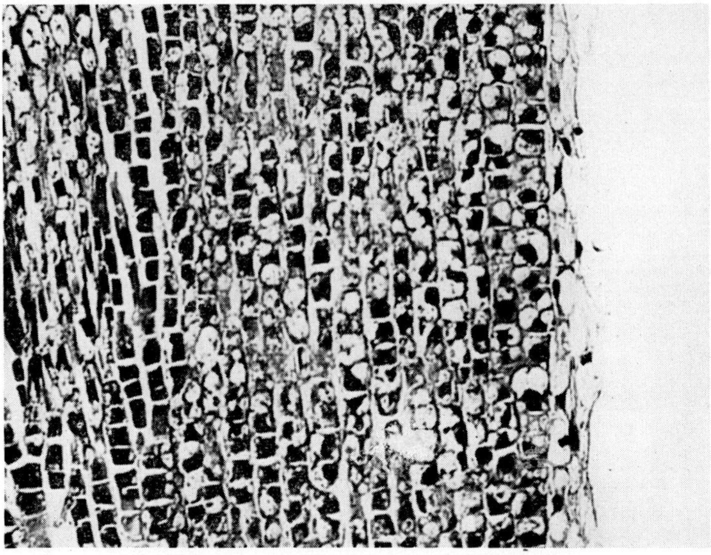

Fig. 7. Edge and center of root as in Fig. 6 (iron hematoxylin, Heidenhain; ×200). (Reproduced with permission from Lehmann, J. F., Baldes, E. J. and Krusen, F. H. Unpublished data.)

contrast to the histologic appearance produced by heat, and from that of cavitation phenomena occurring at lower ultrasonic intensities, a complete and uniform destruction of the root centers was observed. An interpretation that the destructive lesions were not due to heat or cavitation alone might perhaps be suggested by the histologic appearance and also by the fact that the reactions occurred under high pressure. On the other hand, it also has to be considered that the sudden rise of temperature during exposure to ultrasound might facilitate the occurrence of degassing, so that degassing might perhaps be produced by ultrasound in spite of the applied pressure. It must also be noted that no matter what else might have happened to the tissues during the exposure to ultrasound, the temperatures alone that were measured within the tissues during exposure could produce destructive lesions. As a matter of fact, the outer edge of the onion root exposed to high-intensity ultrasound had the same appearance as those roots exposed to high temperatures.

References

Barone, A. 1952. Aspects of the concentration of ultrasonic energy. Acustica *2:* 221–225.

Bergmann, L. 1949. Der Ultraschall und seine Anwendung in Wissenschaft und Technik. Stuttgart, S. Hirzel. 748 pp.

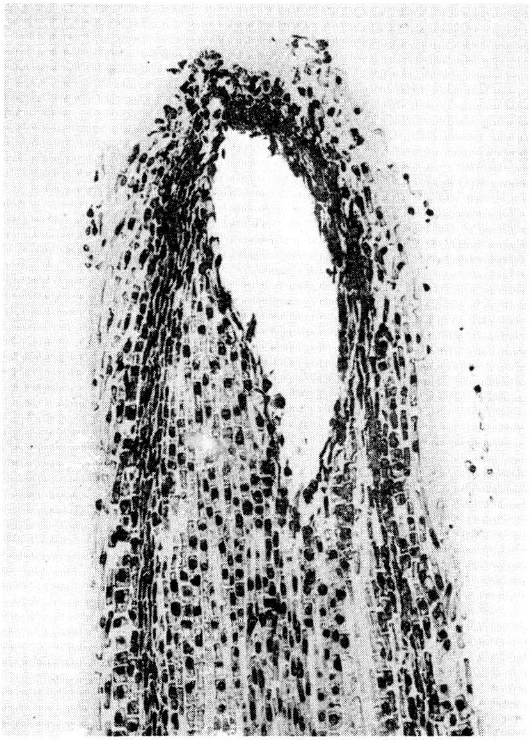

FIG. 8. Shrinkage and vacuolization of nuclei and plasma after exposure to 208° C. Torn tissues in the center of the root with formation of cavity. Tissues partially pushed aside (iron hematoxylin, Heidenhain; ×100). (Reproduced with permission from Lehmann, J. F., Baldes, E. J. and Krusen, F. H. Unpublished data.)

Bronzo, J. A. and J. M. Anderson. 1952. The effectiveness of plastic focusing lenses with high intensity ultrasonic radiation. J. Acoust. Soc. Am. *24:* 718–720.

Fischer, E. 1954. Basic biological effects of ultrasonic energy. Am. J. Phys. Med. *33:* 174–188.

Fry, W. J. 1952. Mechanism of acoustic absorption in tissue. J. Acoust. Soc. Am. *24:* 412–415.

Fry, W. J. 1953. Action of ultrasound on nerve tissue—A Review. J. Acoust. Soc. Am. *25:* 1–5.

Fry, W. J. and R. B. Fry. 1954. Determination of absolute sound levels and acoustic absorption coefficients by thermocouple probes—experiment. J. Acoust. Soc. Am. *26:* 311–317.

Fry, W. J., W. H. Mosberg, Jr., J. W. Barnard and F. J. Fry. 1954. Production of focal destructive lesions in the central nervous system with ultrasound. J. Neurosurg. *11:* 471–478.

Hueter, T. F. 1951. On the mechanism of biological effects produced by ultrasound. Chem. Engineering Progress Symposium, Series *47:* 62.

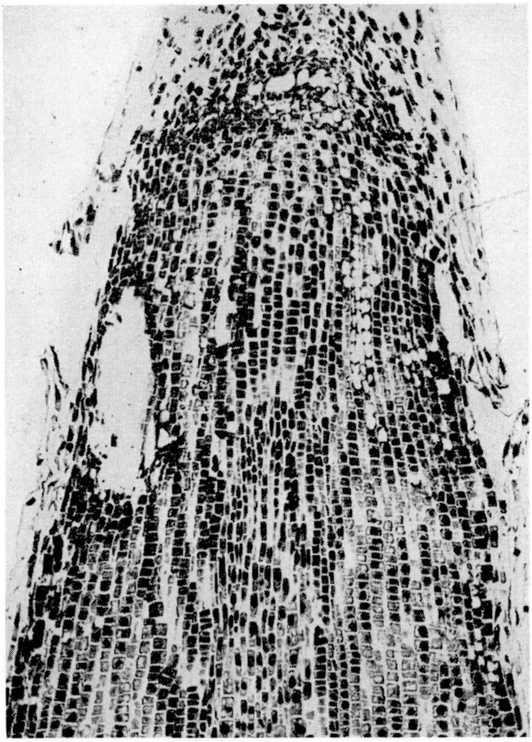

FIG. 9. As Fig. 8 with formation of smaller cavities and more marked vacuolization and shrinkage of protoplasm and nuclei (iron hematoxylin, Heidenhain; ×110).

Hug, O. and R. Pape. 1954. Nachweis der Ultraschallkavitation im Gewebe. Strahlentherapie *94:* 79–99.

Lehmann, J. F. 1953. The biophysical basis of biologic ultrasonic reactions with special reference to ultrasonic therapy. Arch. Phys. Med. *34:* 139–152.

Lehmann, J. F. 1953. The biophysical mode of action of biologic and therapeutic ultrasonic reactions. J. Acoust. Soc. Am. *25:* 17–26.

Lehmann, J. F. and J. F. Herrick. 1953. Biologic reactions to cavitation, a consideration of ultrasonic therapy. Arch. Phys. Med. *34:* 86–98.

Lehmann, J. F., J. F. Herrick and F. H. Krusen. 1954. The effects of ultrasound on chromosomes, nuclei and other structures of the cells in plant tissues. Arch. Phys. Med. *35:* 141–148.

Lehmann, J. F. and F. H. Krusen. Biophysical effects of ultrasonic energy on carcinoma and their possible significance. Arch. Phys. Med. In press.

Lindstrom, P. 1954. Paper read at the Annual Congress of the American Institute of Ultrasound.

Sette, D. 1949. Ultrasonic lenses of plastic materials. J. Acoust. Soc. Am. *21:* 375–381.

Wahim, K. G. 1953. Ultrasonic energy as applied to medicine. Am. J. Phys. Med. *32:* 32–46.

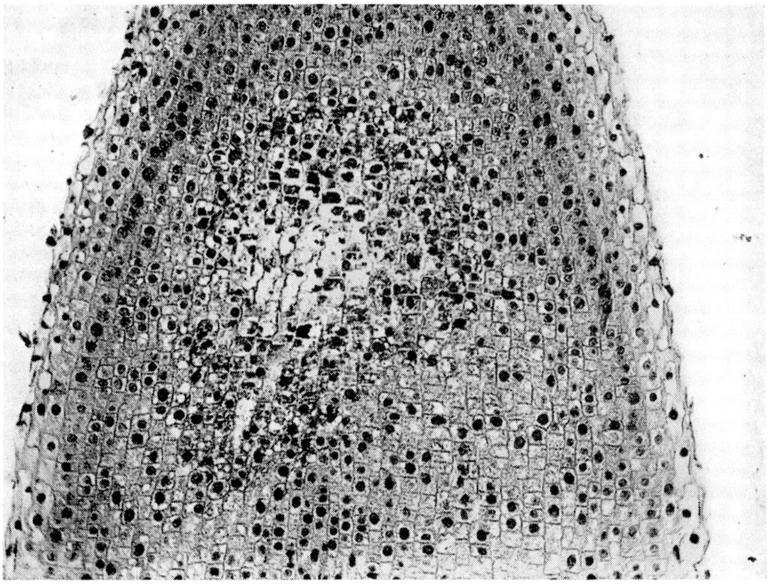

FIG. 10. Reaction to degassing within the onion root. Most severe destruction in the center of the area of reaction. Destructive changes rapidly decreasing with increasing distance from center of the reaction (iron hematoxlyin, Heidenhain; ×125). (Reproduced with permission from Lehmann, J. F., Herrick, J. F. and Krusen, F. H. Arch. Phys. Med. and Rehab. *35:* 141–148. Mar. 1954.)

Wall, P. D., D. Tucker, F. J. Fry and W. H. Mosberg. 1953. The use of high intensity ultrasound in experimental neurology. J. Acoust. Soc. Am. *25:* 281–285.

Wild, J. J. and J. M. Reid. 1952. Application of echo-ranging techniques to the determination of structure of biological tissues. Science *115:* 226–230.

Wild, J. J. and J. M. Reid. 1953. The effects of biological tissues on 15-mc pulsed ultrasound. J. Acoust. Soc. Am. *25:* 270–280.

DR. VON GIERKE: Three years ago at the first Ultrasound Symposium, we had quite a discussion of whether or not it is possible to have an effect from localized heating at a specific point. I believe the calculations of Dr. Fry have shown that, for most tissues, this is at least very improbable. Would you exclude this possibility or not?

DR. LEHMANN: Are you referring to localized heating in the sense that we discussed at that time, i.e., the heating of one or a few cells?

DR. VON GIERKE: No.

DR. LEHMANN: What size of interphase are you talking about?

DR. VON GIERKE: Cellular.

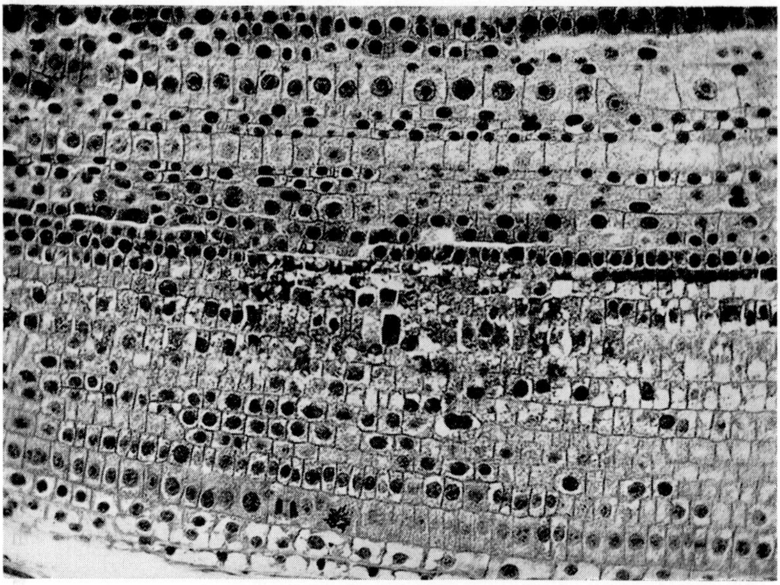

FIG. 11. As Fig. 10 (iron hematoxylin, Heidenhain; ×175). (Reproduced with permission from Lehmann, J. F., Herrick, J. F. and Krusen, F. H. Arch. Phys. Med. and Rehab. *35:* 141–148. Mar. 1954.)

DR. LEHMANN: All right. No, Dr. Schwan has done extensive studies on the question of selective heating in the diathermy field, and his calculations have clearly indicated that you cannot get selective heating as the droplets become smaller and smaller in radii.

When you reach the order of size of the cell radius, I do not believe it is possible to have selective heating. I assume that you are pointing this out, because I mentioned the very high temperatures obtained here. However, the region over which the temperature was measured was not that of a single cell. The diameter was of the same order of magnitude as the diameter of the probes.

Does that answer your question?

DR. VON GIERKE: Not a hundred percent. What Dr. Schwan has shown is that you cannot maintain a higher temperature in some regions, but does that exclude the possibility that the energy is absorbed for a very short time in the interphases?

DR. LEHMANN: In other words, single cell or cellular interphase?

DR. HUETER: Is it not possible that some type of cavitation is present despite the applied high pressure?

DR. LEHMANN: If you heat up the tissues to such a degree, I am sure you will have a solution of gases in the tissues which is close to the saturation point. Now, if you have an addition to the alternating pressure of the sound wave, it is very conceivable at least that bubbles are formed. We have seen, for instance, in the warm-blooded animal that the temperature is an important parameter which primes this tissue for the occurrence of gas bubbles. We have demonstrated that these gas bubble formations depend on the temperature. That is the reason why I am not a hundred percent sure whether or not it is not cavitation in spite of the difference in histological appearance. I feel more experiments should be made in this direction. Unfortunately, I wasn't able to do this.

DR. HUETER: In regard to these strange layer-type lesions which were also discussed this morning in regard to Fry's work, where you have an outer fringe of greater destruction and an inner core of reduced destruction, can this be connected with bubbles which may diffuse out and cause such a fringe?

DR. LEHMANN: I don't know.

DR. FRY: Regarding such layer-type lesions, a possible explanation is that in the outer regions where the early morphological changes in structure are greater, the direct effect of the sound is not so great, and the enzyme systems can carry out the processes of reducing the tissue structurally, but in the center region where, let us say, all enzyme systems or chemical changes are greater, there you have a preserved appearance. The preserved appearance does not imply that the tissues are chemically intact as it is, say, in the normal phase. The structure appears intact because the tissue has no way of carrying out self-digestion, or autolysis.

DR. HERRICK: Is it sort of preserved?

DR. FRY: It has a preserved appearance. The structure remains for five or six days. There is hardly time for diffusion of bubbles. Changes begin to appear in animals sacrificed ten minutes after exposure. There is no evidence of any bubble in the tissue five minutes after irradiation. Regarding the point about "cavitation" without having tension forces, I am not quite clear what is implied, but I assume that what is meant is that some gas cavities and nuclei grow under rectified diffusion. In such an instance, the bubble certainly would not collapse on the positive phase. If the sound is discontinued, the bubble is not going to immediately disappear.

DR. HUETER: It would only be a micron in diameter?

DR. FRY: It isn't like a collapsing cavity. I think in the case that I am suggesting it would be easier to see histologically.

DR. HUETER: That finding of yours may be a significant clue.

DR. FRY: I think pressure is a very important variable in considering the mechanism.

DR. BUSNEL: In regard to the technique you used with boiling water, the pathologists know perfectly well that when you put tissue in boiling water you obtain a good fixation, which is irreversible.

The second point concerns oxidation in the tissue. I remember the experiments before the war by Daniel et al. on the roots of onions. They inject a solution of reduced blue before the treatment with ultrasonic waves. After the treatment with high intensity ultrasonic waves they obtained a blue solution. They produced, therefore, true cavitation in the tissue because of real oxidation.

I recall some publications in the States on work performed by Newcomber and Willis, and also some work in Japan on roots of tulips and onions. Breakdown of the chromosomes was obtained with application of very high energy. Have you observed some destruction of chromosomes or destruction of the cells?

DR. LEHMANN: That is right. Heat is used by the pathologists as a fixative. You get the usual picture of fixation, shrinkage and everything else. We studied these changes in chromosomes and mitotic figures extensively, but since that was done some time ago, I did not mention it. We got the changes that Dr. Newcomber and others observed; chromosome disruption, clumping, increased stickiness and abnormal mitotic figures.

Generating and Measuring High-intensity Ultrasound of Frequencies Between 1 and 68 Megacycles

B. B. Chick

Department of Applied Mathematics, Brown University, Providence, Rhode Island

AT THE OUTSET I would like to indicate that the work I have done has primarily the development of instrumentation for Dr. Bell of the Biology Department at Brown University. In his paper he will discuss the results of irradiating biological material with ultrasound. I am going to talk about some of the instrumentation problems. In particular I would like to discuss some of the problems encountered in developing high frequency generators which could be operated over a range of frequencies between 3 and 100 megacycles. In addition, I will talk briefly about the various indicating devices used, and also about a microapplicator which is now in the process of being developed.

The first high frequency unit, which operates from 3 mc. to 30 mc., used a power oscillator and appropriate matching networks to resonate the transducers. This unit has been used primarily at 27 mc. with a 9-mc. crystal driven on its third harmonic. The total power output obtained at 27 mc. is 85 watts with a plate power input of 240 watts (approximately 35 percent eff.). No major problems were encountered in the construction and operation of this piece of equipment.

In developing the second unit, which was designed to operate from 30 mc. to 100 mc., a power oscillator was also employed. A Colpitts type oscillator was used. Plug-in coils and a variable capacitor provided continuous tuning over the frequency range. A low impedance link was used to couple power from the oscillator tank into a 50-ohm line. This made it possible to separate the oscillator and transducer. At the transducer end of the line another low impedance link was used to couple into a high impedance tank. This tank resonates the transducer at the particular odd harmonic desired.

The most convenient method found to tune the transducer circuit at frequencies above 30 mc. was to use a variable capacitor in parallel with the coil and transducer whereas in the 3–30-mc. unit variable inductors were used. At frequencies below 30 mc. the long leads to the variable inductors did not prevent efficient operation but at higher frequencies it was necessary to make the leads as short as possible and this could be accomplished most conveniently by using a variable capacitor. This type of arrangement worked successfully up to 45 mc., and some indication of output was observed at 51 mc.

The two chief problems encountered above 45 mc. were the following: (1) matching the line so that energy could be transferred from the oscillator to the transducer; and (2) the problem of drag loop effect which may be explained as follows:

If the frequency of the power oscillator is set to the desired harmonic and the frequency of the transducer circuit slowly adjusted to the frequency appropriate for the transducer, the load on the oscillator increases. At first the oscillator will change frequency slowly as the loading increases and may be reset to the desired frequency. Eventually, however, a point is reached where the oscillator tank and transducer tank will suddenly lock together at some frequency other than the desired one. Further tuning of the oscillator will only result in a sudden unlocking of the two circuits and a jump to some other undesired frequency.

The first problem was overcome by adding two more variable capacitors to the circuit, these being in series with the links on either end of the low impedance line. Their function was to lower the effective impedance of the links and make it possible to exactly match the cable. In order to eliminate the second problem, that of drag loop effect, the source of frequency control was removed from the power stage by introducing a separate master oscillator and buffer amplifier and changing the original power oscillator to a conventional tuned power amplifier.

This type of design provides enough isolation between the frequency determining master oscillator and the power amplifier so that as the tank circuit matching the transducer is tuned there is no frequency pulling of the oscillator. With this arrangement we were able to generate sound at 60 mc. by driving a 4-mc. crystal on the 15th harmonic.

Above 60 mc. we again ran into difficulties. Parasitic oscillations were encountered which made it impossible to operate on any desired frequency above 60 mc. The parasitic oscillations were apparently due to the physical layout of the many tuned circuits. It was also difficult to adjust the transmitter for maximum output at and below 60 mc. because of the many independent controls. We therefore attempted to simplify tuning and to improve the physical layout while retaining the same basic design.

The most important improvement was the use of a Mallory VHF inductuner. It is a three section variable inductor normally used for tuning television receivers between 50 and 216 mc. By loading down the inductuner slightly with capacity it can be tuned from 30 mc. to over 100 mc. The first three tanks of the transmitter are tuned with this unit (oscillator, buffer grid, and power amplifier grid). Small trimmer capacitors are connected in parallel with these tanks so that they may be adjusted for maximum drive on the grid of the power amplifier at 100 mc. Because of the excellent tracking of the inductuner sufficient drive on the P.A. grid is obtained over the entire frequency range without readjusting the trimmers. This reduces the tuning problem considerably. Use of the inductuner required straight-line construction of the three stages similar to that which is employed in I.F. strips. This helped to maintain the master oscillator as the primary frequency determining source by eliminating crossed-over ground loops. With this type of design we were able to operate up to 68 mc., however the limiting factor was no longer the electronic circuitry which now operated successfully to over 100 mc. but was the difficulty involved in matching the transducer above 68 mc.

We have been using a 4-mc. transducer of one inch diameter with a capacity of about 40 micromicrofarads. To be able to resonate this capacity requires an extremely small amount of inductance at 100 mc., and we have not been able to couple appreciable power into the circuit. It was previously observed in work done at 27 mc. that approximately the same output could be obtained by using a 3-mc. crystal driven on its 9th harmonic as could be obtained by using a 9-mc. crystal driven on its 3rd harmonic. This suggested to us that a 2-mc. instead of a 4-mc. crystal be used. With a 2-mc. crystal of only one half inch active area the capacity would be reduced by a factor of 8. Such a crystal if driven on its 49th or 51st harmonic would yield output in the vicinity of 100 mc.[1]

In the course of constructing the generators just described, we were constantly faced with the problem of detecting output from the transducer. From 1 mc. to 5 mc. we used the commercial Siemens Sonotest meter. I believe everyone is familiar with it. The Siemens meter, however, is not very useful above 5 mc. We therefore built a comparison-type calorimeter which could be used to make absolute measurements of output at frequencies above 5 mc. It is shown in Fig. 1. The calorimeter consists of a stainless steel chamber (H) about twelve inches long in which the transducer (C) is mounted at one end and a stirring motor and shaft with propeller blades (A) at the other end. In the aperture (D) a thermometer or thermocouple is inserted to measure the temperature rise of the distilled, degassed water which fills the chamber. In addition to the propeller blades

[1] A generator capable of delivering high intensity ultrasound at a frequency of 99 mc. has been successfully completed since the writing of this paper. A 3-mc., 3/4″ diameter crystal driven on the 33rd harmonic is employed. The crystal is mounted close to the power amplifier so that difficulties associated with the use of a low impedance cable are eliminated.

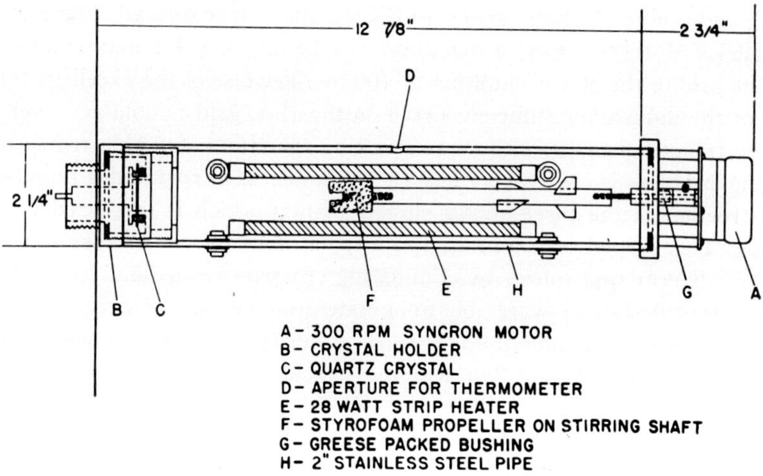

FIG. 1. Comparison-type calorimeter, cross-section view.

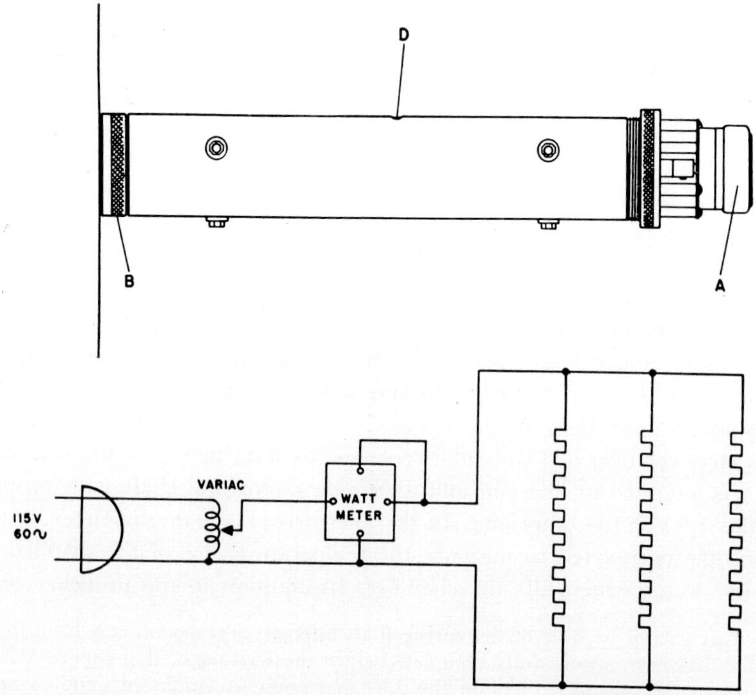

FIG. 2. Comparison-type calorimeter and electrical circuit for energizing strip heaters.

there is also a piece of styrofoam (F) mounted on the stirring shaft. The styrofoam scatters the sound waves impinging on it and also acts as a small propeller. Three 28-watt stripheaters (E), inside the chamber, provide a means for raising the temperature of the water. The stripheaters are energized by a variac, as shown in Fig. 2. The power input to the stripheaters can be measured to ± 2 percent accuracy with the wattmeter used.

The technique employed in measuring the sound output is the following: (1) the temperature rise of the fluid in the calorimeter, due to the introduction of acoustic energy, is measured at the end of a fixed time interval. (At the power level employed the rise is roughly linear.) (2) The same temperature rise is reproduced by introducing electrical energy into the stripheater which in turn heats the medium. The power consumption of

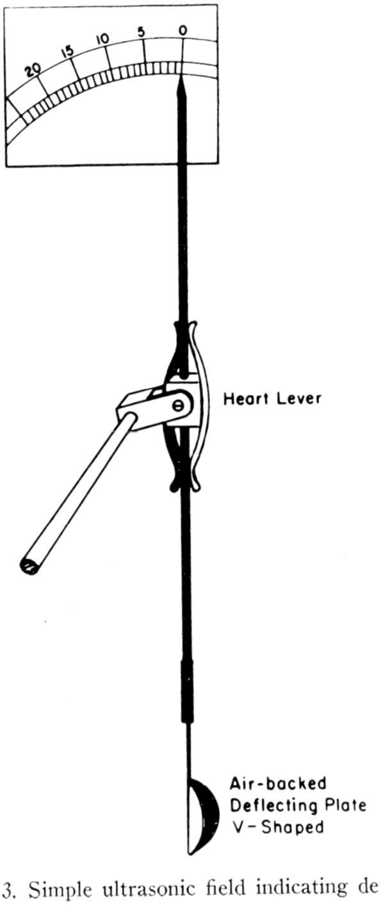

FIG. 3. Simple ultrasonic field indicating device.

the stripheater is read directly from the wattmeter and is a direct measure of acoustic power.

We have used another simple device, shown in Fig. 3, to indicate the presence of ultrasound qualitatively. It is a small, V-shaped, air-backed deflecting plate. When sound impinges on the deflecting plate, which is suspended from a heart lever, the needle deflects along the chart. This device has been used effectively up to 60 mc. It is not practical to use it at higher frequencies because of difficulty in mechanically locating it close enough to the transducer.

The last device about which I would like to speak is a microapplicator, which has been developed for the purpose of irradiating small volumes of biological material. It is hoped that we will be able to irradiate single cells under the microscope and actually watch the sequence of changes due to ultrasound, both during and after irradiation. The microapplicator is shown in Fig. 4. The transducer is mounted in a conventional way with air backing. The crystal holder has been extended in front of the crystal so as to form a built-in water bath. A polystyrene focussing lens is mounted just in

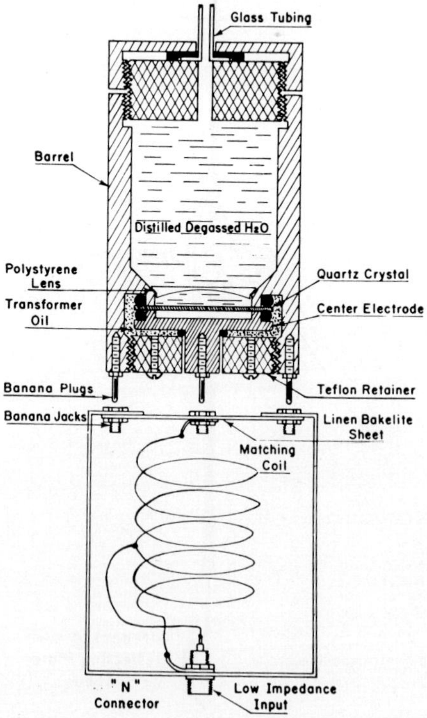

FIG. 4. Microapplicator and matching network, cross-section view.

front of the transducer.[2] The focal point is just at the point where the sound enters the opening in the brass adaptor which is used to support the glass tubing. Although it is not shown the glass tubing is drawn out to a small capillary. We have actually succeeded in passing 4-mc. sound through a capillary only 35 microns in cross-section. An important advantage of the microapplicator is that the entire unit is small and completely portable. Matching coils can be plugged into the probe and a low impedance cable can then be used to couple to the transmitter as a source of high amplitude electro-magnetic energy.

We have run some very preliminary experiments, one of which I might mention here. Frog's eggs were irradiated immediately following fertilization. The capillary used had an exit diameter of one-half millimeter. These eggs were exposed for 5 to 30 seconds at 4 or 12 mc. While about 10 percent of the irradiated eggs developed into acephalic larvae, no acephalic larvae were observed in the control samples. There is still much preliminary work we have to do. We have not determined quantitatively the acoustic output from the microapplicator. We are very much impressed with Dr. Fry's thermocouple arrangement, and it might be extremely helpful for us to use a similar arrangement in actually measuring the intensity of ultrasound delivered by the micro-device. We would also like to know what happens to sound which is passed through a capillary that has been drawn down to an exit diameter small compared to wavelength.

The indicating and measuring devices I discussed have been quite satisfactory for us over the frequency ranges we employ, but we are going to have to make modifications before they are completely useful at 100 mc. As for the high frequency generator, the only problem remaining is resonating the capacity of the transducer. The use of a small diameter 2-mc. crystal should make it possible for us to generate high intensity–high frequency sound.[3]

DR. HERRICK: How do you detect the presence of the sound at the other end of this small capillary?

DR. CHICK: There are several criteria we have used. If the tip of the capillary is sufficiently long, it will vibrate when sound passes through it. Vibrations are recognized by the following sequence of events: As the

[2] Although it is possible to restrict the output from a transducer to an area of small cross-section by interposing an absorber with a small aperture between the transducer and the material to be exposed, the intensity of such a source would be exceedingly low and its usefulness limited.

[3] See footnote 1.

water in the system heats up, a small drop oozes out of the tip of the capillary, and rolls down around the tip; the drop then begins to spin. It spins for awhile and then flies off. Occasionally a very fine stream of vapor may be seen to ascend from the tip of the capillary. This is another indication that we have sonic output.

If the tip of the capillary is immersed into a small vessel containing a dye or a suspension of particulate material the movement of the material under these conditions can be observed readily under the microscope. The tip must be short enough, however, so that the vibrations in the glass wall are damped; otherwise the entire medium vibrates and streaming is difficult to observe.

DR. FRY: A solid rod can propagate a principal mode, and I wonder whether after the diameter of the fluid column becomes of the order of a quarter of a wavelength, it is important to retain the fluid in the capillary. Is the liquid itself much of an advantage when it is such a small fraction of a wavelength?

DR. CHICK: There are two reasons for using the liquid: the first is that there is no problem of acoustic impedance matching when water is the only medium through which the sound is propagated, the second is that if the capillary were closed into a solid rod there would be no place for gas bubbles caused by cavitation to escape. As now used, the gas bubbles can pass through the capillary.

DR. FRY: Where do the gas bubbles occur?

DR. CHICK: They probably originate at a point where the sound comes to a focus in the coupling medium.

DR. FRY: Why not taper the solid rod down and forget about the fluid in it?

DR. CHICK: This may be possible if the taper begins close enough to the lens. This would perhaps minimize the problem of bubble formation.

DR. HERRICK: I was going to call on Dr. Ackerman since he has made a thorough study of measurements by the piezoelectric and the electrokinetic techniques. Dr. Ackerman, have you any suggestions as a result of your extensive measurements?

DR. ACKERMAN: I question whether this focussing did you a great deal of good. I don't have a clear picture of your dimensions, but it looks to me like the lens is focussed at the bottom of the tube, and as far as the focussed wave itself is concerned, it is spread out.

DR. CHICK: The energy is brought to a focus in the coupling medium at the aperture of the brass ring which supports the glass tubing (Fig. 3). By this means most of the energy from the crystal is funnelled into the glass tubing.

DR. ACKERMAN: It looks like the equivalent of using a solid rod from that point on down, the waves simply exciting the tube walls.

DR. CHICK: We have focussed the output of the transducer so that most of the sound will enter the glass tube. Some of the output is probably transmitted through and reflected from the side walls of both the brass piece and the glass tubing.

DR. ACKERMAN: At any rate, it begins to spread out long before it reaches the cells that are being exposed, is that correct?

DR. CHICK: There may be quite a bit of channelling effect.

DR. VON GIERKE: How do you intend to measure the sound at the place of application?

DR. CHICK: We plan to use a thermocouple.

DR. VON GIERKE: If the mechanism which Dr. Fry talked about is operative and which I suspect too, then the whole tube is vibrating, and it might be difficult to do. You cannot attach a thermocouple to the walls.

DR. CHICK: No. The thermocouple would be positioned in the liquid medium, in which the biological sample is contained.

DR. ACKERMAN: How large a volume of liquid do you have this immersed in?

DR. CHICK: Just a small amount, enough to hold the biological material we wish to irradiate.

DR. ACKERMAN: Just the drop that you look at under the microscope?

DR. CHICK: Yes, just enough to accomplish the coupling.

DR. HERRICK: Are you losing some of your sound through the tube?

DR. CHICK: We are getting sound into the side walls of the tube, there is no question about that, but there is air completely surrounding the tube and the coupling to the air is negligible.

DR. FRY: Is the diameter of the tube small compared to the wavelength?

DR. CHICK: At the frequencies we have used (4 mc. and 12 mc.), the exit diameter of the capillary is small compared to the wavelength. Because of high attenuation of the sound in traversing the water path from the transducer to the capillary, it is not practical to operate at higher frequencies.

DR. FRY: You could replace the water with a solid cone.

DR. CHICK: Again, it becomes a matter of impedance matching.

DR. FRY: Quartz might work.

DR. CHICK: We have tried quartz with very little success.

DR. LEHMANN: The use of the solid rod as suggested by Dr. Fry and others might be advantageous from the biological point of view. I remember some time ago Dr. Schmitt, in experiments with amoeba, used such a glass rod to introduce into the protoplasm of the amoeba so that he could work in the protoplasm directly, and I think some changes were observed only locally, whereas the other part of the cell was more or less intact.

DR. HERRICK: At what frequency, do you know?

DR. LEHMANN: It was around 800 kc. or 1 mc.

DR. FRY: I recall reading that article. In this instance, too, one should consider shear waves from the viewpoint of explaining local effects.

DR. HERRICK: There must be some other questions on this interesting new way of transmitting sound from the transducer to the object.

DR. FARRALL: Do you have a difference in efficiency operating on the fundamental of the crystal in comparison to operation at the 9th harmonic?

DR. CHICK: You would expect the output of the crystal to decrease in going to higher harmonics. However, since more inductance can be employed to resonate a lower frequency crystal a much higher step-up in voltage is realized to drive the crystal. Therefore the ratio of input to output power remains roughly the same.

DR. HERRICK: I am interested in reproducibility of results with this method. We have difficulty in reproducibility when our conditions are pretty well known, and now with these other variables introduced, are you having difficulty in reproducing the biological effects?

DR. BELL: We have not done enough to say how reproducible our results are. Dr. Chick alluded to one experiment we conducted with frogs' eggs. We placed the egg on the tip of a capillary, whose exit diameter was half a millimeter. After the eggs were fertilized they were irradiated through the jelly membrane. As sound passed through the egg, both the egg and the membrane were visibly deformed. Following treatment the eggs were allowed to develop and many acephalic larvae were observed in the experimental material. None were observed in the controls. It is too early to speculate about the significance of these results and it will take us some time to work out the details of this problem.

DR. HERRICK: How about the usefulness of Schlieren photographs of the end of this rod? What do you think about that, Dr. Von Gierke?

DR. VON GIERKE: I think you may get interesting results, but one has to be careful in drawing conclusions which one applies to what we usually call compressional ultrasound waves in liquid-type materials, because here you get some kind of point application of the sound, and as Dr. Fry mentioned already you have shear waves which would be very important here from the viewpoint of mechanism. I think it would be quite difficult to define the acoustic stimulus in this case.

DR. BELL: I thoroughly agree. We are dealing with a complex acoustic field.

DR. HERRICK: Still it is very important to be able to make pinpoint applications under the microscope.

DR. VON GIERKE: The velocity amplitude of the tip should be measured.

DR. HERRICK: Would it be possible to use a calorimeter-type of method in any way?

DR. CHICK: This would also tell us what is coming through the walls.

Since we are interested only in the sound available at the tip of the capillary it would not be too useful.

DR. VON GIERKE: You want the velocity at the tip. How much power you get out of the tip depends on how much you load it and that is unspecified. It may be a function of the material which is to be treated.

DR. CHICK: That is right, it is going to be extremely difficult to know exactly what we are doing with this.

DR. HERRICK: I am curious to know how steady a state he has at any time for reproducibility.

DR. VON GIERKE: That depends on the loading, i.e., the mechanical load on the tip. If he treats a big egg it might be different from a small egg.

DR. CHICK: What Dr. Von Gierke says is true but if the biological specimen is small compared to the amount of fluid in which it is immersed, and if the same amount of fluid is used for each exposure the loading should be uniform. In the case of the frog's egg which is balanced on the tip of the capillary and not immersed in a fluid the loading would of course depend upon the mass and nature of the material and would vary from one specimen to the next.

DR. VON GIERKE: You do not have constant power output.

DR. CHICK: We have a constant source of power at the other end but the load may not be constant.

DR. VON GIERKE: That is the thing you have to watch.

DR. NYBORG: This type of source has not been worked with very much, but in acoustics you think of two kinds of elementary waves, plane waves and spherical waves. The approximation usually striven for is the plane wave kind of geometry, or now more recently the focussed spherical wave. It might turn out with further study of such a field as this that it would exhibit a simplicity of its own. There is some hope that it might not be such a difficult geometry to explore.

DR. VON GIERKE: As long as you have spherical waves and you are close to the irradiator, you have shear waves, and complications are thus introduced. Shear and compressional waves are both present.

DR. NYBORG: You have the theory from your laboratory which is going to take care of the situation.

DR. VON GIERKE: The theory is very complicated in this area, because you have both types of waves, and you cannot separate the two.

DR. CHICK: The point I would like to stress here is that eventually we would like to use this device under the microscope. We want to find out more about the nature of the output from the microapplicator, and how best to apply it. That is why we wanted to present it today so we could elicit your comments on it and get further suggestions regarding its use.

DR. VON GIERKE: I have a question which is perhaps a little naive. I am not too familiar with this approach, but is it not possible to use a large crystal and water bath, and put the microscope in the water?

DR. CHICK: Submerging a microscope presents many problems.

DR. VON GIERKE: This way you could expose the material to plane waves, and it seems to me that the use of the microscope under water should not be too difficult.

DR. BELL: It would be possible to expose the material to plane waves, but it would not be possible to expose a very small volume of material to plane waves. If the aperture were made too small over the crystal the output through the aperture would also be small.

DR. FRY: Do you wish to restrict the irradiation to a small volume, or do you want just a high intensity?

DR. BELL: We want to irradiate a small volume of material with high intensity ultrasound.

DR. FRY: Are you interested in irradiating only one portion of the preparation, or the whole thing?

DR. BELL: One portion of it.

DR. FRY: How small a region?

DR. BELL: The smaller we can get it, the better.

DR. FRY: How large is the preparation?

DR. BELL: That depends on the material we would choose. We would like to irradiate single cells; protozoan materials to begin with. *Stentor,* for example, is at times almost a millimeter in length. It would be of interest to irradiate the chain of micronuclei, with the aim of knocking out some or all of them from the outside of the cell. This has been done by microsurgical techniques, but the treatment is quite traumatic as far as the organism is concerned.

DR. FRY: You want to do this without disturbing the other parts of the cell.

DR. BELL: Exactly.

DR. LEHMANN: Is there not a fundamental limit to the size restricting the application of ultrasound? Even with high frequencies corresponding to smaller wavelengths than we usually use, when you consider the diameter of the nucleus of the cell about one micron?

DR. BELL: I do not know that you cannot, if the aperture of our probe is sufficiently small and we can restrict the sound to within the probe. The micronuclei in stentor are not much smaller than the tip of the probe.

DR. FRY: What Dr. Lehmann is saying is that at a certain frequency you are limited by the wavelength as far as the spot size is concerned.

Some Changes in Liver Tissue Which Survives Irradiation with Ultrasound

E. Bell[1]

Department of Biology, Brown University, Providence, Rhode Island

THE FOLLOWING REPORT is a review of cytological and physiological changes which occur in the intact liver of the white mouse irradiated with ultrasound of one or 27 megacycles frequency.

The report is divided into four parts: (1) the disruptive effects of ultrasound on liver tissue, and the nature of necrosis to which they lead; (2) the response of the liver as a whole to damage inflicted with ultrasound; (3) the effects of ultrasound on different cell types of liver; and (4) morphological and cytochemical changes in cells which survive irradiation with ultrasound.

Materials and Methods

Frequencies of one and 27 megacycles are provided by two ultrasonic generators built in the Metals Research Laboratory of the Graduate Division of Applied Mathematics at Brown University. Quartz crystals are used as transducers. Crystal holders are mounted in the end wall of a 10-gallon tank filled with degassed distilled water which serves as a coupling medium for the sound. The over-all experimental arrangement is shown in Fig. 1. A planoconcave lens is used to focus the output from the one megacycle transducer. The lens, made of polystyrene, fits into a recess of the crystal holder and is separated from the crystal by a layer of degassed distilled water ½″ deep. The lens is ground to a center thickness of 0.005″ and has a 1″ radius of curvature. To mark the focal region of the lens in the water bath, a hollow truncated aluminum cone of length equal to the focal length of the lens is threaded over the crystal holder. Positioning of an animal in the focus of the sound beam is thus facilitated. It was not feasible to use focused sound at 27 megacycles since one half of the energy from the transducer is lost in less than 1½ cm. of water. When irradiating livers with sound of this frequency animals were positioned 5⁄16″ from the transducer and irradiated through a small aperture cut in the skin overlying the liver.

[1] Now, Massachusetts General Hospital, Boston, Massachusetts.

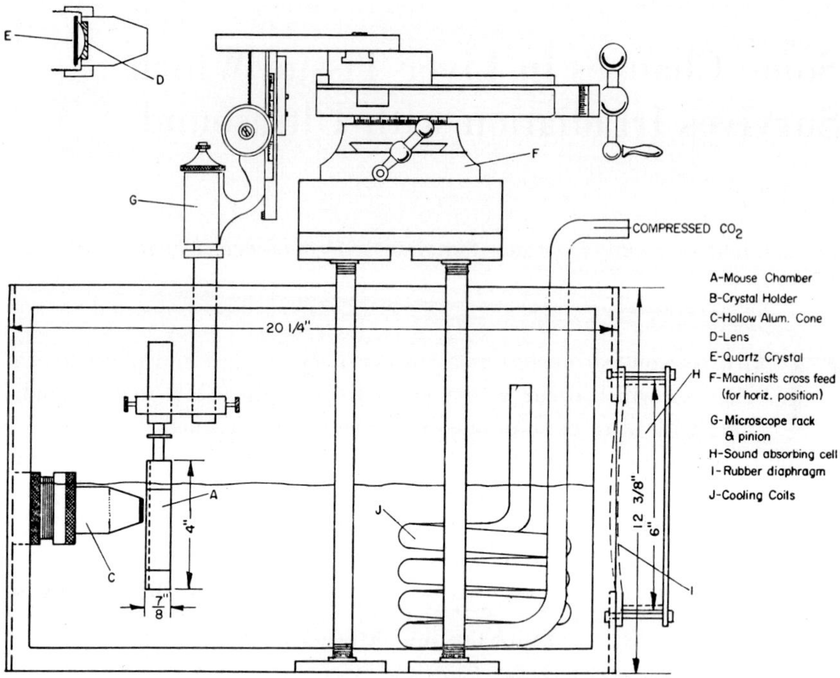

FIG. 1. Over-all experimental arrangement.

Sound intensity at one megacycle was measured with a Siemen's Sonotest meter and at 27 megacycles with a calorimeter. Unless otherwise specified animals are irradiated with ultrasound of 40 watts intensity at one megacycle (total energy delivered to 1st face of lens); and with ultrasound of 35 watts/cm.^{2} at 27 megacycles. The duration of exposure is 15 seconds.

Experimental animals were 3- to 4-month-old BUB and BUC white mice bred at Brown University. Animals were prepared for treatment by shaving the hair on the abdomen. The liver could then be seen below the translucent overlying tissues. Mice were anesthetized with ether and immobilized in a plastic chamber shown in Fig. 1. The chamber is clamped to the post of a three coordinate positioning system and the liver is aligned with the apex of a hollow aluminum cone so that it lies in the focal region of the sound field. The duration of exposure is controlled by an external timer connected to the screen of the oscillator tube.

Histological procedure: Animals are killed by a blow on the head, decapitated and thoroughly bled. Tissue is taken immediately, and fixed in Bouin's fluid for staining with hematoxylin and eosin; in Rossman's fluid for the McManus demonstration of glycogen; or in neutral formalin of demonstration of fat with Sudan IV. The material is oriented for sectioning so that it can be cut in the plane of irradiation. The tissue traversed by sound is thereby revealed in longitudinal section.

Results and Discussion

Disruptive Effects of Ultrasound on Liver Tissue

When the liver is irradiated ventrally with focused sound of 1 megacycle frequency at intensities between 1.5 to 40 watts (total energy delivered to the lens) damage which leads to necrosis may occur either at the ventral or the dorsal surface of the target lobe. In general when livers were irradiated with sound of 20 watts intensity or less, damage occurred at the lobe surface furthest removed from the sound source. This effect is shown schematically in Fig. 2. At intensities above 20 watts, damage occurred sometimes at the ventral surface and sometimes at the dorsal surface of the lobe. If damage occurs at the dorsal surface of the lobe, liver tissue more proximate to the sound source than the zone of damage is traversed by sound but

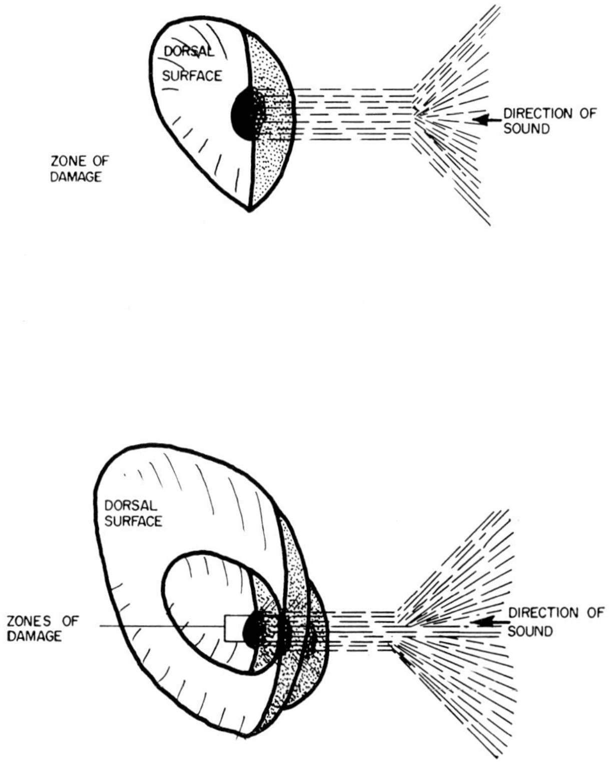

FIG. 2. Occurrence of damage at dorsal surface of liver lobes when livers are irradiated ventrally. Stippled portion of tissue is section cut in plane of irradiation.

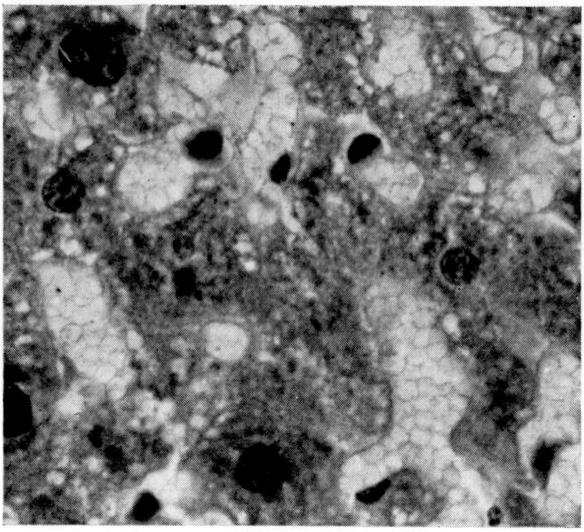

FIG. 3. Distended sinusoids congested with erythrocytes immediately following irradiation with ultrasound of 27 megacycles frequency and 35 watts/cm.^{2} intensity.

not necrotized. Even when damage occurs at the ventral surface one megacycle ultrasound penetrates the entire lobe. If animals are irradiated in the midline and damage occurs at the ventral surface of the liver lobe it is also observed that the spinal cord is injured. This injury is reflected immediately in paralysis of the hind legs. It is apparent then that liver cells adjacent to zones of damage are exposed to sublethal doses of sound, regardless

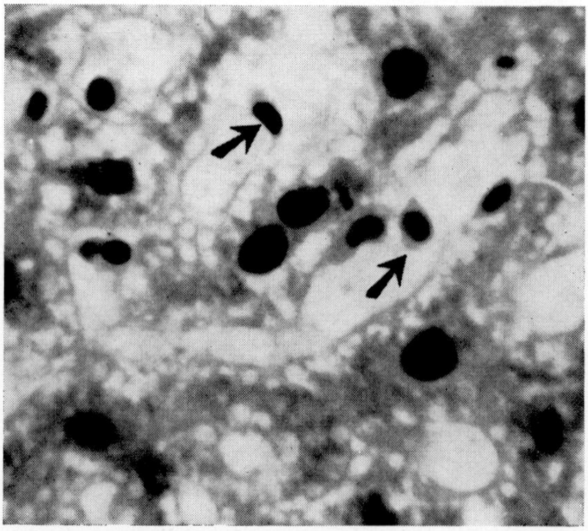

FIG. 4. Arrows point to dislodged macrophages.

of whether the zone of damage is located at the dorsal or the ventral surface of the lobe.

Immediately following irradiation with ultrasound of either one or 27 megacycles frequency, sinusoids in the zone of damage are markedly enlarged. After treatment at 27 megacycles sinusoids are 3 to 6 times larger than normal and after treatment at one megacycle they are 2 to 3 times larger than normal. The distended sinusoids are packed full with erythrocytes (Fig. 3). If thorium dioxide (Thorotrast) is injected intravenously, immediately following irradiation, the most severely injured region of tissue is shown to be completely congested but is not penetrated by thorium dioxide. This is interpreted as evidence of blood stasis in the zone of severest

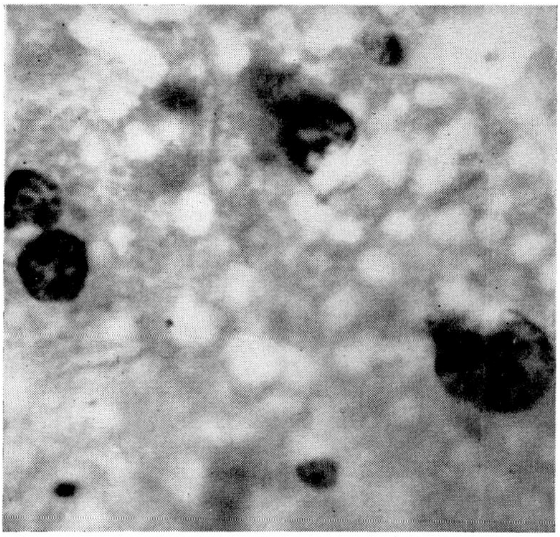

FIG. 5. Ruptured liver parenchymal cell nuclei immediately following irradiation at 27 megacycles.

damage. Blood flow is probably stopped in this region during the course of irradiation.

In the region which is congested, macrophages can be observed floating free in the sinusoids having been dislodged in some way from their attachment to the walls of the sinusoids (Fig. 4). This effect although seen following irradiation at 27 megacycles and not after irradiation at one megacycle is not dependent directly upon frequency. It is probably due to the distention of sinusoids which is greater at 27 megacycles than at one megacycle, and this difference results from more heating at the higher frequency than at the low. When a red-hot glass probe is applied to the surface of the liver the above effect on macrophages is also observed in sinusoids which are 5 to 6 times larger than normal. It appears then that both the extent to which sinusoids are enlarged and the resulting effect upon the macrophages is dependent upon the amount of heat absorbed by liver tissue.

Some parenchymal cell nuclei appear ruptured immediately after irradiation with ultrasound of 27 megacycles frequency (Fig. 5). This has not been observed following treatment at one megacycle or following the application of heat. Nuclear contents appear spilled into vacuoles which are pressed against the nuclear membrane. In fact rupture of the nuclear membrane or milder nuclear distortion always appears to occur in association with vacuoles which are contiguous with the nucleus.

Although rupture of nuclei is not observed in livers irradiated at one megacycle, extensive vacuolization occurs after irradiation with either fre-

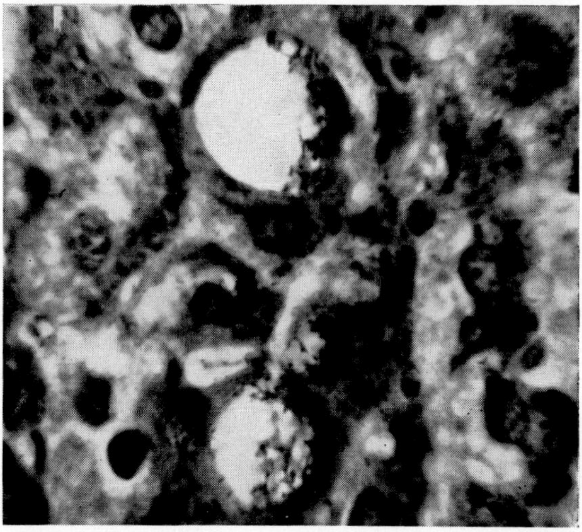

FIG. 6. Holes in liver tissue seen immediately following irradiation at 1 megacycle.

quency in both regions which become necrotic as well as in tissue which survives irradiation. It is not certain to what the vacuoles are due. Neither fat nor glycogen can account for all of the vacuoles observed. It is unlikely that they are the result of cavitation, for if cavitation were responsible for their occurrence, rupture of nuclear membranes should be observed oftener in livers irradiated at one megacycle than in those irradiated at 27 megacycles, but it is not observed at all in livers irradiated at one megacycle.

What do look like cavitation holes, and correspond to pseudo-cavitation which Hug and Pape have observed in livers irradiated with ultrasound of one megacycle frequency are shown in Fig. 6. This phenomenon has not been observed in livers treated with 27 megacycles ultrasound.

The occurrence of glycogen, which is normally not present in the blood,

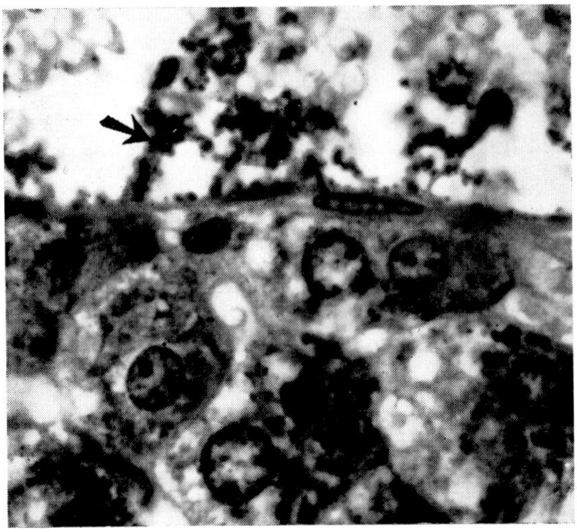

FIG. 7. Arrow points to glycogen granules in blood vessels of liver immediately following irradiation at 1 megacycle. The presence of glycogen in blood indicates disruption of liver cells.

in lumens of small vessels and sinusoids of the liver immediately following irradiation, is unmistakable evidence of cellular disruption in liver tissue. In Fig. 7 the dark specks are glycogen granules in a small blood vessel.

Not only are intracellular materials released into the circulation as a consequence of irradiation, but elements from the circulation are forced into liver cells. A startling effect which has been observed following irradiation

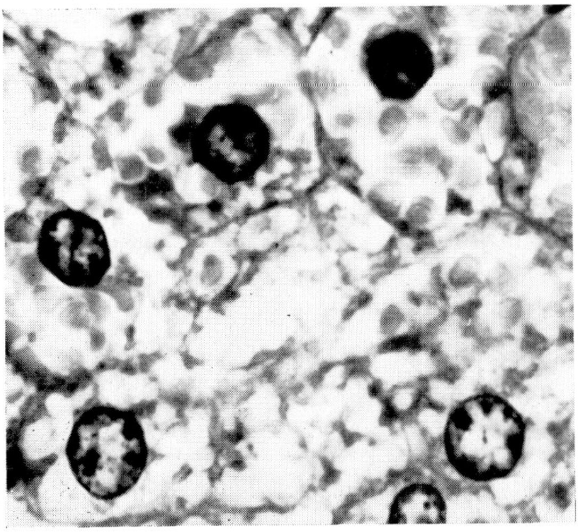

FIG. 8. Erythrocytes in liver cells.

with focused ultrasound of one megacycle frequency as well as with unfocused sound of the same frequency is the occurrence of erythrocytes in parenchymal cells (Fig. 8). It is not known how the erythrocytes enter liver cells or whether all of these cells eventually die. Where the effect occurs in a large number of cells in the same region of the liver the cells become necrotic. However, where isolated small groups of cells or single cells are filled with erythrocytes, there is evidence that some of them survive. This will be discussed later.

The effects described so far are observed in livers of animals sacrificed immediately following irradiation and occur generally in the volume of tissue which becomes necrotic. H and E preparations show the zone of necrosis to be fairly well defined by about six hours following irradiation. The

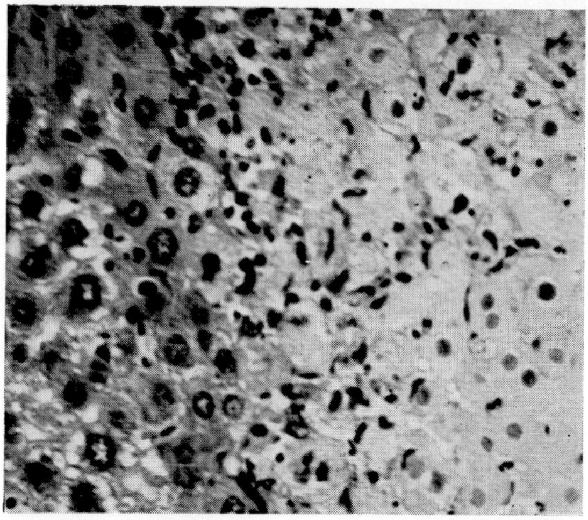

FIG. 9. Liver necrosis 24 hours following irradiation at 1 megacycle with focused ultrasound. Zone of necrosis at left.

cytoplasm of necrotic cells is eosinophilic and nuclei are slightly hyperchromatic. At 24 hours the zone of necrosis is sharply defined and some leucocytes have accumulated at the border between the necrotic tissue and the tissues which has survived (Fig. 9). By 5 days the line of demarcation between the surviving tissue and the zone of damage is a thick connective tissue stroma. Nuclear membranes and cell boundaries in the necrotic region are still visible; nuclei still stain well with hematoxylin and nucleoli are distinguishable (Fig. 10).

By 15 days the necrotized tissue has been sloughed into the abdominal cavity and a well-defined fibrotic scar marks its place (Fig. 11). For as long as 11 days following irradiation structural elements of the necrotized tissue retain their identity. The breakdown of tissue structure occurs only

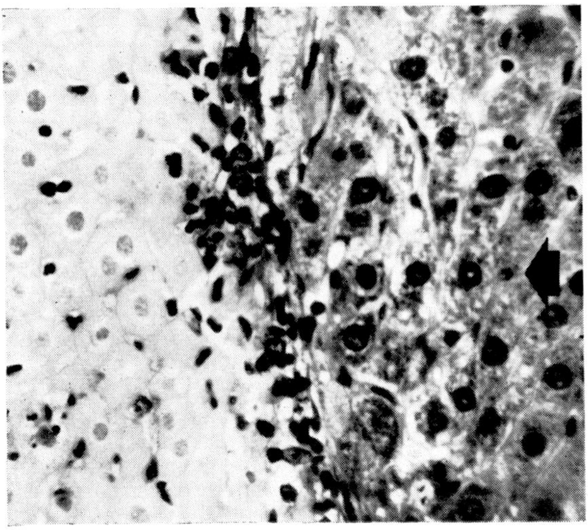

FIG. 10. Liver necrosis 5 days following irradiation at 1 megacycle. Arrow indicates direction of sound. Zone of necrosis at left.

slowly and reflects an equally slow rate of lytic activity. The latter seems to depend on the degree of contact between the necrotized tissue and the blood as well as on enzyme systems within the zone of necrosis. It has been shown that congestion occurs in the tissue probably during the course of irradiation, and that the most severely damaged region is almost immediately deprived of its circulation. These initial events explain the stasis in

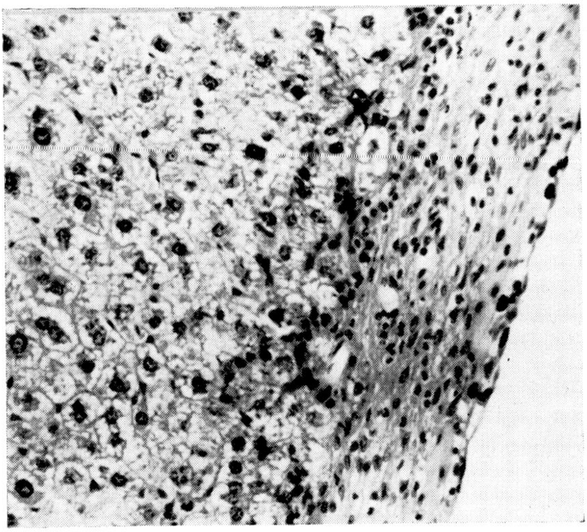

FIG. 11. Fibrotic scar observed 15 days following irradiation at 1 megacycle. Scar marks place of necrotic tissue which is sloughed into abdominal cavity.

lytic activity and the consequent maintenance of structure in the necrotized tissue. The same histological picture can be obtained by ligating small portions of liver tissue with dental tape. Structural breakdown in ligated tissue proceeds slowly, and probably for the same reason as above: that the rate of exchange between the tissue and blood is decelerated. The volume of tissue which is most severely damaged is deprived of its circulation. It cannot be concluded, however, that all of the cells in this volume of tissue have been killed by ultrasound. The effect on some of the cells may be in part an indirect one. Since blood flow through the zone of severe damage is stopped, necrosis of some liver cells could be due to anoxia.

Response of the Liver as a Whole to Damage with Ultrasound

One of the normal physiological responses of the liver is its capacity to repair itself following injury. As much as 70 percent of the liver can be removed or destroyed, and the remaining portion of the organ will proliferate actively until its original size is restored. The lobar architecture is no longer the same but the "new" liver possesses the same volume as that of the "old" one. After ordinary chemical or surgical damage the liver begins to repair itself within two and a half days. That is, cells scattered throughout the uninjured regions of the organ are seen to be in mitosis by that time. The interval between initial injury and the onset of mitosis may vary in the mouse liver depending upon the mode of injury, but it is not less than 24 hours nor more than 72 hours for the various injurious agents which have been studied. For example, following central necrosis due to injection of CCl_4, extensive lysis has occurred by 24 hours and by 5 days the entire process of repair is completed. To determine whether the mouse liver exhibited this regenerative response when it was damaged with ultrasound, and if it did, whether the time interval between injury and the onset of mitosis was the same as for other injurious agents, livers were irradiated with focused sound of one megacycle frequency or with unfocused sound of 27 megacycles frequency. Between 5 and 50 percent of the left lateral lobe was necrotized by ultrasound in each of the intact livers irradiated. The extent of the damage was estimated at the time of sacrifice. Animals were sacrificed serially at 24-hour intervals following irradiation.

Generally distributed mitotic activity was not observed in any of the livers irradiated at either frequency before the 5th day after injury. The interval between injury and the onset of mitosis was the same regardless of the extent of damage.

Since the time of initiation of mitosis might depend upon the volume of tissue damaged, 5, 10 and 50 percent of the left lateral lobe was necrotized by ligation. In all of the sections studied generally distributed mitoses were observed by 72 hours. It is apparent that the mitotic response can be elicited by ligation after the usual time delay even when the extent of damage is small.

Thus cell divisions were observed 2 to 3 days earlier in ligated livers than in irradiated livers despite the histological similarity of the respective necroses. Therefore, the inhibiting effect of ultrasound upon regeneration cannot be ascribed to the retarded rate of lytic activity inferred from histological observations. It is suggested, however, that inhibition might be the result of unique biochemical changes which are not reflected histologically in tissue necrotized by ultrasound. This view is in accord with the hypothesis that the initial stimulus for mitosis emanates from the zone of injury. If the stimulus for mitosis was elicited solely as a consequence of the functional loss of a portion of the liver regardless of events within the zone of necrosis, the interval between injury and the onset of cell divisions would be independent of the mode of cell death. But that this interval does depend upon the mode of cell death is evident from the fact that it is twice as great following damage with ultrasound as it is following ordinary surgical or chemical damage. We have found that cautery as well as ultrasound delays the onset of mitosis. Following cauterization of 50 percent of the left lateral lobe, mitosis is not elicited within 72 hours but the response is delayed until the fourth day after injury, as compared with 5 days after injury with ultrasound, and 2 to 3 days after injury by ligation.

One of the by-products of the foregoing experiment on liver regeneration has been the observation of mitotic abnormalities in liver cells adjacent to

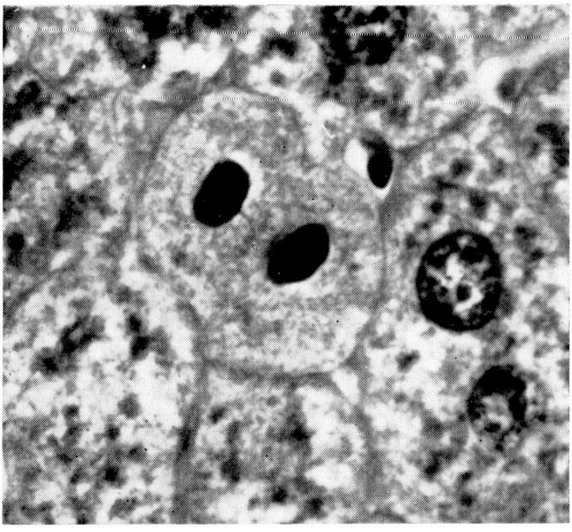

FIG. 12. Chromatin bridge between daughter nuclei in late telophase. Five days following sublethal irradiation at 1 megacycle.

the zone of necrosis which have been irradiated with sub-lethal intensities of ultrasound (Fig. 12). A chromatin thread is seen stretched between two nuclei in a cell in telophase. Lagging chromosomes have been observed, particularly in cells in metaphase. Since these effects occur relatively infrequently, no special significance has been attached to them. The same type of abnormality is observed following damage produced by carbon tetrachloride as well as following damage by other injurious agents.

The Effects of Ultrasound on Different Cell Types of the Liver

Macrophages which appear not to have been damaged by ultrasonic irradiation have been observed in necrotized portions of the liver as long as 24 hours following treatment. Two of the possible explanations for this observation are the following: 1. that macrophages are less susceptible to the damaging effects of ultrasound than parenchymal cells or, 2. that macrophages in the zone of necrosis only appear undamaged but are in fact nonfunctional. Two sets of experiments were performed to test these explanations. In the first set animals were injected intravenously with Thorotrast (colloidal thorium dioxide) prior to irradiation of the liver with ultrasound of one or 27 megacycles frequency, while in the second they were injected with Thorotrast immediately and at intervals following irradiation. Thorotrast is phagocytized by macrophages of the reticulo-endothelial sys-

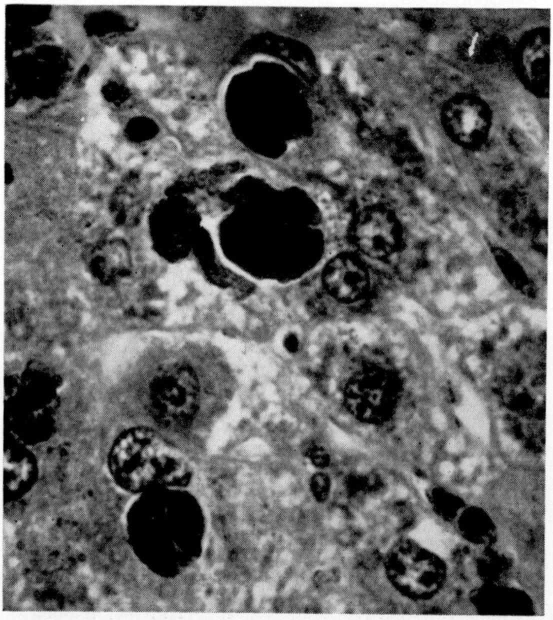

FIG. 13. Macrophages loaded with Thorotrast granules in unirradiated liver.

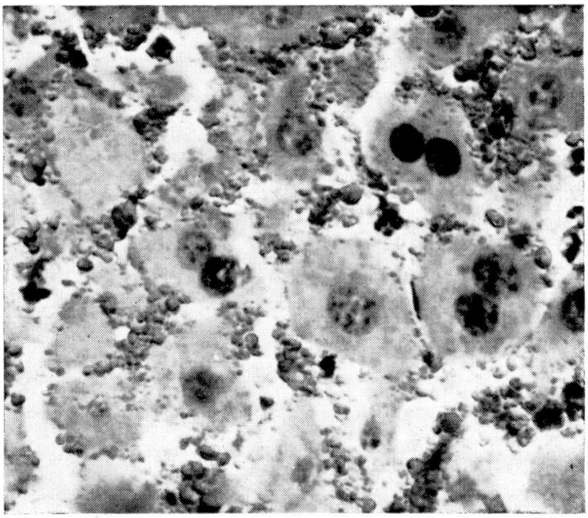

FIG. 14. Break up of macrophages several hours following irradiation with ultrasound of 27 megacycles frequency. Granules scattered between cells.

tem and about 80 percent of the injected material is picked up by the liver. The colloidal material appears in the cells in the form of granules which probably form in the blood prior to being injected by the macrophages (Bell, 1953). Macrophages loaded with ThO_2 granules are shown in Fig. 13.

When livers are loaded with ThO_2 and then irradiated with ultrasound, many of the macrophages are disrupted and granules are scattered through surrounding tissue fluid and blood spaces. The degree of scatter is particularly noticeable several hours following irradiation (Fig. 14). Where the break-up occurs, both the parenchyma and the macrophages become necrotic. In regions where the parenchyma is intact, macrophages are not disrupted. In fact, disruption will not occur unless the acoustic intensity is high enough to produce necrosis in parenchymal cells.

When animals are irradiated prior to injection with Thorotrast, the colloidal material does not flow into regions of severe damage which have apparently become occluded. However, in zones peripheral to the occluded regions macrophages containing Thorotrast can be observed in areas where parenchymal cells are necrotic (Fig. 15). Thorotrast can be injected as long as 22 hours following irradiation, at a time when the zone of necrosis is clearly defined, and some macrophages within this zone can be seen to contain this material.

These experiments suggest that macrophages are less sensitive to the damaging effects of ultrasound than are liver parenchymal cells. It is apparent that the susceptibility of macrophages to damage with ultrasound depends upon their condition at the time of irradiation. If macrophages are laden with Thorotrast at the time of irradiation their cytoplasm is fragmented and Thorotrast granules are released into the sinusoids; however, if they are not laden with ThO_2 at the time of irradiation some of them can still function as phagocytes even after having been exposed to ultrasound intense enough to necrotize parenchymal cells.

Changes in Liver Cells Which Survive Irradiation with Ultrasound

It has been shown that liver cells adjacent to the zone of necrosis are exposed to sublethal doses of ultrasound. Some of the changes which occur in these cells may be due to the unique action of ultrasound; others may be

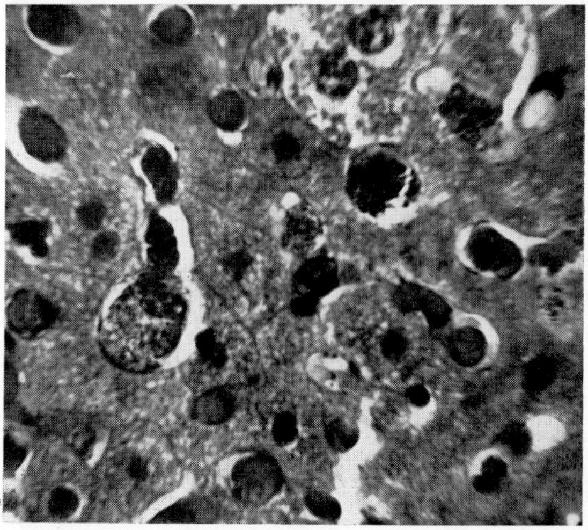

FIG. 15. Macrophages containing Thorotrast in region where parenchymal cells are necrotic. Thorotrast injected 16 hours following irradiation.

non-specific responses which can be elicited by a variety of injurious agents, and still others may be accounted for by the proximity of necrotic tissue which may interact with neighboring cells. It is not yet possible to assign each of the modifications, which will be described below, to one of these classes; some, however, are less ambiguous than others.

For as long as 5 days following irradiation at one or 27 megacycles, some cells adjacent to the zone of necrosis contain inclusion bodies which stain strongly with eosin (Fig. 16). The inclusion bodies are spherical and homogeneous and they vary in size from a few microns in diameter to the size of a liver cell nucleus. They have been observed by others in our laboratory in mouse livers which have been injured with CCl_4.

Many liver parenchymal cells are binucleate. A frequent occurrence in

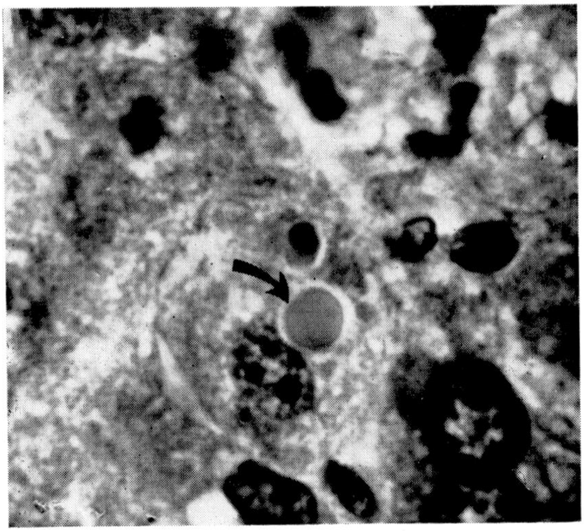

FIG. 16. Arrow points to inclusion in liver cells which has survived irradiation with ultrasound.

such cells which have been irradiated sublethally is the destruction of only one of the nuclei. Fig. 17 shows a binucleate cell in which one nucleus has been injured; the other has remained intact. This effect has been observed at two and three days following irradiation.

Glycogen in the entire band of cells which borders the zone of necrosis is present in reduced amounts as long as 24 hours following irradiation with

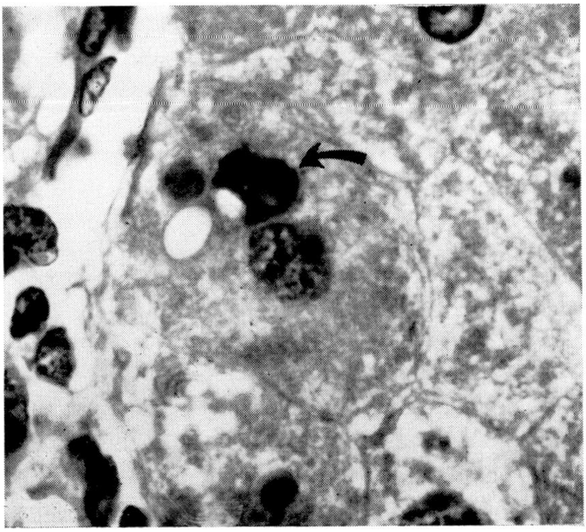

FIG. 17. Arrow points to damaged nucleus in binucleate cell which has survived irradiation with ultrasound.

ultrasound of one megacycle frequency (Fig. 18). A decrease in glycogen in liver cells following treatment of the liver with ultrasound has been reported by several workers. Tsuge (1938) showed that this phenomenon was reflected in an increase in the blood sugar level in rabbits, and Bejdl (1951) has reported that the glycogen content of isolated pieces of rat liver is decreased as a result of irradiation with ultrasound. We have confirmed these observations histologically in intact livers.

It should be noted that if a mouse is handled roughly, glycogen will be released from the liver. The loss of glycogen from the liver is probably an accompanying feature of any traumatic event. However, in cells irradiated sublethally the normal glycogen level has not been restored by 24 hours,

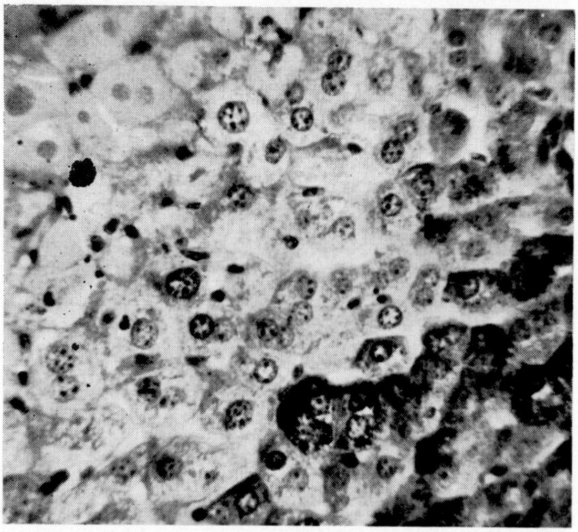

FIG. 18. Decrease in glycogen in sublethally irradiated liver cells. Cells rich in glycogen at upper right. Necrotic cells at lower right.

whereas in other cells it has. This may be an indication that ultrasound has in some way altered normal metabolic function.

There is also an increase in the deposition of fat by 24 hours in sublethally irradiated cells. This too is not extraordinary. Increase in the deposition of fat is observed routinely in cells adjacent to necrotic material, no matter how the tissue has been necrotized.

It was mentioned previously that extensive vacuolization is observed in tissue which survives irradiation as well as in tissue which is necrotized. In Fig. 19 small vacuoles may be observed pressing against nuclei. Apparently vacuolization results in the deformation of nuclei but not necessarily in the death of the cell.

The holes in this figure vary in size, but average about 3 or 4 microns in diameter.

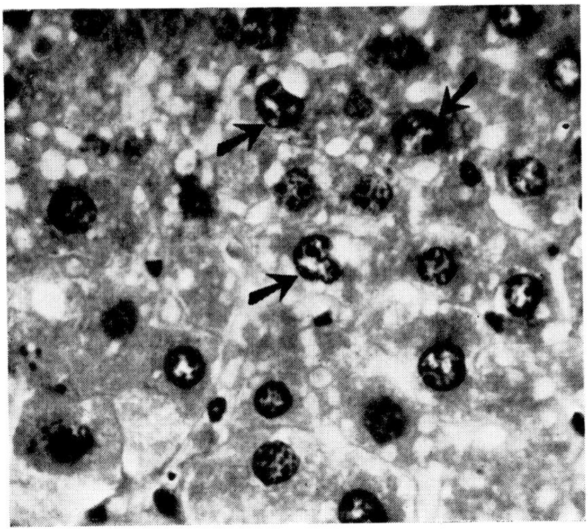

FIG. 19. Arrows point to deformed nuclei in tissue which has survived irradiation.

The occurrence of erythrocytes in liver parenchymal cells following irradiation of liver has already been alluded to. Fig. 20 shows a liver cell 24 hours after treatment with ultrasound which is filled with erythrocytes. The cell is surrounded by normal cells. The nucleus of this cell is only slightly hyper-chromatic and the cell does not appear to be necrosed. The liver of this animal was irradiated with ultrasound of one megacycle frequency at an intensity of 4 watts/cm.^{2} We will study this effect further to

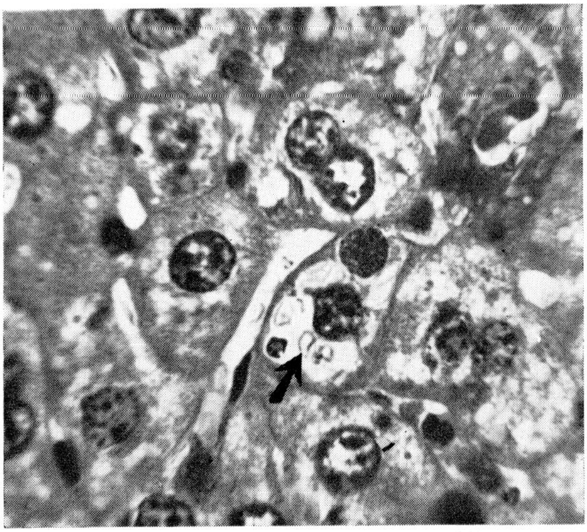

FIG. 20. Erythrocytes in liver cell 24 hours following irradiation of liver with unfocused ultrasound of 1 megacycle frequency and 4 watts/cm.^{2} intensity.

determine whether cells containing erythrocytes are, in fact, viable and for how long. One of the first things to be studied is the character of the cytoplasm which remains in cells filled with erythrocytes. The nuclei of such cells have in a sense been provided with a new environment which may modify their ability to function normally. If these cells are viable what function can they perform? Are they, for example, still capable of dividing? It is thought that this effect is a unique one. It has not been observed in our laboratory under any other conditions.

References

Bejdl, W. 1951. Der Einfluss des Ultraschalls auf das Glycogen der Leberzelle und auf die Kupfferschen Sternzellen. Acta Anatomica *11:* 444–460.

Bell, E. 1953. The origin and nature of granules found in macrophages of the white mouse following intravenous injection of thorotrast. J. Cell. and Comp. Physiol. *42:* 125–136.

Hug, O. and R. Pape. 1954. Nachweis der Ultraschallkavitation im Gewebe. Strahlentherapie *94:* 79–99.

Tsuge, S. 1938. Über die Beeinflussung des intermediären Kohlehydratstoffwechsels in der Leber durch Einwirkung der Ultraakustischen Schallwellen und Ultrakurzwellen auf die Leber. Tohoku Jour. Exptl. Med. *33:* 8–17.

Wilson, J. W. and E. H. Leduc. 1950. Abnormal mitosis in mouse liver. Amer. J. Anat. *86:* 51–73.

Dr. Quimby: Do you consider that the cell walls of the liver cells are intact?

Dr. Bell: Yes, they appear to be intact.

Dr. Krumins: The same picture has been observed following x-irradiation.

Dr. Bell: Under what conditions?

Dr. Krumins: Animals were treated with very high doses, 11,000 R.

Dr. Wild: Dr. Bell, I would like to ask you why you have not considered grading the dose and relating it to the damage? I was wondering if you had that in mind, or whether you do not consider it necessary.

Dr. Bell: Yes, we do. For example, in studying the last effect about which I talked, that is, erythrocytes found in liver cells, we have already altered our irradiation procedure. We have used unfocussed sound at an intensity of 4 watts/cm.^{2} Little necrosis results from exposure to sound of this intensity, but if the entire liver is irradiated at 4 watts/cm.^{2} the animal dies. It may be possible to apply the dose necessary to produce the effect we are looking for by exposing only a small portion of the liver. In other words when we find that a particular effect is significant we will try to quantitate it.

DR. ALDES: Did you do any experiments with what we call therapeutic doses?

DR. BELL: I do not know how you define a therapeutic dose, but we have irradiated some animals at intensities that produce few obvious changes in the liver, and which do not lead to necrosis.

DR. ALDES: What I mean is, say, 1,000,000 cycles at maybe 1 watt/$cm.^2$ on an animal larger than a mouse.

DR. BELL: I have done that, but only in the mouse.

DR. ALDES: And you have found no changes?

DR. BELL: I would not really say that. We have not studied that kind of material sufficiently to say there are no changes.

DR. ALDES: In our study, to be certain we were not getting liver damage, or kidney damage, we ran 24-hour specimens and found no pathology as far as the urine was concerned, or kidney function, or as far as blood count is concerned. We did 24, 28, and 72 of therapeutic doses on humans.

DR. OESTREICHER: Do the lesions grow in relation to the lobules?

DR. BELL: The lesions occur without relation to the lobules. A lesion can involve half of a lobule, or for that matter any fraction of one.

DR. BARNARD: What are some of the earliest sacrifices that you have made after irradiation in the very first stages, and first, what are the very first stages; and second, what are your speculations as to why it is on one surface of it and not in the middle?

DR. BELL: In answer to your first question, Figs. 3–7 are examples of effects which are observed in liver tissue immediately following irradiation; by immediately I mean in tissue removed as quickly as possible after irradiation. This involves killing the animal, opening the abdominal cavity, removing a lobe of liver and cutting off a slice which is placed in a fixative. The tissue is in the fixative within one minute.

As to the second question, I do not like to tackle this problem, but I will say a few words about it. We have performed the following experiment in a model system. Three lobes of mouse liver are placed in contact with one another in a plastic chamber. The ventral surface of the first lobe is contiguous with the underlying tissues of a piece of mouse skin which is stretched over an aperture in the chamber. The other two lobes are positioned directly behind the first lobe with ventral surfaces nearest the sound source. Such a system has been irradiated with focused ultrasound of one megacycle frequency through the aperture in the chamber. When the tissue is irradiated for 15 seconds at an intensity of 20 watts (total energy delivered to the first face of the lens) damage is observed to occur at the dorsal surface of each of the three lobes. This is precisely the effect which is observed in the intact animal. I can only make some guesses as to the reasons for its occurrence.

DR. BUSNEL: Interface?

DR. BELL: Interfaces exist at both the dorsal and ventral surfaces. The question is why does damage occur at the dorsal surfaces of successive lobes and not at the ventral surfaces or somewhere in between the two surfaces? Possibly because incident and reflected energy sums only at the dorsal surface where the capsule might act as a reflecting wall. This summation might create a region sufficiently high in energy density to cause damage. If this is so the effect at the dorsal surface of each of the lobes must occur sequentially in time; that is, it would occur at times t_1 in the lobe nearest the source, at time t_2 in the next lobe and so on. After the occurrences of damage at the dorsal surface of the first lobe, the interface between lobes may be so altered as to no longer constitute a reflection barrier. A further speculation is an alpha for liver which is temperature-dependent.

DR. HERRICK: At what frequency did you do this?

DR. BELL: At one megacycle. When the temperature rises at the dorsal surface of the first lobe where incident and reflected energy is summed, a portion of the adjacent second lobe might be afforded protection as a result of the local temperature rise. This would be so, that is, if absorption decreased as the temperature increased.

DR. CARSTENSEN: What is the geometry of your beam? This is a focused sound field.

DR. BELL: The sound field looks like two cones separated by a cylindrical focal region. Livers are positioned in the focal region of the beam.

DR. BALLANTINE: Did you have any loss of animals, any mortality attributable to the irradiation of the liver?

DR. BELL: I cannot say definitely whether death is due to irradiation of the liver or of the blood in the liver, but when just the liver region is irradiated at 4 watts/$cm.^2$ with unfocused sound the animals die.

DR. BALLANTINE: In what period of time do they die?

DR. BELL: Some of them will last two days, some three or four, and then die.

DR. FRY: How long do you irradiate?

DR. BELL: For one minute.

DR. FRY: At what frequency?

DR. BELL: One megacycle.

DR. BALLANTINE: This is a phenomenon we have observed in mouse spinal cords in which an overdosing of the mouse with ultrasound would produce death of the mouse within eight hours to 3 or 4 days. If you chose the correct dosage, which would paralyze the mouse, they survive almost indefinitely, although paraplegic. This is an interesting phenomenon. I wonder if you observed it.

DR. BELL: No. But I have observed paralysis.

DR. BALLANTINE: I do not mean paralysis. I mean, the fact that the animal dies if he is overtreated, although the lesion seems to be specifically localized to one portion of his anatomy.

DR. BELL: When the lesion is specifically localized in the liver we have never had an animal die. If, however, some part of the gut is hit and if the gut ulcerates then the animal dies from peritonitis.

DR. BALLANTINE: He does not die from an effect that you cannot attribute to ultrasound?

DR. BELL: No, not as far as I have observed.

DR. BUSNEL: Did you make some observation on the physiological movement in the gall bladder after the treatment by ultrasonics?

DR. BELL: No observations. I acknowledge it would be interesting to do.

DR. NAUTA: I should like to ask if there would be a possibility that these curious division figures you had, the nuclei with ultrasonics may not be an expression of amitosis instead of mitosis. Amitosis in the normal liver, I understand is quite a normal phenomenon.

DR. BELL: There may still be some debate as to whether liver cells can divide by amitosis. The chromatin bridge in Fig. 12 can be designated as an instance of pseudoamitosis (Wilson and Leduc, 1950) the occurrence of which cannot be considered a normal event.

DR. HUETER: I am a little bit out of my field here, so permit me to ask what may be a naive question. Do you consider the possibility that through some action on the blood, or through a change of the sugar level you may effect a larger lesion in the region where the focus was placed, i.e., that you destroyed something in a region, and this effect spreads out, so to speak?

DR. BELL: I think that one cannot attribute the effects in tissues which survive irradiation exclusively to the effects upon blood. They are certainly important but one must also consider the direct effect on the liver cell itself. I would not want to stress one without stressing the other.

DR. HERRICK: The liver is a particularly interesting organ because it has venous blood, as well as arterial blood. It has a dual blood supply entering it. There is a definite partition of the circulatory system, so some of these sharp demarcations may be due to interference of certain regions of the circulation.

DR. LEHMANN: I just want to mention that the changes of the mitotic figures, the strand between the nuclei are quite commonly observed after exposure to ultrasound, various modes of action of ultrasound produces these, and there might be instances where mitotic conditions occur.

DR. BELL: It should be pointed out that the effects which Dr. Lehmann is talking about occur in tissues which are exposed to ultrasound while in the process of dividing. The division figures that I showed occur at some later time subsequent to irradiation. The liver was not dividing at the time of treatment. The frequency of cell divisions in the normal liver is about one cell per 20 to 40 thousand, and it is very rare in the course of examining liver sections to see a division figure in liver tissue of a normal adult animal. The mitotic abnormality in Fig. 12 occurred 5 days after the application of sound in tissue which was sublethally irradiated. I am not making the point here that the division figures which occur in general following irradiation with ultrasound of the frequencies employed are abnormal. We have observed only a few abnormalities. Wilson and Leduc (1950) have reported similar abnormalities irrespective of the method by which mitotic activity is induced. I would like to make one more point in this connection. We have induced livers to divide by injecting animals with carbon tetrachloride after irradiating the liver with ultrasound, and we have not observed a higher frequency of abnormal figures in livers of these animals.

DR. CARSTENSEN: In connection with this question of the apparent local absorption of sound energy, I wonder if you might have seen this same sort of thing along other inhomogeneities in tissues such as large blood vessels? I think it is quite likely that microscopic inhomogeneities in the tissue may be a major cause or major source of absorption in the tissues. It seems probable that in this particular model that you make up here in which there are interfaces, although there are similar pieces of tissue, one after the other, that you do have localized absorption. This probably is an important factor to a lesser degree, and for lesser inhomogeneities.

DR. BELL: As I understand your point, you would consider, that because of structural inhomogeneities at the dorsal region of the lobe, absorption in that region might be greater than elsewhere.

DR. CARSTENSEN: Yes, certainly.

DR. BELL: But this is not the case in the mouse liver. The dorsal portion of the lobe looks very much like the ventral portion. There are, of course, differences between dorsal and ventral portions of a lobe in the direction and location (with respect to the source) of larger blood vessels, but this is so no matter where the liver is irradiated. We have not tried turning the whole system around; that is, arranging the lobes in the model system so that the dorsal surface is nearer the source than the ventral surface. If interval inhomogeneities are of no consequence we should still expect that damage would occur at the surface furthest removed from the source, that is, at the ventral instead of the dorsal surface.

DR. CARSTENSEN: Just the mere fact that there is a discontinuity of any kind means that it is possible to produce a reflection, and the reflection may then consist of a small initial component of transverse waves which is very rapidly damped out and produces this localized heating.

DR. BELL: You are talking then about the existence of the membrane, the capsule of the lobe?

DR. CARSTENSEN: Yes.

DR. BELL: Yes, I will agree thoroughly with that. I have no argument. I thought you meant the internum of the tissue, the parenchyma itself.

DR. CARSTENSEN: I am trying to point out this is probably a very nice picture of localized absorption that you get in tissue. It gives a dramatic illustration of a mechanism of absorption which must occur in almost all tissues.

DR. BALDES: Are you planning to make any comparison of your ultrasonic treatment of liver with the work that has been done on gamma radiation?

DR. BELL: We have had no immediate plans to do that. It might be very interesting to compare.

An Ultrasonic Dosage Study: Functional Endpoint

F. Dunn and W. J. Fry

Bioacoustics Laboratory, University of Illinois, Urbana, Illinois

THIS PAPER constitutes an initial report on an elaborate ultrasonic dosage study which has been undertaken at the Bioacoustics Laboratory of the University of Illinois. The completed study will include dosage relationships as a function of base temperature of the tissue, hydrostatic pressure and frequency.

The equipment, both mechanical and electronic, has been developed over the past several years. Instrumentation for such a study must be of a precision nature if quantitative data are to result for elucidation of mechanisms. It is possible to realize accurately reproducible results on a suitably prepared and precisely irradiated biological preparation.

It is the purpose of this paper to describe the experimental arrangement, technique of preparation and accuracy of results obtainable with such a suitably designed system.

The type of results obtainable from such a study will be illustrated with data taken at a base temperature of 10° C., a hydrostatic pressure of one atmosphere and a frequency of 982 kc./s.

The subject used for this study is an intact mouse, approximately 24 hours after birth. The mice used are of the LaFl strain, which is an impure strain, so that brown, white and gray mice are utilized indiscriminately. The mice are cooled to render them inactive so that they can be accurately positioned in the mouse-holder. They are placed in the sound tank which utilizes degassed mammalian saline, as the acoustic transmitting medium. The temperature of the saline is accurately controlled to a few tenths of a degree centigrade.

The mice are positioned in the sound field such that the axis of the beam is centered on the third lumbar vertebra in order to produce motor paralysis in the hind legs. The animals are allowed several minutes, which is sufficient time, to reach their equilibrium temperature before exposure to the sound. The exposure is transcutaneous.

The sound field is calibrated each day, just before the animals are exposed, by the method described by Dr. Fry (Fry and Fry, 1954a; Ibid., 1954b). This makes it possible to precisely determine the acoustic intensity

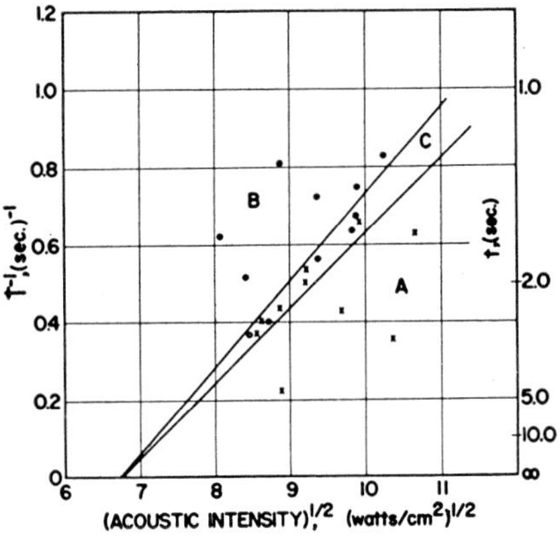

FIG. 1. Scheme for presenting the data. A "dot" represents an unparalyzed animal and an "X" represents a paralyzed animal. Animals which appear in the higher dosage region "A" are always paralyzed. Those which fall in the lesser dosage region "B" are never paralyzed and those which appear in the *threshold region* "C" are distributed between paralyzed and unparalyzed.

at which the mouse is exposed. In this paper, ultrasonic dosage is specified by the acoustic intensity and the time duration of the exposure.

The functional endpoint observed on these animals after exposure to acoustic energy is paralysis of the hind legs; that is, lack of motor response. Anesthesia is also observed; however, correlation between lack of sensory response and ultrasonic dosage is not the subject of this study.

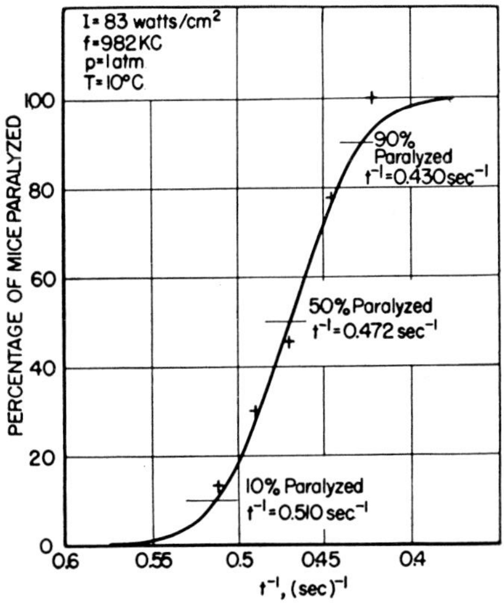

FIG. A–1. Sigmoidal distribution of percentage of mice paralyzed as a function of the reciprocal of the duration of exposure at constant acoustic intensity.

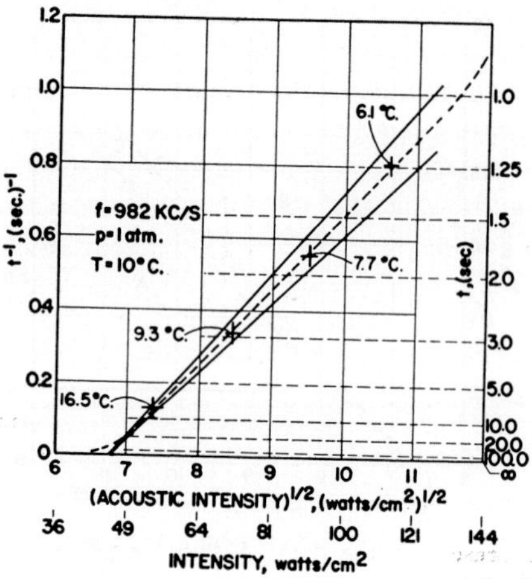

FIG. 2. The ultrasonic dosage threshold curve for base temperature of 10° C. The midline of the threshold region is extended to show the variations at the extremities of the linear portion. The indicated temperature rises were measured by imbedded thermocouples in the spinal cords of irradiated mice.

The results can be plotted on a coordinate system which has the reciprocal of time as the ordinate and the square root of the acoustic intensity as the abscissa (dosage graph), for example, by placing a "dot" at the proper point to represent an unparalyzed animal and an "X" for a paralyzed animal. Fig. 1 illustrates the schemes for presenting these data. When this is done it is possible to place two straight lines, having a common value for acoustic intensity at infinite time, as boundaries for a threshold region. Thus essentially all animals which fall in the higher dosage region "A" are paralyzed and essentially all those which fall in the lesser dosage region "B" are not paralyzed. The animals which appear in the threshold region "C" are distributed between paralyzed and unparalyzed.[1]

[1] This description is readily expressed in more precise terms as follows: If the raw data at one intensity are treated by probit analysis (Finney, 1952), the type of curve illustrated by Fig. A–1 results. The mice considered in this analysis were irradiated at a constant acoustic intensity for various exposure times. The distribution of the number of animals paralyzed is plotted as a function of the reciprocal of the exposure time. Each point represents approximately 20 animals. The standard deviation is of the order of a few percent. From curves such as these, it is possible to define the threshold region in a more precise fashion than stated above. Thus, from a series of curves (at different acoustic intensities) such as Fig. A–1, one can obtain the reciprocal of the exposure time for 10% and 90% of the animals paralyzed. The collection of these two sets of values define two curves on the dosage graph and the region between these two curves is defined arbitrarily as the threshold region.

Fig. A-2 shows the threshold region determined in the above fashion plotted on the dosage graph.

At the present time we have rather extensive data at a hydrostatic pressure of one atmosphere, a frequency of 982 kc./s., and a base temperature of 10° C. These data show that the slopes of these two straight lines differ by approximately eighteen percent. See Fig. 2. In the region of dosages of intensities less than 50 watts/cm.², corresponding to time durations greater than 20 seconds, the slope of the borders of the threshold region appears to increase gradually, probably indicating that excessive temperatures developed at these long exposure times are the primary cause of the effect on the tissue.

The region between 50 watts/cm.², corresponding to 20 seconds time duration, and 120 watts/cm.², corresponding to one second time duration, appears to exhibit a linear relationship between the reciprocal of time duration and the square root of intensity, indicating that in this region a second process has become important. For dosages at intensities greater than 130 watts/cm.², (time durations less than one second) the relationship between

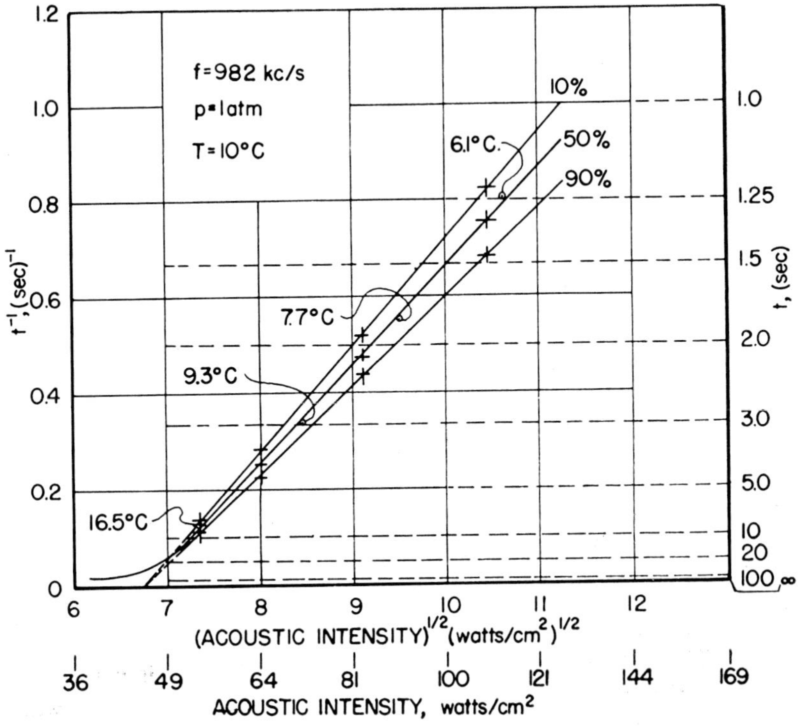

FIG. A–2. Threshold region for paralysis of the hind legs of mice under ultrasonic irradiation. The indicated temperature rises were measured by imbedded thermocouples in the spinal cords of irradiated mice. Time and intensity are also indicated on the coordinate axes.

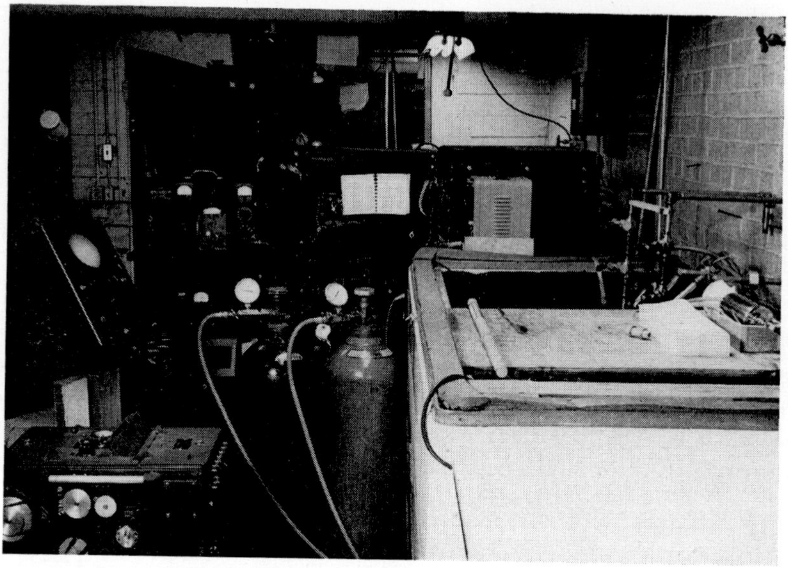

FIG. 3. The arrangement of the equipment showing the deep-freeze unit (which contains the sound tank), the power amplifier, frequency control, timing stages, etc.

the reciprocal of time and the square root of intensity deviates from linearity in that the slope of the threshold region appears to increase further. Thus, it appears that different processes may be involved in the different ultrasonic dosage regions lying in the range from, say 30 watts/cm.^{2} (1,000 seconds) to 250 watts/cm.^{2} (0.10 second).

Measurements have been made of the temperature rise in the spinal cord of the mice as a function of ultrasonic dosage. This was accomplished by imbedding small thermocouples in the cord. The results of these temperature measurements are indicated at the corresponding dosage coordinates in Fig. 2. Considering these temperature increases in the cord in conjunction with the value for the base temperature of the animal, 10° C., it can be concluded that temperature rise is not the primary factor for the observed functional changes in the mice in the linear portion of the threshold region.

An outline of the preparation and technique and a discussion of the instrumentation will now be presented.

The mice are selected for this study 24 hours after birth, plus or minus five hours. They range in weight from 1.2 to 1.4 grams. It is not possible to determine the subsequent color of the mice at this stage so that white, gray and brown mice are irradiated indiscriminately. Males and females are also irradiated indiscriminately. Young mice were chosen for this study for the following reasons: (1) They are essentially poikilothermic, that is, they possess virtually no temperature control mechanism, so that they can be carried through reversible temperature cycles, with the temperature being reduced to nearly zero degrees Centigrade, without producing either morphological or permanent physiological changes. (2) Ossification is not complete. As determined by standard staining techniques, the tissue overlying the dorsal side of the cord is soft tissue, while that over the lateral and ventral sides shows a slight degree of ossification. Therefore, acoustic absorption in the structures surrounding the spinal cord does not result in the large temperature increases characteristic of irradiated adult mice. (3) These animals are small in size so that it is possible to irradiate the desired region with a nearly uniform acoustic intensity with a single controlled ultrasonic pulse.

The equipment comprises a sound tank which is immersed in a deep-freeze unit for maintaining the desired temperature within a few tenths of a degree Centigrade. The overall arrangement of the equipment is shown in Fig. 3. Hydrostatic pressures from one to twenty atmospheres can be developed in the tank. A coordinate system is provided in the tank to accurately position either the calibrator or the mouse. An accurately machined tongue is used to attach either the calibrator or the mouse-holder to the coordinate system. Fig. 4 is a view looking into the tank. The calibrator is shown attached to the coordinate system. A cross-hair attachment can also be fastened to the tongue. The intersection of the cross-hairs has been set so that it coincides with the position previously occupied by the thermo-

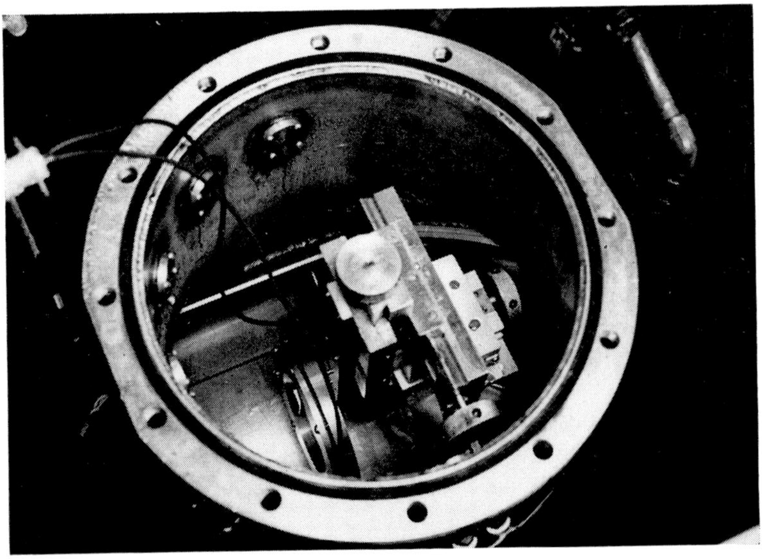

FIG. 4. A view looking into the sound tank. The calibrator is shown mounted on the coordinate system.

couple junction of the calibrator. With adjustments provided on the mouse-holder, together with the tongue and the cross-hair attachment, it is possible to place almost any part of the mouse in the position occupied by the calibrator thermocouple junction in the sound field. Fig. 5 shows the mouse-holder and tongue assembled. Fig. 6 is a close-up view showing the cross-hair attachment in position.

The method of probing and calibrating the sound field is the standard procedure employed at this laboratory (Fry and Fry, 1954a; Ibid., 1954b). A calibration of the sound field is performed daily.

The mice are irradiated at the third lumbar vertebra. Since it is desirable to use as a functional endpoint motor paralysis of the hind legs, the

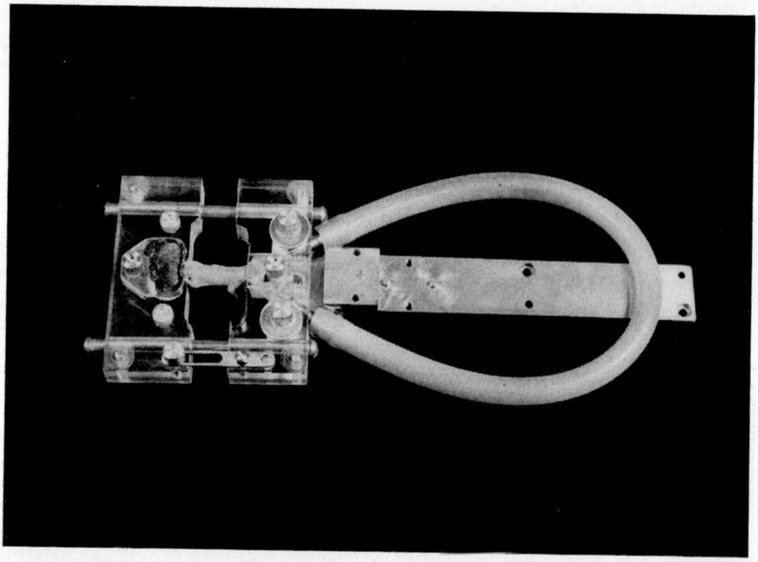

FIG. 5. An overall view of the mouse-holder and tongue assembly. The long tube provides the oxygen for the animal to breathe when submerged in the sound tank.

region of the spinal cord which must be altered is that containing the neurons associated with the femoral, sciatic and obturator nerves. This region, at which the axis of the beam is centered, has been determined by acoustic means.

For a study of this type it is highly desirable to have an acoustic field of almost uniform intensity over the region to be affected. An unfocussed quartz crystal is used to develop the traveling wave field. Fig. 7 shows the transverse and vertical patterns of the beam. At 5 percent below the peak intensity, the vertical beam width (along the length of the cord) is 2.6 mm. At 10 percent down, the beam width is 3.2 mm., and at half-power the beam width is 7.1 mm.

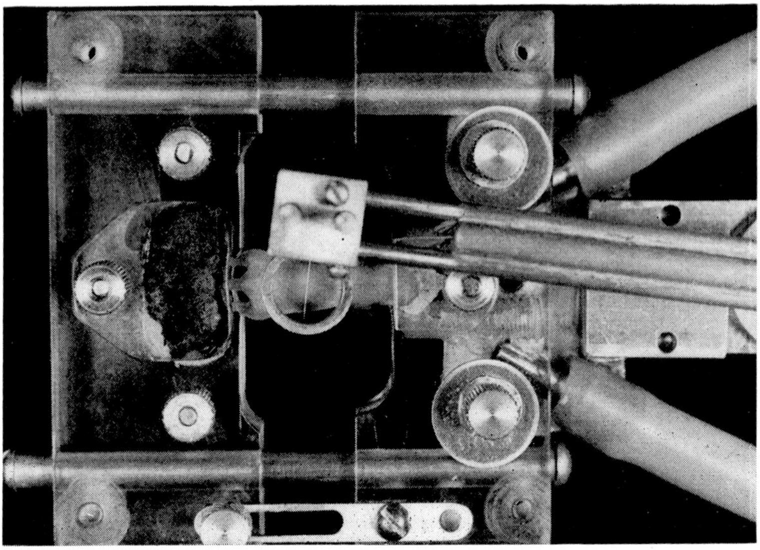

Fig. 6. A close-up view showing the cross-hair attachment in position. The two knurled knobs on the right permit almost any part of the animal to be positioned under the intersection of the cross-hairs.

In the lumbar region, the vertebral segments are 0.67 mm., measured from corresponding edges. Thus, nearly four vertebral segments of the cord are irradiated with an intensity variation of no more than 5 percent.

In preparing the animal for irradiation, the mouse is first cooled down to render it dormant so that it can be properly positioned in the mouse-holder and remain in that position until the termination of exposure. When the mouse is sufficiently cooled, it is placed in the holder which firmly

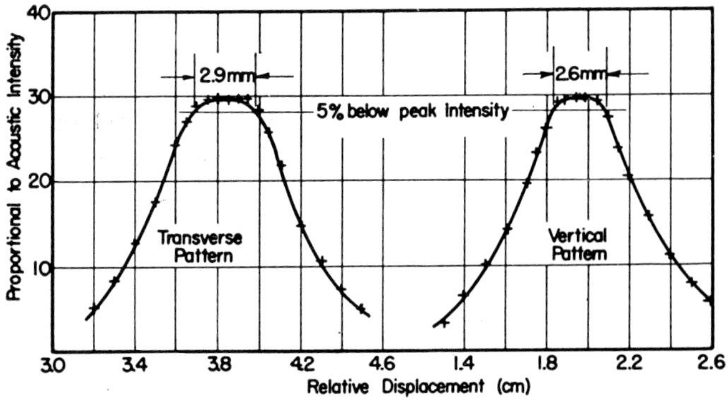

Fig. 7. The transverse and vertical field patterns developed by the unfocused quartz crystal. The cord lies along the vertical direction.

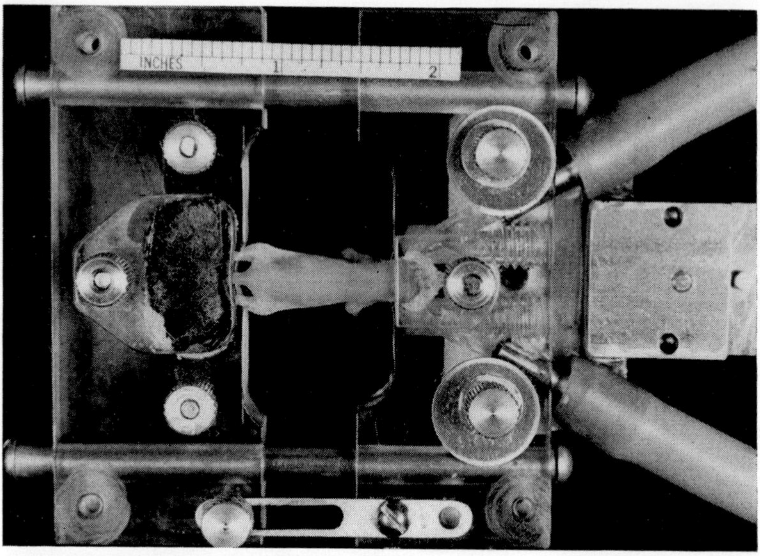

FIG. 8. A close-up view showing a mouse mounted in the mouse-holder.

holds the head, the hind legs, and the tail. The mouse is then fully extended to reduce possible lateral movement. Fig. 8 is a close-up view showing a mouse mounted in the mouse-holder.

The mouse-holder, the tongue and the cross-hair attachment are then assembled (see Fig. 6) and placed over an intense, cool light source. With such an arrangement it is possible to see clearly the vertebrae from the second lumbar through the sacral and caudal regions. The mouse-holder is then adjusted to place the center of the third lumbar vertebra under the intersection of the cross-hairs. The cross-hair attachment is then removed and the mouse-holder supporting the mouse is placed in the sound tank.

Concerning the accuracy of placement of the third lumbar vertebra with respect to the axis of the sound beam, the following statements can be made: (1) The accuracy of the machined parts is $\pm$ 0.002 in. or $\pm$ 0.05 mm. (2) The axis of the beam can be determined to $\pm$ 0.1 mm. (3) The maximum uncertainty in locating the center of the third lumbar vertebra, which is approximately 0.6 mm. in length, is $\pm$ 0.1 mm. Thus the overall uncertainty in the position of the center of the third lumbar vertebra with respect to the axis of the sound field is $\pm$ 0.25 mm. Since the beam width at 95 percent of the peak intensity is 2.6 mm., it appears that the overall accuracy of positioning the animal in the sound field is adequate.

Since these animals are essentially poikilothermic they will come to temperature equilibrium above the temperature of the environment, the exact amount being a function of their age and the temperature of the surroundings. For these animals and the temperature considered here—one day old mice at 10° C.—the equilibrium temperature is approximately 10.2° C. A few minutes times is sufficient for the animals to reach their equilibrium temperature. A single acoustic pulse of rectangular envelope, having a rise time of several microseconds and predetermined acoustic intensity and time duration is then initiated.

After the cessation of the sound, the animal-holder is removed from the tank. The mouse is removed from the holder and rapidly warmed to room temperature. The animals are examined for paralysis or overt movements approximately 15 minutes after exposure and again after 6 hours.

In conclusion, it thus appears that the precision ultrasonic dosage study planned by this laboratory is possible. The instrumentation and technique for obtaining accurately reproducible results with a suitably prepared biological specimen have been developed and demonstrated.

The preliminary results obtained at a base temperature of 10° C., hydrostatic pressure of one atmosphere and frequency of 982 kc./sec., indicates that several processes may be involved in producing changes in the central nervous system in the ultrasonic dosage range from 25 watts/cm.^{2} and 1,000 seconds to 250 watts/cm.^{2} and 0.1 second.

References

Finney, D. J. 1952. Probit Analysis. 2nd Edition. Cambridge Univ. Press. London. 318 pp.

Fry, W. J. and R. B. Fry. 1954a. Determination of absolute sound levels and acoustic absorption coefficients by thermocouple probes—Theory. J. Acoust. Soc. Am. *26:* 294–310.

Fry, W. J. and R. B. Fry. 1954b. Determination of absolute sound levels and acoustic absorption coefficients by thermocouple probes—Experiment. J. Acoust. Soc. Am. *26:* 311–317.

Dr. Hueter: In our dosage study which utilizes adult mice, we have occasionally been troubled with the following problem. We increased the dosage, e.g., the sound amplitude, in order to obtain an additional point on the sigmoid curve. We found that at the higher dosage the experimentally determined point was considerably lower than was anticipated and at a still higher dosage the point appeared in the expected region.

We found that at a certain dosage level cavitation developed in the transmitting medium between the animal and the transducer. We had to increase the dosage in order to get through the cavitation screen with sufficient energy to carry out the experiment.

Dr. Dunn: The experiments which we described were conducted in the absence of cavitation. The degree of reproducibility obtained appears to bear this out. However, we might indicate how we determined that we were not being troubled by cavitation.

In the course of this experimentation, we made a rather extensive set of temperature measurements by imbedding small thermocouples in the mouse cord. The location of the thermocouple was determined after the animal was sacrificed. The soft tissue was cleared and the bone stained with alizarin red. The specimen was then viewed under a microscope and the thermocouple junction was located quite accurately with respect to the vertebral structure.

We irradiated the animals, which contained imbedded thermocouples, at varying dosages. The output of the thermocouple was fed to a recording galvanometer which provided us with a permanent record of the temperature rise versus time function. Now, on some occasions, we did have cavitation present. Figure D–1 is a photograph of such a galvanometer record which shows the type of response obtained both with and without cavitation present.

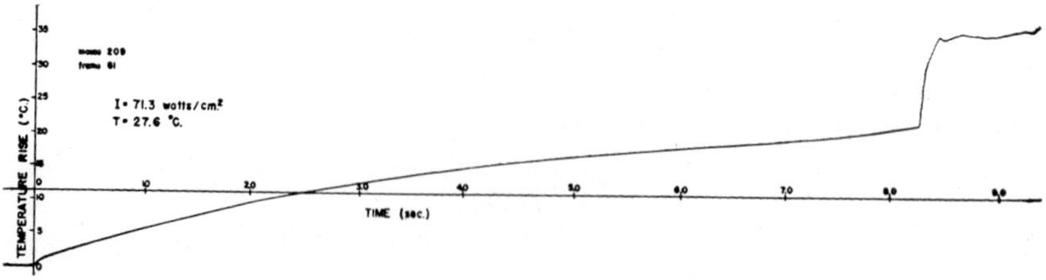

FIG. D–1. Photograph of a galvanometer recording of the response of a small thermocouple imbedded in a mouse cord during irradiation with sound. The record shows the response obtained both with and without cavitation present.

Note that in the absence of cavitation the temperature rise versus time curve has the characteristic shape which Dr. Fry has described, i.e., there is an initial rapid rise due to viscous forces and a subsequent linear rise due to acoustic absorption in the vicinity of the thermocouple. When cavitation sets in, the galvanometer response becomes very erratic with the curve rising to rather high values and presumably high temperatures are developed. Referring to Fig. D–1, after 8.27 seconds of acoustic irradiation at 71 watts/cm.² the temperature rise was 22.2° C. The maximum rate of rise during this time was 10.0° C./sec. which occurred at the start of the irradiation period and which was caused by the viscosity effect. During the initial cavitation blast, the temperature rose 13.4° C. in 0.17 second, for a total rate of 78.8° C./sec.

In our experimental procedure, the vacuum tube voltmeter, which meters a calibrated portion of the voltage impressed across the quartz crystal transducer, is always observed. Now, when cavitation occurs, there is a reaction back on the crystal which is reflected into the electronic circuit.

This is readily observed on the vacuum tube voltmeter. The results which we just presented were carried out in the absence of any phenomena suggestive of the presence of cavitation.

DR. HUETER: In your 4-beam irradiation system, you have an intensity level of 16 watts/cm.^{2} at the transducer. These levels increase toward the dura and it would appear that you should at least develop occasional cavitation or gas bubbles.

DR. FRY: Such gas bubbles are observed when the water in the transmission path becomes gassy which means that it is being forced to serve its purpose too long. Our experiments are performed in the absence of such undesirable conditions. We are careful in our preparation and handling of the degassed water.

DR. BALDES: What temperatures did you actually get in your thermocouple recording at 10° C.?

DR. DUNN: The temperatures measured, of course, are highly dependent upon the dosage, i.e., the time duration of irradiation and the acoustic intensity. For example, at 54 watts/cm.^{2} and 7.70 seconds irradiation time, the measured temperature rise was 16.5° C. At 112 watts/cm.^{2} and 1.25 seconds irradiation time, the temperature rise was 6.1° C. Both of these values are in the threshold region. High temperature rises can certainly be obtained. For example, at 54 watts/cm.^{2} and 20.00 seconds time duration of irradiation the temperature rise was 29.0° C. This is well beyond the threshold region where all animals are paralyzed. Conversely, in the lesser dosage region where animals are never paralyzed, at 54 watts/cm.^{2} and 1.00 seconds irradiation time, the measured temperature rise was 2.43° C. These values are observed at the positions in the cord of highest temperature rise, i.e., the ventral side of the cord.

It is interesting to compare these temperature rises in the mouse cord with those in onion roots previously described by Dr. Lehmann. Dr. Lehmann observed temperature increases in onion roots of the order of 150° C. when irradiated with 1 mc./s. ultrasound at 110 watts/cm.^{2} for five minutes. His experiments were carried out under a high hydrostatic pressure.

DR. CARSTENSEN: I wonder if someone would comment on the reason for the time lag between the onset of this cavitation effect and the application of the sound field which was just described. Is it presumably that there is a minimum time requirement for the bubbles, or whatever we have here, to grow to the proper size to produce an observable effect or is there perhaps a time rate of production of bubbles which requires a particular time interval to reach a sufficient concentration to produce an observable effect?

DR. NYBORG: I think Dr. Leonard's experiments are illuminating. He used focussed sound and studied the cavitation at the focus. He found that considerably greater sound pressures were necessary to produce cavitation under these conditions than were necessary under other experimental conditions. He explained this by the fact that in the focal region, the fluid in the region of high sound pressure moves at very high velocities. This is a kind of acoustic streaming which means that part of the fluid does not remain in the focal region very long and consequently the bubbles do not have sufficient time to grow to the proper size to produce an effect.

DR. ROSENBERG: I personally feel that the time required for the bubbles to grow to a particular size to be able to produce the effect is most important. In the plane wave case it is definitely the growth time that is important. This is also true of acoustic streaming. Concerning the population, I feel that unless one employs a focussed beam with an extremely small focal region, the population, in all such cases, is large. In the case of a focussed beam of exceedingly small focal region, one may have to allow adequate time for both the growth of the bubbles and the build-up of the population before the effect can be observed.

DR. HUETER: With respect to your mouse data, you indicated that the threshold region displays three different shapes, a linear region sandwiched between two non-linear regions of increasing slope. I wonder if one could not argue that the entire threshold region has a parabolic shape.

DR. DUNN: One may, of course, argue this, however, the experimental evidence appears to be otherwise. We should like to point out, in comparing your mouse data with ours, that with respect to the duration of time of irradiation, there is a reasonable correspondence. Our data, for single shots of sound, shows a deviation from the linear portion beyond approximately 10 seconds of exposure to the sound. Our data covers irradiation times from one second to beyond 1,000 seconds. For your data, let us consider the length of time for which the sound is actually on, e.g., for 10 pulses, each of 0.4 second duration, pulsed at the rate of one per second. Now, your data covers total irradiation only from 4 seconds to 24 seconds, i.e., 10, 30 and 60 pulses. While your data seems to follow a parabolic relationship, the greatest curvature appears to occur beyond approximately 8 or 10 seconds of time during which the animal is actually exposed to the sound. Perhaps if your data extended over a wider range especially to shorter total exposure times you might have found a linear range as we did.

Thermocouple Probes

W. J. Fry

Bioacoustics Laboratory, University of Illinois, Urbana, Illinois

The talk by Professor W. J. Fry on thermocouple probes was not recorded. The following is a synopsis of the presented paper.

THE SHORT WAVELENGTHS characteristic of ultrasound in liquid media in the frequency range above one megacycle per second require probes of very small size if the structure of field distributions, generated, for example, by focusing irradiators, is to be determined and if "point" values for the acoustic field variables are to be measured. In addition, very small probes designed for routine rapid field measurements are extremely useful especially if they can serve to determine absolute sound levels independently of any other calibration procedure. The thermocouple probe developed by the author and his associates at the Bioacoustics Laboratory realizes these desirable features.

It should be emphasized that the thermocouple probe which is the subject of this talk is completely different from other thermocouple probes which have been and are currently being used by other investigators to detect the presence of an acoustic field. All these other probes utilize essentially the "equilibrium" temperature rise principle—that is, the thermocouple junction detects the *maximum* temperature change produced by the sound field in a mass of absorbing material in which the thermocouple junction is imbedded. The value of this maximum temperature rise is thus dependent upon the size and shape of the absorbing mass and the field distribution within it. Since the mass is usually not less than about one millimeter in diameter, the minimum probe size is thus of the order of a millimeter in linear dimensions. Such probes interfere with the sound field, they are not capable of high accuracy, they cannot be used for absolute determinations of sound levels without previous calibration and their calibration is dependent upon the field configuration in which they are immersed.

By contrast, the thermocouple probe which has been developed at this laboratory does not suffer from these limitations. This probe consists of a thermocouple junction imbedded in an acoustic absorbing medium which closely matches in density and acoustic propagation velocity the values for these quantities characteristic of the medium in which the sound field exists. The method of operation consists of producing a pulse of sound with, for example, a rectangular envelope and observing the electrical output of the thermocouple in response to the initial time rate of the temperature rise of the absorbing medium (or in response to the temperature rise a short interval of time after the initiation of the pulse). This quantity is independent of the size, shape and configuration of the absorbing medium in the acoustic field. (This assumes that the transmission path of the sound in the absorbing medium is not so long that there is an appreciable reduction in sound level at the junction because of absorption along this transmission path.) This situation obtains since heat conduction processes are not involved in the determination of this initial time rate of temperature rise or the value of the temperature rise after a short interval.

We will now illustrate these ideas by describing the specific design of such a thermocouple probe which has proved extremely useful for studying the fields and determining the sound levels produced by focusing irradiators used in the research at this laboratory on the production of changes in the central nervous system by ultrasound. Fig. 1 is a photograph of such a probe. This type has been in use here for the past several years. The device consists of a fine thermocouple which can be seen in the photograph as a fine horizontal line lying along a diameter of the device. The thermocouple is constructed from 0.003″ diameter iron and constantan wires which are etched to a diameter of 0.0005″ in the neighborhood of the junction. The circular ring members support two thin (0.003″) polyethylene diaphrams which enclose a disc of an absorbing liquid such as, for example, castor oil. The ring opening is of such size as to permit the entire sound beam to pass through without reflection from the ring members. The particular probe shown in the photograph is fitted with a supporting bar which can be fastened to a positioning system. The thermocouple wires are supported from two Kovar seals which are soldered to one of the stainless steel rings. These Kovar seals constitute the electrical lead-throughs for the electrical connections. In order to reduce the effect of external shocks from breaking the thermocouple junction or wires, a short spring is incorporated in the constantan wire. The spring portion of the constantan wire lies beneath the stainless steel rings and is not visible by viewing through the membranes.

We have published an extensive analysis of the theory of operation of such thermocouple probes and have also indicated in the literature the type of experimental results which are obtained (Fry and Fry, 1954a; Ibid., 1954b). I would, however, like to discuss briefly several aspects of the theory of the operation of the device and also illustrate the type of response obtainable. As indicated previously, an electrical output voltage is produced in response to a short pulse of sound (for example, one second duration.) The duration of the pulse is chosen so that the effect of heat conduction processes in the absorbing material and the thermocouple wires are unimportant during the time of exposure of the probe to the sound. When a pulse of ultrasound falls on the probe the temperature change detected by the thermocouple junction is caused by two distinctly different mechanisms. One source of heat results from absorption of sound in the

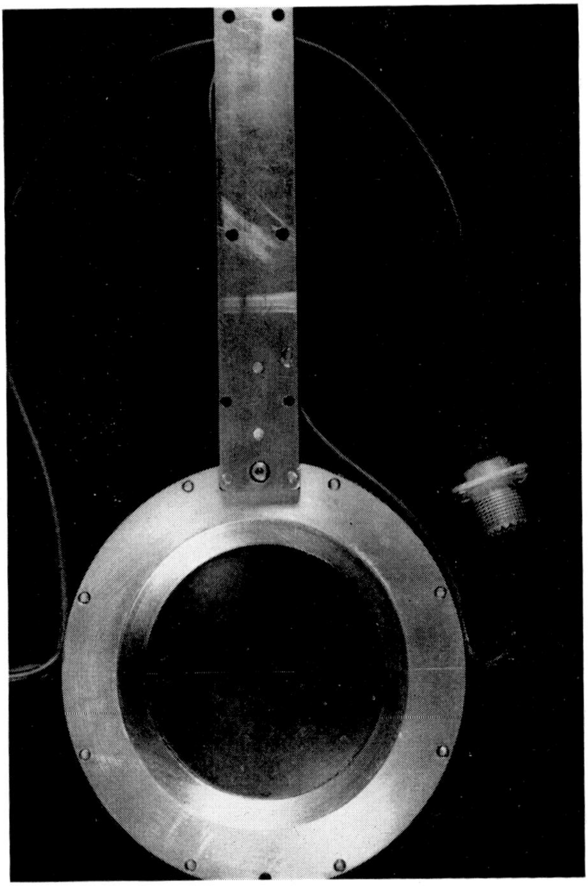

FIG. 1. A thermocouple probe, membrane window diameter three inches.

acoustic absorbing medium which surrounds the junction. The time rate of temperature increase is proportional to the absorption coefficient and the square of the acoustic pressure amplitude. A readily derived theoretical formula relates the acoustic pressure amplitude to the time rate of temperature rise, the acoustic pressure absorption coefficient, and the heat capacity per unit volume of the absorbing medium. The second heat source, which contributes to the temperature rise, results from the action of viscous forces between the wires and the imbedding medium. The viscous action is caused by relative motion between the wires and the liquid. This contribution to the temperature rise, which is proportional to the square of the particle velocity amplitude, would, of course, be absent if the wires were not present. The viscous source of heat is localized to the immediate neighborhood of the wires and junction and therefore the resulting temperature rise exhibits a rapid approach to an equilibrium value as compared with the rate of approach of the temperature change, resulting from acoustic absorption in the liquid medium, to its equilibrium value. When such a probe is subjected to a sound pulse of rectangular envelope of one second duration at a frequency of approximately one megacycle per second, the response recorded on a magnetic oscillograph is shown in Fig. 2. The

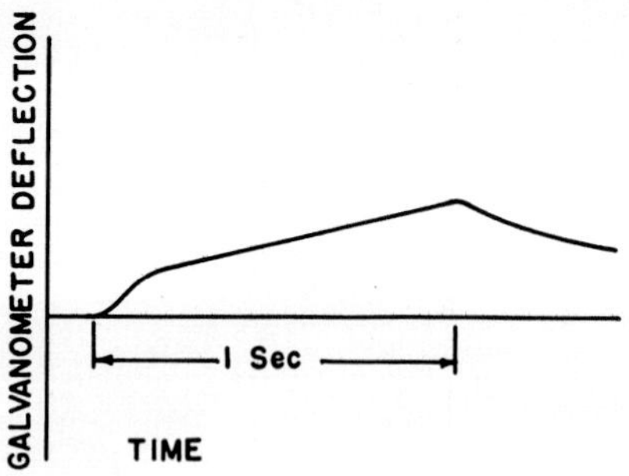

FIG. 2. Response of a thermocouple probe to a one-second pulse of 1.0 mc./s. ultrasound. The galvanometer deflection is proportional to the temperature rise at the junction.

initial rapid rise is caused by the viscous force action. The subsequent slow rise results from absorption in the acoustic absorbing medium in which the thermocouple junction is imbedded.

It might be well to mention that another mechanism, in addition to the two just discussed, contributes to the temperature rise at the junction. This contribution results from a lag which occurs during each cycle of the acoustic disturbance in the heat conduction process at the liquid-wire boundary. The periodic transfer of heat at the fluid-metal boundary gives rise to a term in the function describing the periodic temperature change in the fluid which is not in phase with the pressure. Acoustic energy is thus transformed into heat. This mechanism contributes only about 1/1,000 of the heat contributed by the viscous mechanism for the probe construction which we have been using.

It should be pointed out that resolution of fine structure of a field as well as the accuracy with which absolute determinations of acoustic pressure amplitudes can be made are functions of the diameter of the thermocouple wires and the junction. Theoretical expressions have been derived which permit a choice of wire size to be made consistent with the required accuracy and resolution.

In summary, thermocouple probes which operate on the principle of the initial time rate of change of temperature in response to an acoustic pulse have proved extremely useful, at this laboratory, in studying complex sound fields at ultrasonic frequencies. These probes can be used for rapid determinations of acoustic field configurations, for adjusting and studying focusing irradiators of both the single and multibeam type, and for determining absolute sound levels of ultrasound fields without recourse to any other calibration procedure. The devices are rugged and are stable over long periods of time. This type of thermocouple probe is a precision instrument for use in the ultrasonic frequency range in the neighborhood of one megacycle per second and above.

References

Fry, W. J. and R. B. Fry. 1954a. Determination of absolute sound levels and acoustic absorption coefficients by thermocouple probes—theory. J. Acoust. Soc. Am. *26:* 294–310.

Fry, W. J. and R. B. Fry. 1954b. Determination of absolute sound levels and acoustic absorption coefficients by thermocouple probes—experiment. J. Acoust. Soc. Am. *26:* 311–317.